PARENTHOOD
THE WHOLE STORY

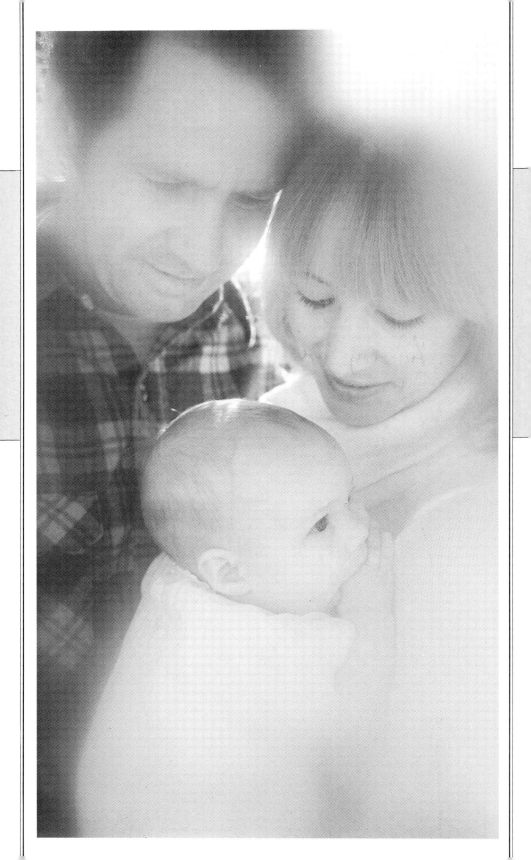

DOROTHY EINON

PARENTHOOD
THE WHOLE STORY

BLOOMSBURY

For those who have shared parenthood with me

First published in Great Britain in 1988
Bloomsbury Publishing Ltd, 2 Soho Square, London W1V 5DE
Copyright © Dorothy Einon 1988
Copyright © Duncan Petersen Publishing Ltd 1988
ISBN 0 7475 0158 0

Conceived, edited, designed and produced
by Duncan Petersen Publishing Ltd,
5 Botts Mews, London W2 5AG

Filmset and originated by SX Composing Ltd,
Rayleigh, Essex

Made and printed in Britain by Butler & Tanner Ltd,
Frome, Somerset

All matters involving a mother's or a child's health require some degree of medical supervision. The ideas, procedures and suggestions in this book are intended to enable parents to collaborate effectively with health professionals, not to replace their services. Any applications of treatments suggested in this book are made at the reader's own risk.

All illustrations are by **Sandra Ponds** and **Will Giles**
except those on pages 38-41 and 105, which
are by Tony Graham; and those on pages
112-3 and 190-1 which are by Michael Woods.

(A full list of photo credits appears on page 352.)

The author would like to thank the many people who contributed to *Parenthood – The Whole Story* by being ready to discuss, give opinions and disagree, but especially her mother, sisters and close friends; and her children for being so tolerant of the long hours spent writing.
   She is also particularly grateful to Dr. Elizabeth Budge and to Jamie Nichols for their help in compiling the medical section.

Editorial director
Andrew Duncan

Sub-editor
Gwen Rigby

Assistant editors and research
Cindy Creedon and Carol McGlynn

Index
Rosemary Dawe

Art director
Mel Petersen

Designers
Chris Foley and Beverley Stewart

About **Parenthood – The Whole Story**

'He' or 'she'?
In childcare books, as in life, it is a shame to call a baby, or a child, 'it'. So, in this book, the imaginary baby (and child) around whom my text is written happens to be a girl and is referred to throughout as 'she'. I have chosen not to complicate matters by using 'he' and 'she' alternatively. She has an elder brother.

The paragraph numbering system
This has been used because to tell the story of parenthood so many different threads, which don't necessarily mesh chronologically, must be wound together.

You will probably want to read parts of the book as a continuous narrative, and you will find that large portions read on from one numbered paragraph to the next, as in a conventionally organized book.

Equally, you will want to dip into the book for guidance on specific topics. Here the paragraph numbering system comes into its own – the index is based mainly on the paragraph numbers so that you can home quickly in on your problem.

You may also want to trace a specific theme forwards through the text, leaving out chunks. The cross referencing system also enables you to do this with ease, but bear in mind that it concentrates on the book's secondary themes, rather than principal strands. 'Secondary themes' are issues such as the role of the father; changes in the parents' relationship and division of labour in childcare. 'Principal strands' are essentially the mother's progress through pregnancy and birth; the baby's development and baby- and childcare. These naturally tend to run on at greater length than the secondary themes.

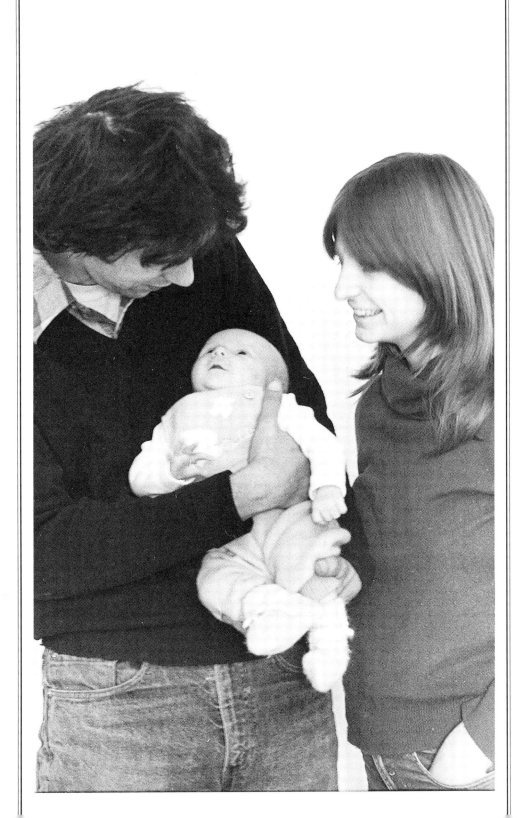

Contents

Parenthood – The Whole Story
is in four main sections, and a
medical section at the back:

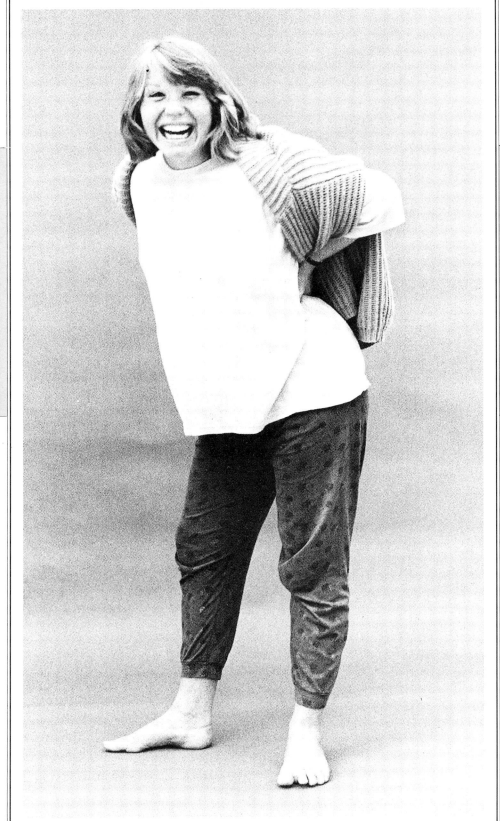

Pregnancy

1-321

Fundamentals

1 An approach to writing childcare books

This is a book about having and making a family, written by a firm believer, who has got it wrong as often as she has got it right.

I never for one moment considered a life without children. But neither, it must be said, did I really consider life with them.

The books I read as I awaited the birth of my first child reinforced the pleasures and wonders of creating a new life; the delights of motherhood; the bloom of pregnancy. They must have mentioned men, but as rather shadowy figures in the background. I know they did not say I would see myself differently, or view my husband and parents in a different light. I think they mentioned morning sickness, and sleepless babies, but nothing prepared me for the unbelievable tiredness of those early months of pregnancy and motherhood, or the difficulties that three individuals have in adjusting to each other as life begins for one and changes so dramatically for the other two.

If nothing else, this book is meant to be more down-to-earth – more relevant than its counterparts to the needs of all the players. One that deals even-handedly with the realities of pregnancy and childcare as well as the ideals.

Life will be turned upside down by the arrival of your first child. You will not be in the best state to cope with all the changes. It is a time of stress: a major event in your life.

My hope is that this is a book which reassures you in the testing times; which helps you understand your feelings at the same time as mastering the practicalities of having and caring for a child.

2 Not that easy

This is not a book that tells you childcare is easy, because if it is, I have never found it so. It is rewarding; it is delightful, but it is also hard work. Don't imagine you will never regret it. The 24-hour-a-day demands of small children go on, day in, day out, and there are moments when even the most loving parent longs to escape.

If all this sounds negative as you contemplate pregnancy, it is, in a sense, deliberately so. Any magazine can show you pictures of tranquil mothers and contented babies. We all know it is rarely like this.

A sleeping baby can fill you with love and contentment. But so can the sticky face and the muddy boots of your toddler. Love sweeps in at the most unlikely moments. If one day you find yourself in the chaos of your kitchen, looking at your children and feeling unbelievably happy, so have countless others. And if you find yourself one night screaming at your crying baby, countless others have been there too. Occasionally, anger is natural. We feel it towards our parents and towards our partners. It is natural that at times we should also feel it towards our children.

3 Don't try to be perfect

I have written this book from lessons I have learned, from successes as well as failures. It is a book for fallible parents, who hope to do the very best for their children, yet believe that it is not good to sacrifice everything for them.

I do not pretend to have all the answers; but I can tell you how I have coped, and what others have suggested when faced with similar problems. At the very least, a book such as this can provide the background information which will enable you to make decisions.

You will make mistakes. Console yourself, as I do, that life without mistakes would be a dull and unrealistic model to place before children. Who could live with, or live up to perfection? We have to fit our children for the world, not a fairytale.

4 What is a family?

Mother, father, son and daughter is the obvious answer. But families come in all varieties. You may be a single woman or already have step-children. But however small or large the unit, the essence of a family is that it shares life and love. It is mutually supportive. See also 7, 19-20 and 28; single parents see also 740 and 752.

5 Changing attitudes to pregnancy

In the nineteenth century, a lady was not pregnant: she was in an interesting condition. Even as recently as the 1950s, advertisements showed pregnant women without bumps, even when they were advertising smocks. So ingrained was this view that a loose dress almost made the statement 'I am pregnant'. Today we are allowed to be proud of our bumps: but only our bumps. There is still something unreal about how society views pregnancy.

6 A woman's view of herself

In 1977, a group of women were asked what they understood by words such as feminine, sexually attractive and motherhood. Feminine meant young and sexually attractive. Motherhood and femininity did not mix. Nor did motherhood and being sexually attractive.

Times have not changed. "I cannot imagine you writing about children and parenting", I was told by a man who tried to chat me up at a conference. "I didn't expect her to look like that", said the designer working on the layouts for some PR work I was doing. I am just one of millions of mothers who does not look homely or motherly.

So where do the values come from? A feeling that once she has produced children, a woman should hide her attractions and sexuality from the world, bringing them out only in the marital bed? Do we really still think like that?

Will pregnancy alter how you think about yourself? How you feel about what you are?

7 Mothers and fathers

The English language has a number of telling phrases about families. Take, for example, the verb to father or to mother a child. Both refer to parenting, but the meanings are very different. Fathering a child is a biological event and not something a woman could ever do. It refers not to a lifetime of support and caring, but to the donation of sperm at the time of conception.

Father figures, heavy fathers, Victorian fathers, most of the phrases associated with fathers depict a stern (or benign) figurehead. A protector, a disciplinarian. Someone to look up to and respect, perhaps even someone whose love has to be earned. There are men and women today who reject this view.

Mothering, on the other hand, means caring. It can be done by men, but in our society, as in most societies, mothering is women's work. Women spend more time with children, have primary responsibility for them, and form the major emotional ties with babies. When no biological mothers pass care on to others, it is invariably women who take over. Men can mother, men do mother, but it is the exception, not the rule. Women's mothering is one of the few enduring and universal facts in the sexual division of labour.

What do you think about this state of affairs?

8 Changing views of family roles

It does not have to be so. There is little biological evidence for maternal instinct (see 29), or any hormonal predisposition to mother. And if we watch small children with babies, boys are often as loving and gentle as girls. So why do women take the initiative?

Maybe we are reluctant to share our children: not quite trusting anyone else (even fathers) to care for them properly. Or perhaps we are just holding on to one of the few areas where women are presumed superior, where their authority is not questioned. Or perhaps we are simply fulfilling the role for which nature and society has fitted us.

However you feel about this, and you may be perfectly happy with the existing division of labour, you should be aware that if you do decide that your baby will be the equal responsibility of both parents, society's expectations will mean that this is only achieved by conscious striving.

If a baby is screaming in public, or a child wanders off as you lie on the beach, the reaction of most of us is that she should do something about it, and that she should have taken more care.

Society does not make taking equal responsibility easy for men. Maternity leave is commonplace, paternity leave is not. Parenting has to be learned. For a mother to have the newborn baby with her in the hours and days after birth is known to be important for the development of a strong emotional bond between her and the child, a bond that means she tunes into her child's needs, grows with it to form a family.

The bond also means that the baby comes to recognize a mother's smell and voice. Few fathers can be with a baby in the hours after birth, or spend as much time with his child as mothers can. Breast feeding, while it is desirable on all counts for mother and baby, puts a further barrier between father and child. Inevitably, fathers are behind in bonding, and not surprisingly many babies seem to prefer mother. This cannot help a man working

against the social conditioning that fits women – and women alone – to be mothers. See 110.

9 Some views of pregnancy

Man's main aim in life is to copulate. Woman's is to bear children.

Pregnancy is a time of suspended animation before full womanhood; a time of calm before a life of burden.

Pregnancy is a period of illness; but only for nine months. Then you get back to normal.

Pregnancy and birth are a right of passage.

Morning sickness, swollen ankles, you drag yourself around. Birth is painful (and mine was worse than most). Stitches, you can't sit down for a week. Don't let anyone tell you it is easy.

Women suffer. It makes them women.

Pregnancy is a duty.

Pregnancy is the gateway to real life.

Pregnancy is growing up.

Pregnancy is an opportunity to grow and develop.

10 Making the decision

There are no *good* reasons for having a baby – except that we cannot imagine doing anything else. There are many bad reasons. Yet it is in the nature of babies that whatever the reasons for having them, once here, few of us could envisage life without them.

A child is your responsibility for 18 years or more. For longer, in fact, than many of us will stay with our partners. You can think of having a child as entering into an arranged marriage without the possibility of divorce. We choose only the other parent for our children. After that we must take what is given.

11 Some questions to ask yourself

The American National Alliance for Optimal Parenthood (NAOP) recommends that you ask yourself the following questions BEFORE you go ahead and have a child:

What do I want out of life for myself, what is important?

How would a child interfere with my growth and development?

Do I want a boy or a girl child? What if I don't get what I want?

Would I try to pass on to my child my ideas and values? What if my child's ideas and values turn out to be different from mine?

Does my partner want to have a child? Suppose one of us wants a child and the other doesn't? Who decides?

12 You will both change

Becoming a parent changes you: changes how you think and feel about yourself and about your partner. It changes your view of friends, parents, and your job. It makes you less tolerant of some people (and this includes your partner) and perhaps more tolerant of others – (and this can include your partner). Time and space become more important. You will have less of both. How will you organize it? Who gives up the time, who gives up the space? Do you mind? See also 110.

13 Talking about it

Talk to your partner about why you want a baby; how you think it will change your lives; how you intend to divide the responsibilities. Talk about your own childhood and what you feel about it. What would you like to be the same for your children; what to change?

Talk about how your parents treated you. Will you act in the same way?

How will the baby fit into your lives, how will you both change? Talk about jobs. Will you both work? Whose job is the baby? What is the role of grandparents? What is interference? What is help?

Talk and think about your own feelings and relationship with your parents. Will your child feel like this about you?

14 But why do it?

The interesting question, a friend said, when I told her I was writing this book, is not just why we do it, but having done it once why we ever do it again. Three months pregnant, feeling tired and sick, she was dragging a bad-tempered four-year-old around the supermarket. In the last two years she had had two miscarriages. With a challenging job, and a seemingly happy marriage, one wondered what compelled her to risk yet another pregnancy.

Once there was no choice. Women married and pregnancy followed marriage as night follows day.

Now other avenues are open to both men and women. We actively choose to have babies, to become pregnant, to interrupt or to give up careers. There must be something in it.

15 But could it be a mistake?

Making a family is, for many of us, the most wonderful and creative experience. It can also be unbelievably boring, unbearably confining and bring even the mildest parents close to violence.

But surely, that is also true of all human relationships. Living alone has its freedoms, but sometimes, as the song says, *that is just another word for nothing left to lose.* Having children is not for everyone. Nor is marriage. But if it is for you, there will come a time when you feel it is right. It could be after years of planning, or on finding yourself unintentionally pregnant. After you have made the decision, you will probably change your mind a thousand times. That is normal. You are about to change your life drastically: to have no doubts, to see no problems, would be unrealistic, even unhealthy.

It *could* be a mistake. Marriage, after all, is often a mistake.

16 Depression

Mothers get depressed. In most developed countries about 16 per cent of all mothers suffer from post-natal depression. Few of us think that it could happen to us. It can.

The months after childbirth are not the time to start from scratch in coming to terms with changing roles, lifestyles and relationships. If you have sailed through pregnancy, avoiding all negative thoughts, the post-natal blues (from which all women suffer to some extent) may hit you with a reality which it is almost impossible to face. If you have never talked through your problems, it will be difficult for you and your partner to start now.

Women who do not feel (or do not admit to feeling) anxiety in pregnancy are more, not less, likely to have problems after their child is born. It is natural to feel that pregnancy and childbirth are taking you over. Working through these feelings is part of your adaptation to a changing life.

But too much anxiety and stress in pregnancy can also affect you so that you are unable to cope. Panic makes it difficult to come to terms with change.

Part of a woman's preparation for childbirth must be psychological; so must part of any family's preparation. Understanding your emotions and feelings will not guarantee freedom from depression, but it will help. Neither will it cure depression, but it will help this too.

17 How can you know when to have a baby?

You cannot. Having a baby is something one can decide in a moment, or agonize over for years. Only our children can finally judge how well we chose the moment and even they can be wrong. Many of us are good with small babies and hopeless as they grow up; most of us are less than perfect at all stages. Don't let it worry you: could you have coped with perfect, infallible parents? The best we can hope for is that our children will be glad, in the long run, that they had us for parents. Warts and all.

18 The unknown in the equation

How you cope, how well you do, is a three-way equation. You know two of the elements before you start. The third is luck of the draw. Look around your family. Who has not got a relative to whom they would not give house room? In that moment when one sperm and one ovum meet, you are not there to select Aunt Meg's beautiful hair and Uncle Jim's fine nose, any more than you can reject Grandma's foul temper, or your own insecurity. Of course, the environment you provide colours and alters that basic endowment, but anyone who has had more than one child will tell you that children are different, and something of what they are, what they become is there from the beginning. Some children are easy, some you can say with feeling you

should have strangled at birth. Except, of course, you would not and could not. Other people's horrors you can blame on them; yours, alas, you are stuck with. Most have redeeming qualities. As indeed do most parents.

19 Why have children?

● 'It was never a conscious decision. More a feeling that one ought to have a family.'

● 'All our friends are having babies. I never questioned that we would too.'

● 'It seemed the obvious next step. We were approaching thirty. It was somehow the right time.'

We admire the family unit. It has taken some knocks, but most of us still believe in it. If we can get it right, it is still what we want.

20 A judgement

Jim and Sue have three children under five. They have just won first prize in a national lottery and decide to put their children up for adoption, buy a boat and sail around the world. It is something they both dreamed of doing before they had children.

All three children are adopted by a childless couple who can never have their own.

Your reaction?

Do you commend their generosity in providing a young family for the deprived couple?

Do you say, 'What an adventure – I wish I could be as certain about what I want from life'?

Do you say, 'How thoughtful and considerate not to confine toddlers on a small boat for 12 months'?

Of course not. Like most people, you think them selfish, and odd. You wonder why they had children if they were not prepared to raise them. You would probably not say so, but deep down you would feel they were breaking a sacred institution for a whim. See 89.

21 Conforming to social expectations

Conforming to society's expectations puts us in the mainstream of life. This is not necessarily a belittling conformity.

Collectively, we form society; together we guide and change its opinions. And it in turn forms us. Doing what is expected can be seen as doing what is right for most of the people, most of the time.

Of course, the 'accepted view' can be wrong for some individuals, and we may want to fight for change. But most things, including the instinct to raise a family, are as we want them, given the right timing, and give or take some adjustment.

22 Personal fulfilment

Children affirm a woman's femininity; yes, they reinforce the expectations raised by playing with dolls in childhood.

Children make men virile, masculine; turn them into provider and protector.

A child will make a parent feel whole and complete; at one with his or her human heritage; at one with him or herself for having passed on the gift of life.

These clichés are not universally true, but they contain a great deal of truth.

23 Personal identity

Life before children can lack focus: a job leading nowhere; enough money, enough dates, trips out, or sitting around in bars and cafés. You get a new kitchen, a new sofa, and your home changes until it looks like those in the magazines. But then what? Next year you will try Kenya for a holiday. And then?

You have taste, you have holidays, your job is satisfactory. But with children you could be mother to Jessica. Father to Mark. Life would have an additional meaning.

You may never be an interior designer, a travel writer or the world's best secretary. You may never make it as a top banker; but Jessica's face lights up when you come through the door.

Don't knock it. Good parenting is no small achievement, as those of us who are its products know only too well. The skills of loving and caring are greatly undervalued.

24 To please

● 'I wasn't wild to have children, but he wanted it so, and in the end I said "Well, why not? But you are going to have to get up in the night."'

● 'Dad wanted to be a grandfather so much. He went on and on about it, and so did Paul's mother. And in the end we sort of said "Well, why not?" Lots of our friends were doing it.'

25 For immortality

If you have children, then grandchildren, and great-grandchildren, there will always be something of you around for posterity. You will see the family looks reappear in each generation; pass on the business; keep the heirlooms in the family; have a daughter just like her mum.

26 For God

Most religions perceive having and raising children as basic to the purpose of life. To have children and bring them up in the knowledge and love of God is the very basis of marriage. It gives meaning to the union.

Catholicism and Judaism are perhaps the two most obviously family-oriented religions, but all religions, since they regulate life, also see a role for children within marriage. And in some, the absence of children is grounds for divorce.

27 For country

Today, our historians and politicians think in terms of regiments and dreadnoughts: the time will come when they think in terms of babies and motherhood. We must think in such terms too, if we wish Great Britain to be much longer great.
– Sir Frederick Truby King, 1921

28 For ideals

Raising children within a family is still, for most of us, the ideal. Even if, in the end, we leave it to others.

Most of us grow up in families. When talking of people who did not, we are inclined to add words such as unfortunate to any description of their upbringing. The feeling that the nuclear family of mother, father and children is how it should be is deeply ingrained in most of us.

29 Motherhood as instinct

A view we often ascribe to 'other people', but one that persists, is that life goes on because we all have an uncontrollable

Round faces, wide eyes: designed by nature to awake the mothering instinct.

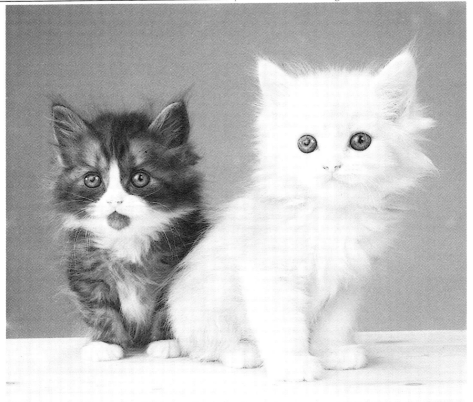

drive to reproduce. I find this a simplistic view; a more sophisticated version points out that there is in all of us a tendency to love the helpless, to say 'Ah' and 'Oo' when we see the young of any animal, including our own. See 124.

If you think you are immune, ask yourself, honestly, if you could walk past a kitten crying because it is stuck up a tree.

30 Getting it wrong

I can, I thought as I sat pregnant before the typewriter, finish my thesis, carry on in full-time research, cement the present harmony with my husband (a harmony often a little shaky prior to my pregnancy) and live happily ever after.

I wanted to make, as my parents had made, a close and happy family. Why? I think, for many of us who come from happy families, the love of a family becomes idealized into love without questions. For others, especially where love has been difficult, the love of a child for its parents is enormously attractive. We will love a child, and it will love us

whatever we are or do. 'Love for myself alone and not my yellow hair,' to misquote Yeats.

But of course it is not like this. Love, even mother-love, has to be learned. But the myth is strong, and the temptation seductive, especially when marriage, friendships and career do not live up to expectations. For myself, I know that in spite of being aware, at one level at least, that the tight, loving nature of my large, extended family appalled my husband, I set out to recreate it. It was, for me, security and comfort. I did not see the dangers, the selfishness of my actions. I would have said I understood what children meant (I am, after all, the eldest of five); so would he. Sadly, they meant different things to each of us.

I found myself, one year later, alone with a baby who slept no more than six hours in 24, a thesis still unfinished, a job badly done, little money to pay both baby sitter and mortgage, and unemployment looming. I understood, as I had not before, that it was possible to feel violence as well as love towards children. And if this violence was never expressed physically, it could be felt, at times, in an overwhelming desire to scream 'This is not what I meant.' And yet I would, and did, do it all again, because for me, life without children amounts to life without depth.

31 A change of life

Children do not guarantee happiness. Nor do they bring peace and harmony. They certainly interrupt careers, cost money, and alter the pattern and structure of your life. They will not solve your problems, or make a failing relationship work.

From conception to first words takes almost two years, about the same time as puberty, and it is at least as difficult. Like puberty it is, for a woman, a time of enormous hormonal changes. You will feel tired, depressed and elated. You will, if you are lucky, feel that you could take on the world, and at other times find it impossible to even cross the road. Your body can, in turn, give you enormous pleasure, both sexually and in feeding your child, or leave you wondering what you ever saw in sex, or for that matter how anyone could suggest that having a baby sucking at the breast gives pleasure.

32 The right age

If there is a rule of thumb, it is that probably the best time to embark upon parenthood is when you cannot imagine the future without children. This could be after years of coming to terms with the idea, or on finding yourself accidentaly pregnant. It could be at 17 or at 47, with no guarantee of success at either age.

I had my first baby at 28, my last at 37. Two of my sisters had babies as teenagers, and my mother had two babies in her forties. Was any age right? Any wrong?

33 The very young mother

Having a baby when you are under 20 brings a slightly increased risk of hypertension (see 270-273), premature labour (see 318) and having a 'small for dates' baby.

Taking on the strains of childcare when you are little more than a child yourself can make you feel trapped, that you are missing out as friends travel and have fun while you lack the money to pay a baby sitter.

Conversely, pregnancy and childbearing

is not so physically daunting for the very young. It is easier to get back into shape and to keep up with the children.

In her thirties, with her family ready to leave home, a woman still has the chance to develop a career which will not be disrupted by young children.

34 The middle route

I had my babies and established my career at the same time. Whether or not I would have been more successful as a mother had it been otherwise, I cannot say. I like to think sometimes that my career would have been more successful had I not had to cope with babies who did not sleep, or had I been able to work in the evenings and at weekends. But somehow I doubt it. At least this way I have an excuse for not achieving all that I thought I might.

Biologically, the twenties are perhaps the best years to have children. They are certainly the time that most of us choose.

For a woman whose career is her children, there will be other friends, other women of the same age doing much the same thing. It is a time when friendships are easily formed, the support of other women easiest to find.

35 Unemployment at 40

But having babies in one's twenties and early thirties can leave too many years of unemployment. Starting a new career at 40 is not easy. Nor is the redundancy faced by a career mother' when, in her early 40s, the children leave home.

36 Older mothers

Some women circumvent these problems by collecting their old age pension and family allowance at the same time. There are many advantages. You are mature, surer of what you want and can be more relaxed in your dealings with others. Your earning capacity is higher, making it easier to pay for childcare if you wish to return to work. Of course, it takes longer to get back into shape, and fewer of your friends have young children, but I find it hard to think of any real disadvantages.

All of us can see advantages in what we have done, and disadvantages. Perhaps we should view life as giving us what we need, when we need it. For some of us that is having a last-minute child; for others it is the first thing we do on reaching adulthood.

Medical Considerations

37 The father's age

Men over 36 years of age are more likely to produce sperm which are faulty and carry genetic disease; see 43. Why this is so no one fully understands, but the longer we have been around, the more chance we have of being exposed to harmful chemicals and other substances which can cause genetic mutations. This should not alarm you unduly. There is an increase in the number of early miscarriages when the father is older, and an increase in certain rare genetic disorders. But most of these, such as Alpert's Syndrome, in which the child has a deformed skull, are so rare (one in 160,000 births) that they can be discounted.

38 The mother's age

This also influences the rate of genetic disorders. The incidence of all chromosomal disorders rises from one in 527 births at the age of 25 to one in 23 at the age of 45. Of these, Down's syndrome – mongolism – is the most common. The probability of having a baby with Down's syndrome is one in 1,923 at 20, but one in 12 at 49. We can easily think of one in almost 2,000 as 'not us'; it is much harder to think of one in 12 this way. Add to this an increasing likelihood of other chromosomal disorders, which probably reduce the odds to somewhere in the region of one in nine babies at 49, and it would be foolish to think 'it could not happen to me'.

39 Age factors

Whether the father's age plays any Graph of incidence ofpart in causing Down's syndrome is difficult to judge. Studies in Japan, Denmark and Germany suggest that the incidence of Down's syndrome increases when fathers are over 41. Another study in the U.S.A. suggests that the father's age plays no role. It is possible to discover whether or not the child you are carrying has a chromosomal abnormality before birth, and abortion is normally offered to any woman in this position; see 232 and 238.

40 Preparation

Some of us plan well in advance; some of us get careless about contraception,

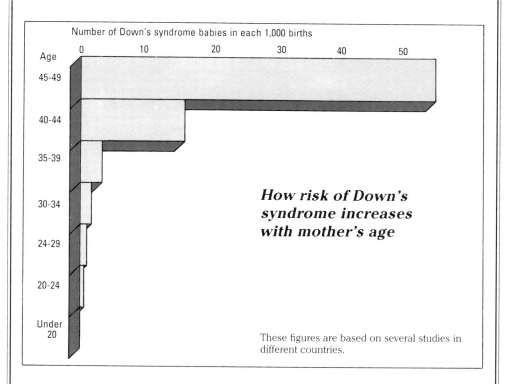

Number of Down's syndrome babies in each 1,000 births

Age		
45-49		
40-44		
35-39		
30-34		
24-29		
20-24		
Under 20		

How risk of Down's syndrome increases with mother's age

These figures are based on several studies in different countries.

saying "if it happens, it happens". Others have no intention of having a baby until they find that they are. But whether you plan or not, there are things you can do to ensure the health of your child.

41 Risks in proportion

By the time you are sure that you are pregnant, the embyryo is starting to take shape. It is delicate and vulnerable. Drugs, diet, smoking, and exposure to chemicals may influence its development.

The main organs of the body develop between the third and eighth weeks, with the brain and the gonads (the sex organs) developing a little later. Before the embryo begins to take shape at three weeks, any damage caused by chemicals (including drugs) will probably make you miscarry. After these critical three weeks, chemicals, and diseases such as *Rubella* (see 65), can cause certain organs to develop abnormally. Sometimes the abnormalities are so severe that the embryo cannot survive; again, the consequence is usually miscarriage. At other times the abnormalities, although serious, do not cause death and the baby will be born with a serious handicap.

The chance of serious abnormality, whatever the cause, is about two in 100 babies. Although, with care, you can

reduce the risks to your baby, you cannot eliminate them. Before you begin to panic, perhaps because you have been dieting, smoking or had too much to drink at a party, remember that everything that follows in the next few pages is about reducing that 2 per cent risk. There are few factors which increase the risk by a substantial amount. *Rubella* (German measles) does. Thalidomide did, and certain other chemicals might. Most risk factors carry only a slight probability of damage to the foetus. They are worth heeding *if you can.* They are not, worth panicking about if you cannot.

42 Maintaining sound general health

Health in pregnancy is like health at any other time. Eat sensibly, take exercise, don't smoke or binge on alcohol and coffee and take drugs sparingly or preferably not at all. By 'drugs' I mean over-the-counter preparations, prescription medications and 'street' drugs. If you are on any regular prescription drug, you must discuss the implications of this with your doctor before getting pregnant.

It is sensible to control feverish temperatures with paracetamol and to avoid harmful substances at home or work; see 50-62.

19

43 Genes and chromosomes

Genes are codes, sets of instructions which tell the developing embryo what to do. Each of us has the same set of genes, which is why we all look much the same. However, there are slight variations and it is these that make us look different. The more closely we are related, the more genes we have that are the same. So Irish people all have a certain look, which is different from a Greek look. You probably look more like your mother than I do.

You can think of genes as houses arranged along a street; the street is the chromosome. We have 23 different types of chromosome, which come in pairs. Each one of the pair is built with identical houses, so that, for example, in each instance number 27 is just before the bend and number 58 is next to the pub.

The key fact to grasp about chromosomes is that my streets are just like yours. In fact, everyone who has ever lived has had two streets in which 58 is next to the pub and 27 is just before the bend.

Although the houses never move, over the years people make changes: a new door here, a wall knocked down there. So the houses vary a little.

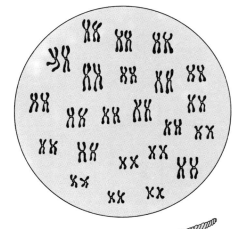

Top, the set of 23 chromosomes carried in a human cell. **Below**, chromosomes are made of the complex chemical compound DNA. 'Unravel' a chromosome, as in the illustration, and the beautiful spiral structure of the DNA molecule chain is revealed. **Opposite**, electron microscope photograph of human chromosomes magnified many thousands of times.

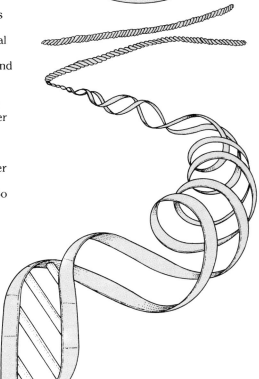

Genes can change in the same way; the changes are called mutations. We all have the same genes in the same places on the same chromosomes; but our mutations are different.

It is these mutations that make us all slightly different: they are responsible for some people being tall and others short, some fair and some dark. And it is mutations which produce genetic handicaps.

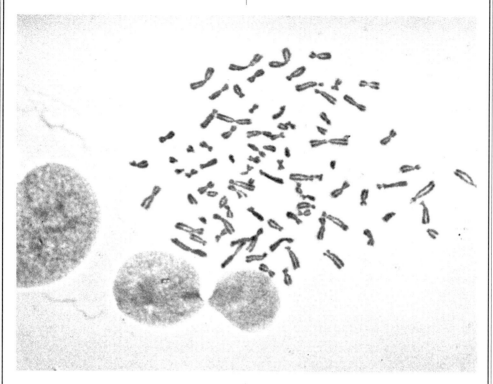

The fact that 'the houses' always stay in the same place makes it possible for scientists to look at our genes and see if we carry a mutation that will give our baby a handicap. Or to see if the baby who is growing in the womb has that handicap.

Once they know the address, scientists can, as it were, go in and see if you have knocked a wall down; see also 71.

44 Do I need counselling?

You should ask for genetic counselling if you or a close relative have a child handicapped by a genetic disease; if a genetic disorder, such as haemophilia, runs in your family; if you have had more than three miscarriages; or if you belong to certain racial groups (and your partner belongs to the same group); see 73. If you work with potentially harmful chemicals, counselling is also strongly advised.

Experts can now tell whether you and your partner are carriers of certain genetic disorders, and whether the baby you expect will have that disorder. But this does not mean they can give a guarantee that anyone is free from genetic disorders. There have been amazing leaps in the understanding of heredity in the last few years, but finding where a particular gene lives on a chromosome is like finding the house of a friend in a big city when you do not have the address. At present, science has managed only to locate the postal districts with varying degrees of exactitude.

However, if we do not know exactly where some genes are, we can at least say which street they are on, and at which end. And because houses in some terraces tend to stay much the same, science can state with a high degree of certainty that if some things are inherited, others will follow. We are at this stage of knowledge with many genetic diseases, including Huntingdon's chorea and cystic fibrosis. Screening every single person for every possible genetic defect would be an impossible task, and it will probably always be the case that many of us will only ever know that we carry a rare genetic disorder when we have passed it on to our child.

Heredity is, in any case, complex. Spina bifida does run in families and so does club foot, but it seems that even if a child has a genetic predisposition to spina bifida, it will not necessarily be handicapped in this way. In all these cases, genetic counselling can tell you the type of risks you run.

If you suffer from any chronic condition (epilepsy, diabetes, coeliac disease, heart disease or allergies), you should ask your doctor's advice on whether genetic counselling is necessary. See 71.

45 Can one usefully prepare for pregnancy?

Some doctors believe that pregnancy should be prepared for well in advance of conception, that the body, male and female, should be in good condition, free from drugs and correctly nourished. Some even claim that this would reduce the number of malformed babies and early miscarriages, and that many of those who have difficulty conceiving would benefit. As far as I can see, there is little firm evidence to support this.

Antibiotics, for instance, influence gut flora (microscopic organisms that aid digestion) for weeks after we stop taking them. Hormone balance is important in the maintainance of pregnancy in the first few weeks; it is in turn influenced by nutrition; and nutrition is affected by the flora in the gut. So, in theory, miscarriage could be induced by drugs taken in the month before conception. But there is no irrefutable evidence that it is, and whether any of this has a major influence on the average pregnancy is another matter.

Which leaves the question of whether sperm, or egg, can be damaged by outside influences in such a way as to result in a malformed foetus.

In theory, what a man eats, chemicals, X-rays or radioactivity, can affect sperm in two ways. They can damage the 'blueprint' – the germ cells – from which sperm are made, or rather copied; or they can damage the sperms themselves while they are stored in the testes. In the first instance, all sperm copied from a damaged cell will be faulty; in the second, only those sperm that were produced or stored at the time will be harmed.

Fortunately, most damage seems to be of the second type. Since sperm are stored for only about three weeks (after which they die), three weeks before conception would appear to be the critical time during which a man should take care of his sperm – if indeed that is possible. Put it another way: a normal, healthy life style and common sense precautions, such as avoiding X-rays in the weeks before conception, will make it more likely that a healthy sperm will win the race to the waiting ovum.

Much the same applies to the female ova. They are copied from 'blueprint' cells, the division taking place in the weeks before conception, during which common sense precautions are worthwhile.

46 Timing conception

If your periods are regular, you will conceive a fortnight before your period is due. See the chart.

47 Don't eat for two

What you eat and drink, the baby shares. This does not mean you have to eat for two: think of how little food a baby takes in the first few weeks of life – just a few ounces of milk at each feed. In the first weeks following conception, all you carry is a few extra cells, smaller than a pimple on your chin. It can easily share your normal food intake.

Fertility, day by day, over an average menstrual cycle of 28 days.

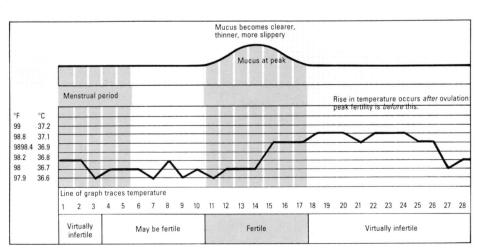

Mucus becomes clearer, thinner, more slippery

Mucus at peak

Menstrual period

Rise in temperature occurs *after* ovulation; peak fertility is *before* this.

°F	°C
99	37.2
98.8	37.1
9898.4	36.9
98.2	36.8
98	36.7
97.9	36.6

Line of graph traces temperature

1 2 3 4 5 6 7 8 9 10 11 12 13 14 15 16 17 18 19 20 21 22 23 24 25 26 27 28

Virtually infertile	May be fertile	Fertile	Virtually infertile

48 Malnutrition

Malnutrition can influence your ability to conceive. Many women suffering from *anorexia nervosa* ('slimmer's disease') stop menstruating and cannot become pregnant. If they do still ovulate and have regular (or irregular) periods, they suffer an increased likelihood of miscarriage. This is not because they are starving their baby, but because the correct hormone balance needed to maintain pregnancy depends upon adequate nutrition. Drastic and prolonged dieting, though falling short of anorexia, may have similar effects. If you think you should lose weight, do; but plan to stop the diet at least a month before you become pregnant.

Once you are pregnant, your baby is relatively immune from the effects of too little food. In the first six months of pregnancy only the severest malnutrition is likely to influence development. Your body will put the baby first and, needing so little, the baby will almost certainly receive enough to develop normally.

In the last three months, the baby demands more, but in the Western world undernutrition is still highly improbable – unless the mother goes on a prolonged crash diet, or suffers from anorexia. If by some unlikely chance there is genuine malnutrition, the consequences are increased miscarriage, premature birth, stillbirth and neonatal death. Low birth weight is common, but there is no evidence of any increase in the number of malformed babies.

As a result of malnutrition, there may be fewer cells in certain organs of the baby's body, including the brain, but it is not clear what effects this has on the child's well-being or intellect.

Malnourished children are small and often physically inert, but not necessarily dull. Indeed, it is difficult to show that children who have suffered from malnutrition *alone* (for example in times of war) have any persistent problems once food becomes available. They grow up to be as intellectually capable as those children who have not been malnourished if they grow up in a stimulating environment. The problem for many Third World babies is that malnutrition affects parents and children alike. How can a child be stimulated when all around her are inert for want of food?

49 Diet

Although it is difficult, in the developed world, to suffer from undernutrition or malnutrition, it is easy to eat the wrong food, or not to get enough of certain nutrients.

At least, make sure your diet has plenty of whole grains and green leafy vegetables, which contain folic acid (see box). Too little of this may increase the chance of spina bifida if you carry the genetic predisposition. Britain, especially South Wales and Northern Ireland, has the highest frequency of spina bifida in the world. The lowest incidence is in black, Asian and oriental peoples.

If you are at risk, it is wise to increase your intake of folic acid and other vitamins in the second half of each menstrual cycle: it is in the two or three weeks before you are certain of pregnancy that the risks can be lowered.

If you are taking folic acid, you may as well do so along with other useful vitamins. Capsules are available which include folic acid, vitamins A and D, thiamine, riboflavin, pyridoxine, nicotinamide, ascorbic acid, ferrous sulphate and calcium phosphate. Do not overdose. One tablet three times a day is normal.

Folic acid sources

Folic acid, as one of the vitamin B group, is merely one of several constituents of the diet necessary for normal functioning of various body organs. It is difficult not to get an adequate supply, even in pregnancy, when the body's demand for folic acid increases considerably. It is in all foods except fats, sugar and spirits. Folic acid deficiency, resulting typically from chronic alcoholism, can result in anaemia.

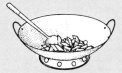

Prime sources include:
Liver, kidney, brewer's yeast and yeast extracts, spinach, parsley, beetroot, broccoli, watercress, lettuce.

• 50-90 per cent is destroyed by cooking vegetables, so eating raw, or quick stir-frying, make sense.

Other useful sources:
Cauliflower, cabbage, orange juice, rice

Useful but not so rich sources:
Oranges, carrots, bananas, potatoes, cheese.

Even if you do not want to take these capsules, it is certainly wise for British women of child-bearing age to increase the folic acid content of their diet.

Similarly, zinc in the diet may offer some protection if harelip runs in your family.

Since it is known that the correct balance of nutrients, trace elements and vitamins can affect a woman's hormone levels (and thus both conception and maintainance of pregnancy, as well as development of the embryo before the 14th week), it is in any case wise for any mother-to-be to switch to a diet rich in fruit, vegetables and whole grains, to eat less processed food, and to avoid fad diets and junk food. Lean meat and fish provide all the necessary proteins.

If you are a vegetarian, you should make sure that you get a variety of different proteins each day. As long as you include dairy products in your diet, you will not need to take any supplements. Vegans do need to watch their diets more carefully, and may need to take supplements.

50 Avoid excess caffeine

Caffeine is known to produce various congenital malformations in animals. In humans there are studies that show increased miscarriage, prematurity and congenital malformations; and there are studies which fail to confirm any of these. Until one can be certain, it is probably wise at least to cut down coffee and tea: both contain caffeine and eight cups in a day is probably excessive. Remember, too, that 'cola' drinks and certain other soft drinks can contain at least as much caffeine as coffee. Look at the list of constituents on the label.

You may find that nature cuts your consumption for you: going off tea and/or coffee is common in early pregnancy.

51 Avoid megavitamins

A normal dose of vitamins may be beneficial, but massive vitamin and mineral supplements are unwise. Women who take the oral vitamin A derivative, isotretinoin (also called accutane and used to treat acne), are 25 times more likely to have a miscarriage or a baby with congenital malformations of the cardiovascular and nervous systems. Other vitamins and minerals taken in large

doses are known to have similar effects in animals, although the picture is not clear in humans. Again, it is probably best to play safe, only taking these supplements on medical advice.

52 Are food additives safe?

There is little evidence to prove that food additives are harmful to the developing foetus, and little evidence of their safety, either. Since they can often be avoided, it is wise to do so when you can. Red food dye 2 (amaranth) is known to be harmful, and coal-tar dyes used in drugs and cosmetics are of questionable safety. Artificial sweeteners have been widely studied and are, for the most part, safe (some people have doubts about saccharin); and monosodium glutamate does not seem to be harmful in small quantities.

53 But isn't it all in the genes?

A child is always a product of its genetic inheritance (see 43) and the environment in which it develops. It is like cooking a cake. You take the ingredients: the genes and the environment; you mix them and bake them, and in the end you have a child. Once she is there, you cannot isolate the ingredients and state with certainty that such-and-such a defect is bound to be the result of such-and-such a deficiency or excess or congenital fault. What can be stated with certainty is that children born to mothers who smoke are smaller, that drinking too much alcohol, or having a high fever in early pregnancy, can produce problems. But however careful you are, there is no guarantee that pregnancy will be trouble-free.

Put like that, true or not, it is probably worth the small amount of effort required to put 'safety first' into practice during pregnancy.

54 The vulnerable embryo

The human embryo is most vulnerable to drugs and other chemicals in the first 12 to 16 weeks after conception (see 40-41), but if you find yourself pregnant unexpectedly there is no need to panic. During the earliest stages of development, the cells of the embryo are considered by many to be fairly resistant to harmful chemicals; or to put it more correctly, harmful chemicals will produce early miscarriage rather than a baby with deformities. Such a miscarriage may even occur before you realize you are pregnant.

If you have been exposed to any drugs prior to missing your first period, or in the time before your pregnancy is confirmed, consult your doctor. He can reassure you if the dangers are minimal, or advise on abortion if they are significant. You should also tell him if you have had injections of live vaccine during this period.

Once you know you are pregnant you will want to reduce any risk. Anything which is potentially harmful in the first three weeks is likely to be more harmful in the next six. But the risk is, nevertheless, often only slight.

Drugs in pregnancy: summary

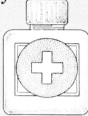

Unless specifically given a safe substitute, ALWAYS AVOID the following:

Analgesics, including aspirin

Recently introduced antibiotics

Anti-coagulants (for blood clotting problems)

Hormones/hormone replacement therapy

Anti-emetics (against nausea) and antihistamines

Immunizations/vaccinations

Best avoided:

Antacids

Laxatives

Tranquillizers

Antidepressants

Steroids

Thyroid drugs

See 55-65

Anti cancer (cytotoxic) drugs are always forbidden in pregnancy.

55 Medicines in pregnancy

Before taking any drugs in pregnancy it is wise to remember that most drugs, chemicals and chemical substances have not been adequately studied. Science may well have established that a drug could influence the foetus, but not how much, nor in what circumstances. Few drugs can be guaranteed safe.

Remember it took a number of years before the effects of thalidomide were known; it was frequently prescribed to pregnant women and caused major and unusual birth defects.

You are advised to follow these rules when taking any drug:
- If you can avoid taking it, do.
- If the doctor does not tell you it is safe to take in pregnancy, ask.
- Read the information on the package. This will tell you if the drug is known to be harmful during pregnancy.
- If you are still nervous, check before taking the drug.

Libraries and medical bookshops have books advising doctors what can and cannot safely be prescribed in pregnancy. There may also be a local telephone advice line: some cities in the USA have them. If you cannot get a quick and satisfactory reply from your doctor, you could try the pharmacology department in your nearest medical school. You might also like to try the departments of obstetrics, embryology, neonatology and medical genetics at the local hospital.

Unless a new drug is the only thing which can maintain your health, avoid it.

If you are dependent on 'street drugs', it is essential that you treat this before having children. Dependency on heroin and barbiturates can be passed on to your child. If you are not dependent, the risks (even if small) are not worth taking. Street drugs are often cut with other (unknown) substances which may carry their own risks.

56 Occasional use of street drugs

If you are an occasional user of street drugs (and one of those occasions was in early pregnancy), be assured that the chances of this causing any serious damage are extremely slight. No one has studied occasional users, and even studies of heavy users are not clear cut. Many of the people studied do a number of potentially harmful things apart from drug-taking. They drink alcohol, smoke cigarettes, eat poorly, have untreated illnesses, and live in poor housing. All of these factors are known to affect the unborn child.

57 Over-the-counter drugs

Few over-the-counter drugs are known to be harmful, but it must be said that few of them have been tested. They were in use long before adequate testing was introduced. Remember that many of these drugs, particularly cough medicines and cold remedies, are mixtures. Some of them contain iodine, and these should be avoided: iodine can harm the foetus. Large doses of aspirin have been associated with harelip and midline body defects. If you can avoid taking aspirin or medication which includes aspirin, do. Although some of the evidence is disputed, there are safer alternatives such as paracetamol. Later in pregnancy, aspirin can cause foetal bleeding, including brain haemorrage, and can increase the likelihood of pre- and post-delivery haemorrage.

However, all the surveys have been carried out on women who took large doses of aspirin. If you have to take large doses for a pre-existing medical condition, you will need to consult your doctor. For the rest of us, it is worth remembering that high fever is associated with birth defects, and that here the evidence is probably clearer. If you do get a high fever, you must lower it as quickly as you can. Take paracetamol if you have it to hand, and back this up by sponging with ice cold water or sitting in a cool bath (get out before you become shivery). If you have no paracetamol or no access to a cold bath, aspirin is almost certainly safer than the fever.

Antacids are also best avoided, but if you suffer from heartburn late in pregnancy, your doctor may be able to prescribe a relatively safe one for you.

58 Antibiotics

New antibiotics are being developed all the time. There is no evidence that they cause foetal abnormalities in the early stages of pregnancy, but serious maternal reactions do occasionally occur, and these could be harmful. Your doctor will advise you. Later in pregnancy, certain antibiotics can cause deafness in the child. (See 278.)

59 Anti-cancer drugs

Because these kill dividing cells, all anti-cancer drugs must be regarded as potentially harmful to the developing foetus.

60 Anticoagulants

Many of these are harmful, resulting in miscarriage, foetal death and neonatal death in approximately 20 per cent of cases. They should be taken only under specialist supervision.

61 Anticonvulsant drugs

Many of these cause problems, but not all are unsafe. If you need to take them, it is wise to consult your doctor before becoming pregnant. He can then make sure that you are taking the safest variety, and that the dose has been adjusted to suit you. You may need to watch dose levels carefully throughout your pregnancy. See also 85.

62 Hormones

Many of these may cause problems later in pregnancy, but in the early weeks most of them are safe although oestrogen (DES) should be avoided. The sex hormones (testosterone and oestrogen) should never be taken during the period in which the baby's sex organs are developing.

The contraceptive pill causes an increase in cardio-vascular and skeletal defects. Many doctors feel the risk is high enough to advise abortion, others disagree. It is therefore best to stop taking the pill a few months before you intend to become pregnant.

63 Other contraceptives

There is a report from the U.S.A. that the use of spermicide creams after conception may increase the chances of having a handicapped baby; more studies are needed before we can be sure of this. Until then, it is probably wise if your pregnancy is planned to avoid these creams in the month prior to conception. Many people think that fears about these creams have been exaggerated (see 216).

64 Psychodynamic drugs
It is sensible to avoid monoamine oxidase inhibitors, and lithium carbonate (both used in the treatment of depression), since both carry considerable risks. But it is extremely foolish to stop taking them abruptly. If you are taking any of these drugs, you should discuss pregnancy with your doctor before going ahead.

There are also doubts about diazepam (Valium) and chlordiazepoxide (Librium) taken during pregnancy.

65 Vaccination
You should not have a vaccination using live serum when you are pregnant. Nor should you have a child vaccinated against German measles *(Rubella)* if you intend to get pregnant in the near future. *Rubella* is serious if it is contracted during pregnancy. Tell your doctor at once if you come into contact with the disease. He can test your immunity.

66 If you are seriously ill. . .
Your child is dependent upon your survival, now and throughout her early life. Putting yourself at risk is selfish and short-sighted. Children need mothers for at least 18 years, not just safe vessels to carry them to birth.

If you are seriously ill and suspect you are pregnant, see your doctor at once. If you know you are on drugs essential to you but dangerous to a foetus, you should not be considering pregnancy until you are well.

67 Alcohol
Between 30 and 50 per cent of the babies born to alcoholic mothers who continue to drink during pregnancy will have some birth defects. Up to 80 per cent will have foetal alcohol syndrome, which includes mild or moderate mental retardation, as well as a range of other serious malformations.

Even small amounts (four units – see panel) of alchohol taken daily can produce slight effects.

The conclusion is simple: if you avoid nothing else, avoid drinking.

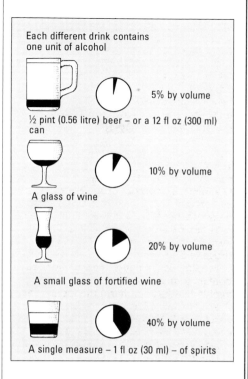

Each different drink contains one unit of alcohol

½ pint (0.56 litre) beer – or a 12 fl oz (300 ml) can — 5% by volume

A glass of wine — 10% by volume

A small glass of fortified wine — 20% by volume

A single measure – 1 fl oz (30 ml) – of spirits — 40% by volume

68 Cigarettes
For a heavy smoker, the risk of spontaneous abortion is increased by almost 2 per cent. There is also a risk of still birth, prematurity and low birth weight.

If you always meant to stop smoking, pregnancy gives you the opportunity to see it through.

69 Radiation
Although large doses of radiation are certainly harmful, exposure of the foetus to 1-3 rads (the amount used in an single X-ray) does not seem to be dangerous. Obviously, unnecessary exposure should be avoided, not least because the effects of radiation can last a lifetime. People exposed to radiation at work may develop cancer many years later. It is possible (and there is a small amount of evidence for this) that although your baby is perfectly normal at birth, she could develop cancer in childhood because she was exposed to radiation in the uterus.

70 CAT scans
Computerized tomography – body scans – also known as CT or CAT scans are not known to be harmful.

27

71 Family history

A genetic (see 43) disease is one which can potentially be passed on within families. There are different types, each with a varying risk of recurrence.

Perhaps those we understand best are chromosomal disorders. The genes are arranged along the chromosomes like houses along a street; see 43. A chromosomal disorder occurs when a child inherits an extra chromosome, part of a chromosome, or one with a major rearrangement. For example, imagine that the houses at the top of the street had been lifted up in a hurricane, twisted around and dropped further down the street. This is what is known in genetics as a translocation. Down's syndrome (mongolism), the chromosomal disorder we probably know best, can be caused by a translocation of chromosome 21 (which can run in families); by an extra chromosome 21 (most Down's children are of this type); or, more rarely, when a child has a mixture of normal and abnormal cells.

The most common diseases with a genetic component are called multifactorial or polygenic, meaning they are controlled by more than one gene. Coronary heart disease is one, cancer another, severe depression, schizophrenia, and hypertension are others. Alcoholism is yet another.

Looking at this list, one can, however, see more than one factor at work. Yes, it does seem that some families have more than their fair share of cancer. But we also know that cigarette smoking increases lung cancer, that the genital wart virus (commonest in the promiscuous) plays some role in cervical cancer. In other words, the life style or even the temperament of the individual also plays a role.

If both your parents suffer from schizophrenia, you have a 40 per cent chance of inheriting the disease. But we know there is more than genetic inheritance involved because the identical twin of a schizophrenic patient has only a 40 per cent chance of developing

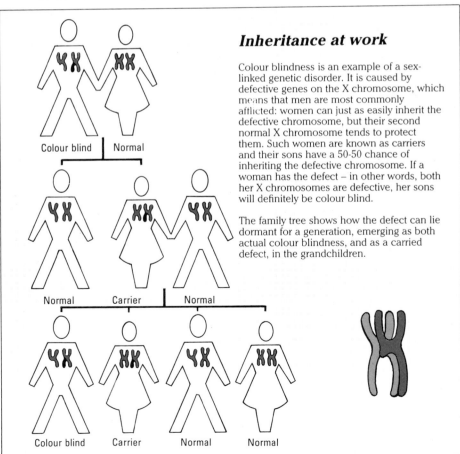

Colour blind | Normal

Normal | Carrier | Normal

Colour blind | Carrier | Normal | Normal

Inheritance at work

Colour blindness is an example of a sex-linked genetic disorder. It is caused by defective genes on the X chromosome, which means that men are most commonly afflicted: women can just as easily inherit the defective chromosome, but their second normal X chromosome tends to protect them. Such women are known as carriers and their sons have a 50-50 chance of inheriting the defective chromosome. If a woman has the defect – in other words, both her X chromosomes are defective, her sons will definitely be colour blind.

The family tree shows how the defect can lie dormant for a generation, emerging as both actual colour blindness, and as a carried defect, in the grandchildren.

schizophrenia at any time in her life, even though she has all her genes in common with the patient. Many aspects of your child's intelligence and temperament are probably inherited in a similar way: the genetic background is enhanced and changed by the environment in which the child grows.

It is, perhaps, easiest to imagine how this works if you think of something as seemingly fixed as the way a person looks. Personality, dress sense, style, flair, can all combine with a basic physical endowment to make that person rather ordinary or exceptionally pretty.

Other, rarer, genetic diseases result from the action of a single gene which is transmitted according to the laws of Mendelian inheritance. This means that if you carry the gene, you have a 50 per cent chance of passing it on to your child. Your partner has exactly the same chance if he carries the gene.

What does that mean? If the gene concerned is dominant, it means that if you carry the gene and pass it on to your offspring, the child will have the disorder. In order for your child to inherit a genetic disease carried on a dominant gene, one of the parents must have that disease. Huntington's chorea, a type of senile dementia that occurs in men and women in early middle age, is carried on a single dominant gene. You will almost certainly know if any such diseases run in your family.

Most single-gene disorders are probably recessive. This means that in order to inherit the disease, a child must have two genes which code for the disorder. In other words, both you and your partner must be carriers. Most of us carry a number of genes such as this, and most of us never know about them. Sadly, until we produce a child with the disorder, we often have no way of knowing.

Sickle cell anaemia, beta thalassaemia, Tay-Sachs disease, and cystic fibrosis are examples of single-gene genetic disorders. You are more likely to carry the first three if you belong to certain racial groups. One in 22 people is a carrier of cystic fibrosis: one in 400 couples is at risk of producing an affected child.

72 Sex-linked disease

A sex-linked disease is carried on the X, or female, chromosome: women are carriers, men sufferers. Women may have the disease, but this is very rare. If they do have it, they will hand it on to all their sons. A man with the disease cannot pass it on to his children, but his grandchildren can inherit it from his daughters. Colour blindness, haemophilia and Duchenne's muscular dystrophy are carried in this way. If a woman's brothers are affected, she has a 50 per cent chance of being a carrier, and may pass the disease to her sons. If her father was affected, she will certainly be a carrier.

In some sex-linked diseases, such as colour blindness and Duchenne's muscular dystrophy, it is often possible to tell whether or not a woman is a carrier, since she is mildly affected by the gene. With haemophilia the woman is usually affected, as also with alpha and beta thalassaemia and with sickle cell anaemia. See also 109.

73 When to seek advice

Although it is often impossible to say whether someone carries a disorder, in certain instances it is important that you ask advice.

Jewish couples have an increased risk of producing children with Tay-Sach's disease and the infantile form of Nieman-Pick's disease. Black people of African origin are more likely to carry sickle cell anaemia; Afrikaners are at increased risk with cystic fibrosis and Huntington's chorea; and people of Mediterranean origin have a tendency to beta thalassaemia. Among Cypriots, as many as one in six people are carriers, and the incidence is also high in Greeks, Italians and Indians. In all these cases, it can be established whether you might pass the disease on to your child. If you belong to one of these groups, you should ask for genetic counselling.

74 How common are genetic disorders?

About one infant in every hundred is affected. Many of these are minor disorders, few are life-threatening. More and more genetic disorders are recognized each year. There were thought to be 1,487 in 1966; by 1983 this had risen to 3,368. Some of these are sub-types or sub-groups of diseases that are already known.

75 Inherited asthma

Three in every hundred people suffer from asthma at some time in their lives. But your family, like mine, may have more than its fair share. Some of the causes are genetic.

If there is a history of bronchial asthma in your family, the risk to all first-degree relatives is about 5 per cent. However, if some of your relatives have allergic rhinitis, hay fever, or eczema, then the risk that your child will have asthma or one of those allergic problems is increased. If a brother or sister is affected, the risk rises to 10 per cent. If one parent is affected, it rises to 26 per cent, and if both parents are affected, to 34 per cent.

These are 'life span' risks: they could occur at some time in your child's life. It does not mean the child will be asthmatic. It could mean she will have hay fever as an adult or get a rash from touching cats.

76 Inherited diabetes

Diabetes is not one disease, but several, and some forms are more heritable than others.

If a member of the immediate family (mother, father) has juvenile onset insulin-dependent diabetes, the risk to a child is between 1 and 2 per cent. If you already have one child with this form of diabetes, it rises to between 5 and 10 per cent for subsequent children.

If either parent has mature onset non insulin-dependent diabetes, the risk is between 5 and 10 per cent.

If either parent has maturity-onset diabetes, the risk is 50 per cent. But although this risk is high, the condition itself is mild.

77 Inherited hypertension and heart disease

There are many causes, some of which have a definite genetic component. Risks cannot be assessed until the type of hypertension is known. The same goes for heart disease. Your doctor, or hospital, will be able to tell you what the risks are for your child.

78 Inherited epilepsy

The chances of passing on epilepsy are about 5 per cent if one parent is affected, rising to 10 per cent if both suffer from the condition. It is 5 per cent if one of your previous children is affected.

79 Inherited multiple sclerosis (MS)

About 3 per cent of children develop the disease if either parent suffers.

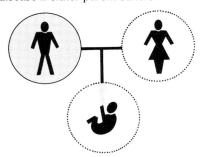

80 Inherited cancer

Certain forms of cancer also seem to run in families, breast cancer being the obvious example. Some studies suggest that the risk rises from one in 12 to one in 5 if one's mother has had a breast tumour. The risk factors for most cancers have not, however, been assessed; nor is it clear whether all, or even most, cancers have a genetic component.

81 Inherited mental disorders

Schizophrenia and manic-depression do run in families; quite how heritable they are depends on which survey you believe, and what one considers as schizophrenia. The figures which follow are conservative. (Depression in this context means clinical depression, or depressive psychosis, not just feeling low or having premenstrual tension.)

If either parent has schizophrenia the risk is 13 per cent; if both parents have it, it is 40 per cent; if a brother or sister is affected, it is 9 per cent; and if a cousin is affected, 3 per cent. Again, these are lifespan risks. If an individual has shown signs of schizophrenia by the age of 30, the risk is halved, by 50 it is exceedingly small.

The risks for depressive disorders can be divided into those which involve only depression, and those which include manic episodes. Manic-depressive psychosis is more heritable than depressive psychosis. The figures are similar to those found in surveys of schizophrenia.

82 Inherited alcoholism

The harsh truth is that drink problems are easily inherited.

83 Risk summary

84 Occupational hazards

The panel lists possible hazards to working women during pregnancy. It is not exhaustive (how could it be?), nor is there any firm evidence that everything in the list is harmful. It is best regarded as a list of things to avoid if possible. If you belong to one, ask your union if it has any information about the dangers to pregnant women working in your industry.

85 Mother has long-term medical condition

- Asthma should cause a pregnant woman no problems, it may even get better in pregnancy. If the asthma is severe, you will need careful management. If you are short of breath, so will the foetus be. Check with your doctor that your asthma medication is safe in pregnancy – not all of it is risk-free.
- Epilepsy: There is no reason why women with epilepsy should not become pregnant; but pregnancy must be carefully managed, since in a small number of cases it can lead to an increase in the number of seizures. You may need to change your current medication for a safer one, and to take additional folic acid; see also 63.
- Diabetes: It is safe to become pregnant, but careful management is required. Some oral diabetic medicines may increase the

Possible occupational hazards in pregnancy

Occupation	Substances
Anaesthesia	Anaesthetic gases
Clerical workers	VDUs, trichloroethylene, carbon tetrachloride, cleaning agents, asbestos in air conditioning
Dentists and dental hygienists	Anaesthetic gases, mercury, X-ray, solvents, cements
Domestic cleaners	Soaps detergents, alkalis, solvents, hydrocarbons
Dry cleaners	Industrially contaminated clothes, perchloroethylene, trichloroethylene, benzene, naphtha
Electronics	Epoxy resins, methylene chloride, trichloroethylene, methylethyl ketone, tin, lead, antimony
Hairdressers, beauticians	Hairspray resins, halogenated hydrocarbons, hair dyes, benzyl alcohol, ethyl alcohol, acetone, nail polish solvents
Doctors and paramedics	Infectious agents, radiation, X-ray, anaesthetic gases, drugs, chemicals, radioactive isotopes, blood products
Laboratory workers	Chemicals that may be carcinogens, mutagens, and/or teratogens, radiation
Opticians	solvents, iron oxide, hydrocarbons, coal tar pitch volatiles
Photographic processing	Bromides, iodides, mercuric chloride, caustics, pyrogallate acid, silver nitrate
Clothing manufacture	Common and synthetic fibre dusts, formaldehyde, organic solvents, asbestos

risk of foetal abnormality, but insulin injections and diet management are safe; see also 222 and 223.
• High blood pressure: a successful pregnancy is possible, given careful management; see also 246.
• Heart conditions: don't become pregnant without consulting your doctor first.
• Thyroid therapy: avoid becoming pregnant.
• Cancer treatment: avoid becoming pregnant.

86 Lifestyle

Putting your feet up was what doctors often used to advise. But this was always a fantasy for most women: as if anyone with two or three small children and a home to run could rest most of the day.

Exercise can be continued during pregnancy; see 94-95. You certainly should not think of giving it up before you conceive. Exceptionally intense athletic exercise (for example, training for a marathon), may occasionally produce a temporary loss of periods (and thus temporary infertility), but even this is unlikely. You can travel, work (unless you work with hazardous materials) and continue all your normal activities.

The U.S. Federal Drugs Authority suggests that pregnant women should not lean against microwave ovens. You may want to go further and avoid using them altogether in the early stages of pregnancy.

Toxoplasmosis is an infection you can catch from cats and uncooked meat. It is rare – one in 8,000 people is likely to catch it – so it is not worth giving up your cat; nor however, is this the time to get a new one. You can also catch it from raw meat and raw fish. If you are worried, ask your doctor for a blood test.

Saunas, hot whirlpools and indeed any prolonged hot bath is unwise in the early stages of pregnancy. Gin and a hot bath was, after all, an old recipe for abortion. Sun-ray lamps should also be avoided, not because ultraviolet rays are dangerous but because of the possibility of overheating.

Perming your hair is fine, colouring may not be if coal-tar based dyes are used – there have long been suspicions that these are carcinogenic. If cells are dividing rapidly, as they are when a baby develops, carcinogens may be especially dangerous.

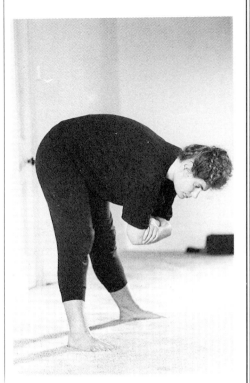

87 Home birth? Plan now

In hospital used to be the only answer, at least in recent years. But there are other choices. The main alternative is, of course, to have the baby at home. It is often easier said than done, since many doctors have an aversion to home delivery. There is no basis for the prejudice: for most women it is at least as safe as a hospital delivery. If you intend to have the baby at home, you need to start planning and organizing now, not because it is actually difficult to have babies at home but because it is difficult to get many members of the medical professions to agree that you have a choice and that it is perfectly safe.

Start by asking your doctor and midwife if it is possible, and if they will attend you in these circumstances. If they will not, you have to find someone who will. Many countries have organizations promoting home confinement which should be able to help you find someone qualified to attend a home birth. The local health authority should also be able to advise.

If you have any strong opinions about the way the baby is to be born, you should also ask the hospital about its birthing policy. Say how you would like the baby delivered and ask if this is possible. If it is not, ask around. There may be another hospital within reach that might be more receptive to your requests.

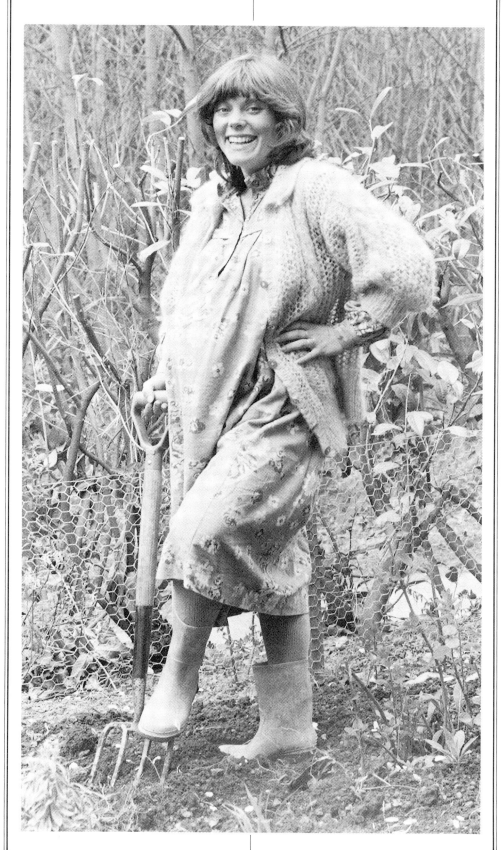

Being Prepared, Body and Mind

88 Planning work

For the majority of women, the birth of a first child marks at least a temporary end to paid employment. But it is a slim majority: about 40 per cent of women who work during pregnancy are back at work by the time their baby is eight months old. Know your rights to employment: the legislation that protects a woman's job while she gives birth may not apply in certain countries (including the UK) if you have recently changed jobs. Nor does it protect the jobs of those working in small concerns. Of course, you could find that your union has negotiated a favourable agreement with your employer, and that there are subsidized childcare facilities available for your return to work. In most countries, however, the odds are against this. If you think you may continue working after the child is born, childcare facilities should be investigated now. There are often long waiting lists for places in daycare nurseries; see 647.

Pregnancy rapidly becomes obvious. It is not an illness, but do not assume you will be able to carry on as normal. In the first months you may feel tired and sick; in later months you may be forced to rest because of complications. Your work could suffer. Your workmates are the people most likely to be affected by this, and it is only fair to let them know before they guess for themselves. You should also give plenty of warning to anyone who will be affected by your taking time off work when the baby is born. You cannot be sacked because you are pregnant; but this is hardly the point. If you intend to continue working after the baby is born you need the goodwill of colleagues.

Sleepless nights, sick children, childminders with a sudden dose of 'flu: however well you plan your cover, there are simply more things to go wrong when you add a baby to your life. Any woman working while her children are small needs her work colleagues on her side. See also 279.

89 Right to a home

If you are pregnant and living in some countries, including the U.K., there is probably legislation giving homeless persons the right to housing, but not the right to housing in which it is suitable to rear a child. If you live in a large city the chance of waiting a long time for such subsidized accommodation is probably higher than elsewhere.

90 Moving house

Small babies take up a great deal of space. Just visit a friend who has a baby; better still, ask them to stay for the weekend. Once the pram is in the hall, the chair in the kitchen and the cot in the bedroom, you may begin to feel you need a bigger place.

Taking on a bigger mortgage as you loose one salary (or start having to pay for childcare) puts added strain on your adjustment to parenthood. But you may feel it less of a strain than being short of space.

The most organized will move before pregnancy, the less organized while pregnant. Only the foolhardy will move into a new home with a new baby, especially if that home needs work done on it. DIY with a baby in tow can be hell, and getting people in to do the work does not really solve the problem.

91 Local support

Life with a small baby can be lonely, especially if your life was filled by a busy job and social life. Four-hourly feeds (the maximum gap, not the norm if you breast feed) restrict you, and days seem long without the company of another adult. You may never have seen neighbours as friends before, but they can be: the quick cup of coffee between a load of washing and feeding the baby can restore your sanity on a bad day. Cultivate a local support group.

92 New friends

The whole basis of life changes in the months as you await a baby, and it is not surprising that you look for others to share the experience. Pregnancy, particularly the middle trimester, is a time when many couples make new and lasting friends.

It is often difficult for those without children to understand 'baby obsessions', or, to be fair, to know how to react to them.

Few people want to be accused of being sexist, or to be seen to patronize women. Does talking about the baby fall into this class? The acceptable position is that women have careers, thoughts, opinions and interesting things to say. Having and rearing children is a rather old-fashioned thing to do, something you mention, like the weather, before the real conversation.

You may intend to give up your job, but it might be thought sexist for anyone else to make this assumption. You will find that people tread warily, unsure how to react to your pregnancy. They may even pretend not to notice.

This can be carried to ridiculous extremes. I once applied for a job in which there was a seven-month delay between application and interview. I wanted the job, and thought that saying I was pregnant would imply that I did not. I can only assume that the ten men on the interview panel thought it sexist to mention my obvious condition (I was seven months pregnant). The result was that although no one mentioned my bulging stomach, avoiding the subject actually dominated the whole interview.

Even close friends may feel that pregnancy and babies are taboo subjects unless you start the conversation. When you feel the need to share baby obsessions, other pregnant women are, in the end, often the best companions.

93 Body image

Slim is beautiful. Fat is ugly. So can you really be pregnant and beautiful? No woman can have a baby and keep her waistline. If you are naturally slim, you may be unaware of your own prejudices against fatness until you find you can no longer squeeze into your jeans. If you already despair of your uncontrollable tendency to plumpness, you may find yourself very unhappy with your body once you cannot do up the waistband of your skirt.

Faced with a thickening waist, you may resort, as many women do, to the biscuit packet or cake tin for comfort; increasing your inches, and your problems.

One of the major advantages of the current vogue for exercise and fitness is that it has changed the fashionable body image from super-thin to super-firm. Slimness is out of the question for the next nine months, healthy muscle tone is not. Indeed, even without work, the stomach and leg muscles will become firmer and stronger. Fitness can help you feel pride, not despair, at your changing body shape.

94 Keeping fit...

Firm muscles and the ability to run a mile will not guarantee a trouble-free pregnancy, an easy birth, or a healthy baby. But you will feel good, look good

35

and be better equipped pysically and mentally to face your changing lifestyle.

Exercise increases muscle strength, stamina and body flexibility. It is the first two of these which are most important in pregnancy. Flexibility makes it harder to damage muscles, but learning to do the splits or to put your head between your knees can wait. There is no need to stop being flexible. Jane Irwin was three and a half months pregnant when she won a bronze medal for platform diving in the 1952 Olympics.

Doubt is often expressed about the wisdom of stamina exercises when women are pregnant. But if you are fit, there is no problem. Andrea Mead Lawrence won two skiing medals at the 1952 Winter Olympics while pregnant; Mary Jones completed a half marathon in 2 hours 5 minutes in 1976

when eight months pregnant; and the jockey Mary Bacon won three races the day her daughter was born. All without ill effects.

These are, of course, exceptional instances. Marathon running, learning to ski and horse racing would be unwise for the average pregnant woman. It is not what you do, but the way you do it; not the exercise that is dangerous, but the side-effects of breathlessness, overheating and exhaustion if you are unfit.

Never push yourself until you are overheated; high temperature, however produced, can be dangerous in the first few months of pregnancy.

You should not run or swim until you are panting for breath. If you are short of breath, your baby will be too. But if you are fit, and sensible, avoid hot humid weather, and slow down on the hills, none of this should happen.

A warming dozen

Always start at the top of your body and work down. Stand with your feet hip-width apart, back straight, bottom tucked in.

1 Touch your left ear to your shoulder eight times, repeat to the right.
2 Try and point your chin to the ceiling, holding for a count of four. Repeat four times.
3 Lower your chin to your chest for another count of four.
4 Roll your shoulders forward for eight, then back.
5 Next screw up your face as small as possible. Hold for eight.
6 Now open your mouth as wide as possible.

You should feel these exercises stretching the muscles of the neck and those that support the breasts.

7 Grip each wrist with your hands. Holding your arms out in front and level with your breasts, push the skin up towards your elbow, hold and relax. These are small quick movements. You should feel the benefit in the muscles supporting the breasts.
8 Next, lean forwards from the waist, holding for a count of eight.
9 Now put your hands behind your head and lean to the left, then the right, eight times. Move from the waist, keeping the hips and legs still.
10 Put one hand on your hip and raise the other in a curve over your head. Stretch to the side, pointing the upper hand towards the floor. Hold for eight and repeat to the other side. Keep hips and legs still. Now move your hand on to your thigh and repeat. You should feel the stretch in your waist.

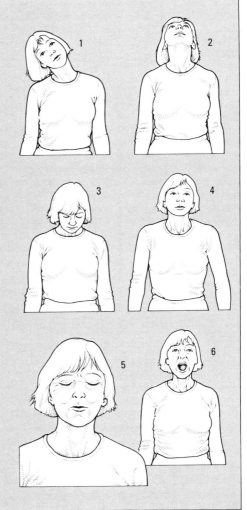

Even if you are less than perfectly fit, a gentle 20-minute jog or a brisk walk will not cause problems: indeed many pregnant women find swimming or energetic walking the most comfortable way to take exercise. Sports requiring fine balance may be uncomfortable during pregnancy.

95 Exercises

Because of humans' upright stance, we carry babies rather low, and out in front. This can, and often does, put considerable strain on the back. If your abdominal muscles are weak, and/or your posture bad, you may be prone to backache. It is advisable to tone up these muscles and to work them gently throughout your pregnancy.

This does not mean you should do daily sit-ups and leg-lifts. Both are potentially dangerous, and can cause difficulties for anyone prone to back trouble. A beneficial exercise will seem easy and will not cause strain. It will work the muscles by the repetition of small movements; you should feel it doing good, not hurting, and should build on this day by day. Cold muscles are easily damaged. Before starting any exercises, warm up with some gentle stretches and a little jogging on the spot.

Most warm-up programmes include plenty of toe touching: not necessarily a sensible idea for the heavily pregnant. I found it easier when pregnant to bend my knees while touching my toes (or the floor in front), and to stretch by bending and straightening my legs from this position. Flex your knees as you come up from this bent position. Remember the extra weight out front can strain your back if you lift yourself from the waist.

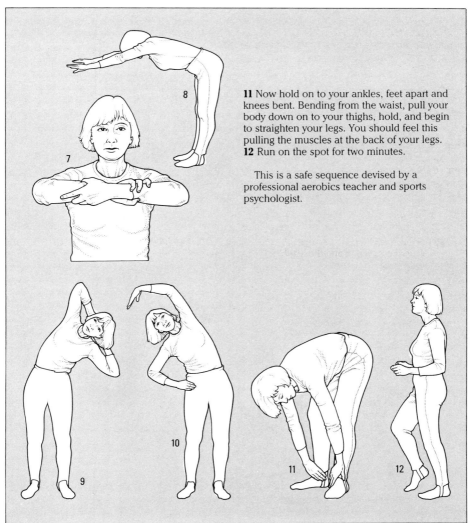

11 Now hold on to your ankles, feet apart and knees bent. Bending from the waist, pull your body down on to your thighs, hold, and begin to straighten your legs. You should feel this pulling the muscles at the back of your legs.
12 Run on the spot for two minutes.

This is a safe sequence devised by a professional aerobics teacher and sports psychologist.

The pelvic floor muscles
The unseen muscles

A little back ache is one thing. Gynaecological problems are quite another.

However out of condition a woman's body gets, her pelvic floor should be well exercised before, during and after pregnancy. Few of us get through life without gynaecological problems: a sagging pelvic floor makes them more likely to occur. Standing upright means that the muscles around the vagina are under pressure for much of pregnancy, and after a vaginal delivery they will be very stretched indeed. If you do no other exercise, at least use this daily routine, preferably for the rest of your life.

If you do not keep to this, promise yourself at least that you will pee haltingly, as described below, between now and the time that the baby is six months old. Ignore this advice and you may find yourself, like many mothers, with stress incontinence: a tendency to wet your pants when you run, jump, or cough.

It is easiest to find the muscles in question when you urinate. Wait until you have a full bladder, pee with full force and halt. No dribbling. Start the flow again, and stop. The muscles you are using are the ones you need to exercise. (You may also know them as the ones you move voluntarily, and involuntarily, when you make love.)

If they are in good shape, you should be able to stop the flow of urine from a full bladder while standing with your legs apart. Or, with a full bladder, do 20 'jumping jacks' without leaking.

If you are still unsure that you have the right muscles, imagine you are caught short. You need a loo, but there is not one around. Stand with your knees relaxed and imagine you need to pee. Stop yourself. Now imagine you have diarrhoea; hold it back. Lastly imagine that a tampon is slipping out. Try to draw it back in.

Those are your pelvic floor muscles. They are arranged in a figure of eight around your anus and vagina. They support everything in the pelvic cavity, including the uterus, and because of your upright stature they are, like your back, easy to stress.

Having located the pelvic floor muscles, try to draw them upwards. Draw up, hold, count to ten slowly, relax and repeat. Do this ten times every time you think about it. Once you can do it, try pulling up in stages like a lift stopping at different floors. It is much easier in a standing position. I started doing this in the queue in the supermarket, when my eldest son was a baby. I still do. No one can tell you are doing it.

You can check you have got it right by placing a finger inside your vagina and a thumb on the pubic bone. As you squeeze, you should be able to feel the muscles relaxing and contracting around your finger.

(There are, of course, other, more pleasurable ways of checking this out.)

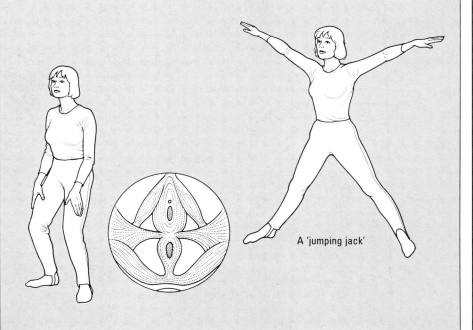

A 'jumping jack'

38

Pelvic floor exercises

1 I find this exercise useful for both the pelvic floor and the inner thigh. Sit on the floor. Cross your ankles, squeeze your thighs together, and try to push your ankles apart at the same time. Squeeze tight, lift the pelvic floor and try to hold for as long as you can. Aim for 12 seconds, repeated ten times.

2 Then try placing something solid between your knees and squeeze and hold; as you hold, raise your pelvic floor. Hold this position for as long as you can.

3 These exercises work wonders on the bottom as well as on the pelvic floor. Lie on your back, knees bent and waist pushed into the floor. Lift your bottom about 2 inches (5 cm) off the ground. (You will need to support it with your hands later in pregnancy.) Squeeze your bottom and thighs tight, lifting your pelvic floor at the same time. It should feel as if you are trying to draw a thick rope through your thighs. Start by doing it about 20 times and build up to about 50.

4 Now open your knees and repeat.

5 Then put your feet apart and your knees together and repeat once more.

You may find it easiest to do these exercises to music. Together they will ensure that your pelvic floor, bottom and thighs are firm and ready to support your baby. Used after the birth, they will rapidly rid you of the bottom sag, thigh flab and vaginal slackness which inevitably (and depressingly) follow.

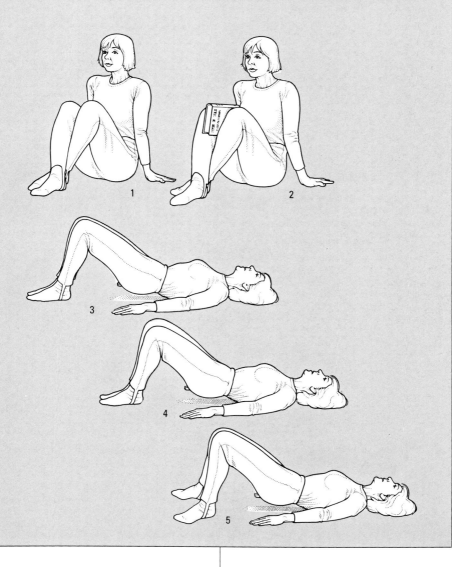

Exercises for the legs and thighs

1 Stand with the legs apart, knees bent, back straight, as if perched on the edge of a high bar stool. Raise your arms out to the side, level with the shoulders. Swing arms forwards slightly and push back. It is quite a small movement. If you cannot feel it in your legs, sit down a little. Work up to about two minutes of pushing.

2 Lean forwards, resting your elbows on your knees and bounce slightly. Again, aim at two to three minutes. If your legs start to ache, stop.

3 Going back to the bar stool position, with arms by your sides, tense your bottom tight, tense again and release. That is all. If it seems too easy, sit down a little lower and hold the tension a little longer.

4 Finish by stretching the muscles with numbers **8** and **11** from the warming dozen illustrated on page 37.

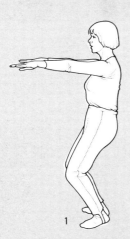
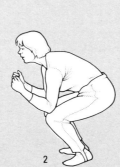
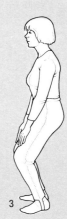

Exercises for the abdomen

If your muscles are weak, you need to build up slowly. The aim is to reach 50 of each of these in one session, but even ten will help.

1 Lie on the floor, waist pushed in, bottom tilted up and legs bent at the knee. Place your hands behind your head and lift your head and shoulders off the floor. Your elbows should cradle your head. Now lift your shoulders up an inch or two, pulling from the stomach, drop back a little, and pull up again. Repeat, moving shoulders back, breathing out as you come up, and in as you go down. It is only a small movement, but you should feel it in the top of your stomach. Now place your left leg on top of the right and repeat. Then the right on top of the left and repeat.

2 Staying in the same position, lift your feet off the floor and cross your legs. Your knees should not come forward. Lift from the waist as before. You should feel the strain a little lower down in the stomach.

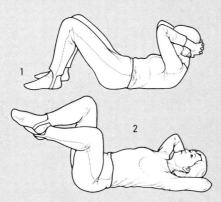
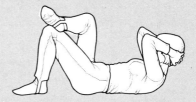

If you feel any strain in your back or shoulders at any stage, stop. Check that your back is pushed well into the floor and that you are using the abdominal muscles to pull yourself up. If you feel cramp, pull your knees up on to your chest and hold tight.

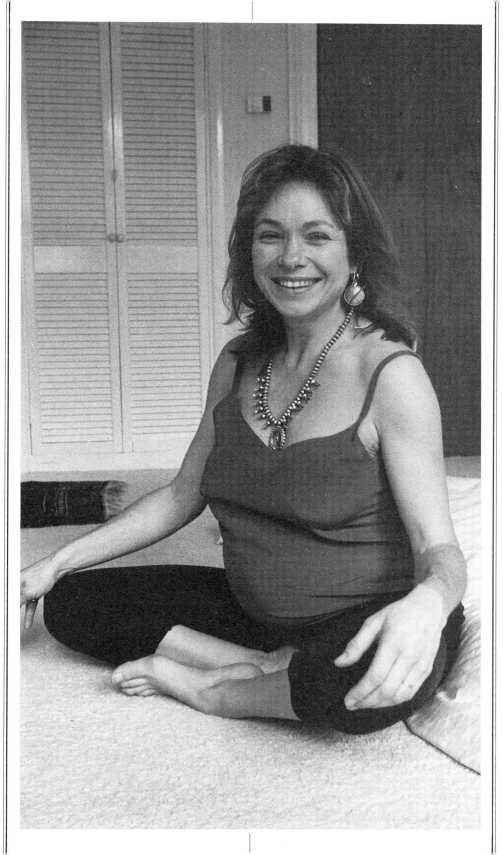

Conception

96 Day one

The day when sperm and egg meet is the day when a potential human being becomes a reality: the first day on the way to his or her life; the first day of the rest of your life, in which nothing will ever be quite the same again.

Some women say they know they are pregnant from this first day, but there is no evidence that they really do. Yes, you may feel it, but how often before have you been sure before when it has not, in fact, been true?

97 The social reality

Man is a social animal. He shapes the rules of the culture in which he lives. but he is also a product of that culture. History and society are made, generally speaking, by individual action, but individual action is also framed by history and society. Values, it cannot be denied, are made by people, but at the same time we have to concede that these values make people what they are.

Society's goals and values influence the way any group of people lives. We share a special understanding with others who grow up in the same culture, even if we later abandon its values.

When a cat has kittens, it is a biological event. She cares for them in an instictive way: the ties are not social, there is no cultural tradition in which to raise the offspring. There are no expectations of their future lives, or of how soon she should become pregnant again. After the kittens depart, she may be lost for a day or so, but there is no lasting concern. The birth of a human baby is a social event: how we feel about the birth and how we care for the child is the result of cultural, not biological, pressures. These social pressures begin at conception.

98 A solemn rite

Among men and women, the transition to parenthood is viewed as a solemn social act. In all societies it is treated with reverence and marked with ceremony and fanfare. We have lost some of that sense of ceremony, as the availability of contraception has separated the celebration of marriage from the birth of the first child.

Nevertheless the goals, values, and beliefs of society still mean that people who become parents are treated differently by almost everyone. They are, in one sense, the caretakers of our culture and, in another, the agents of change. It is, after all, children who will make tomorrow's society.

99 An institution

Parenthood is a social institution; to which, in a way, all parents feel they belong. We see ourselves as different from people without children. We have a different status, a different standing, often different values and priorities. As with all institutions, there is a sense in which parenthood exists above and beyond us. It has a coercive power of which we may not be fully aware before embarking upon it. If you doubt the potency of the social values surrounding parenthood, consider the attitudes implicit in the usual responses to these questions:

• What do you think of the woman who leaves her three small children to live with her lover?
• What do you feel about the two 14-year-olds who have just had their second child?
• What do you feel about the woman who says her career is more important than her two daughters?
• What do you feel about the 80-year-old man and his 48-year-old wife who have just declared that they expect a baby?
• What do you feel about the man who feels young children should be banned from planes, trains and restaurants?
• What do you feel about the couple who cannot have a child?
• What do you feel about the mentally handicapped couple who expect a child?

Having conceived a child, you and your partner will become the custodians of these values. If, as individuals, either of you wishes to deviate from them, you will meet fierce opposition. Minor adjustments are possible, but even then other parents may feel they have a right to suggest that you justify your actions.

100 Understanding your body

It is your body, every inch, every feeling, and the better you know it, the easier it will be to recognize what is happening to it. As the baby grows inside you, and doctors and nurses prod and poke at you, you may sometimes wonder if you still own it. You do. No one should do anything to it you do not understand. Pregnancy may seem like a miracle, but it need not be a mystery. Feel your body, look at it, find out what happens inside and out.

Know your feelings and accept them. Do not be surprised if your mood swings wildly, your temper rises and tears fall. It will happen. If you have longed for pregnancy, you may be alarmed by your negative feelings. Don't be. They are normal. Worrying about yourself, the baby and your ability to cope, are normal too.

You do not have to hand over your body to anyone. It is not unreasonable to expect doctors and nurses to explain why and what they are doing. They may be better qualified, but they are not in *your* body. They may have seen 30 other women in the clinic that morning, but not you.

Your feelings are yours too. You do not have to feel happy just because others expect you to be so.

There is only one individual who can make unreasonable demands. That is the baby. It is obliged to share your body, and as long as it does so, it has a right to ask that you do not abuse the body you share.

101 The politics of menstruation

For most of us, a missed period is one of the first signs of pregnancy. Aristotle believed that the seed of the male caused the menstrual blood to coagulate into an egg from which the baby developed. A very male view of conception, this: woman is seen as a glorious seed bed, a nourishing plant pot. Men are an arrogant lot, but one has to admit they are clever. It is a view that at once over-estimates the male role in fathering children and puts a woman firmly in her place.

Since women do not usually menstruate when breast-feeding, it was also thought that milk came from menstrual blood. There were other roles for the blood too: warding off evil, curing diseases, extinguishing fires, tempering metals, and protecting men from wounds in battle.

But such views were rare. Mostly it is, and was, regarded as unclean. Hindu women are not supposed to prepare food for their husbands when menstruating, Moslem women cannot pray in a mosque, and some Buddhists must keep out of the temple. In the Jewish and Christian religions there are rituals for cleansing after menstruation. No wonder it is called the curse.

The curse of Eve; the badge of womanhood, when a woman's body was thought to fill up with an excess of blood which had to be discharged once a month.

The menstrual cycle

At birth, a baby girl has 500,000 eggs or ova, more than enough to fulfil her reproductive needs for a lifetime. From puberty to menopause, one will ripen each month. At the beginning of each cycle, a small number begin ripening. By ovulation (usually 14 days before menstruation), one will have reached full ripeness and be ready to be shed from the ovary into the Fallopian tube where fertilization takes place. Sometimes more than one egg ripens fully (the tendency runs in families), and if that happens, and both eggs are fertilized, twins may develop.

The timing of egg ripening and release is controlled by hormones which interact in a complex pattern known as the menstrual cycle. In most women, the cycle lasts for about 28 days, and is quite regular. It begins when hormones released by the pituitary (situated just above the roof of the mouth) begin to build up in the blood stream. The first of these, the follicle-stimulating hormone (FSH), starts the ripening process. As FSH builds up, the ovary begins to release oestrogen (another hormone). This tells the brain to stop releasing FSH ('we have an egg maturing, thank you'); it also tells the womb to start preparing its lining in readiness for the forthcoming pregnancy. As oestrogen builds up, the brain begins to release a second hormone known as LH or luteinizing hormone. It starts slowly at first, but as soon as oestrogen levels reach a certain level, it is as if a dam has burst. There is a sudden surge in LH and ovulation follows.

After ovulation, when the egg is released from the ovary, and starts to move along the Fallopian tube, levels of another hormone, progesterone, start to rise. The wall of the womb thickens further. If conception takes place, the fertilized egg embeds itself into this thickened wall; if conception does not occur, the levels of all four hormones fall, and the thickened womb lining sloughs off during menstruation.

Hormones' role in determining sex
The menstrual cycle in women is controlled by the brain. Men release FSH and LH too, but not in a cycle. At about six weeks after conception, the internal and external sex organs begin to develop and at this time a male embryo will begin to secrete the male hormone testosterone. When this happens the brain, as well as the sex organs, are exposed to testosterone, and this stops the adult brain releasing FSH and LH in a cycle. So the rules for male and female hormone release are written into the brain long before they are ever needed.

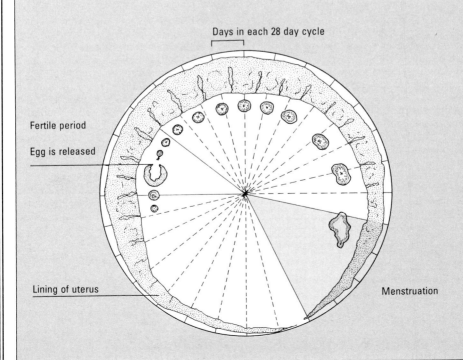

Days in each 28 day cycle

Fertile period

Egg is released

Lining of uterus

Menstruation

This notion was disproved 150 years ago, but the idea persists. We still think of menstruation as ridding us of something undesirable. Yet we do not question why this 'cleansing' happens only to women.

102 Oestrus

At oestrus we release an egg, or ovum, ready for fertilization by one of the sperm which swim (barriers permitting) high into our Fallopian tubes. The female of most species only accepts the male at this time, when she is 'on heat'. Women are different, and there is not even an increase in sexual desire at ovulation. But like all other animals, women have a short period of fertility and a much longer period of infertility. So well do we hide our fertile time that it was not until 1930 that it was known for certain to be mid-cycle.

Oestrus comes from a Greek word meaning a gadfly, a fly whose buzzing drives herds of cattle crazy during summer months and makes them 'gad about'.

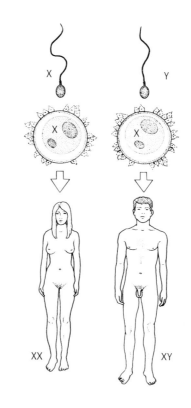

103 Boy or girl?

It is unwise to set your heart on a boy or a girl, but there is no harm in trying to influence the outcome. There is no infallible method of ensuring the sex of your baby, but you may be able to adjust the odds slightly.

More boys are born than girls, and studies show that the more you make love, the more likely you are to have a boy. So, early in a relationship or when babies are conceived after a long parting, they are more likely to be boys. This probably explains the odd finding that more boys are conceived in times of war.

Douching before intercourse is another option you might try. The received wisdom is to use an alkaline douche for a boy (one tablespoon of bicarbonate of soda in half a pint of warm distilled water). Buy the water at a garage and boil it before use. For a girl, put one tablespoon full of white vinegar into *distilled* water. Douches are available from chemist's shops.

The French believe in diets. For a girl, you should have a low-salt diet rich in starch and milk, with calcium supplements. For a boy, plenty of salt, meat and fish, no dairy products and potassium supplements.

Another option is to time intercourse. This theory is based upon whether the sperm meets the ova or the ova the sperm. At ovulation, the ova is released and moves slowly down the Fallopian tubes towards the uterus; it will be fertilized at some point on this journey. The sperm are released into the vagina when a man ejaculates, and subsequently swim up through the cervix and the uterus into the Fallopian tubes. See page 49.

There are two sorts of sperm: 'X' sperm (girl-makers) and 'Y' sperm (boy-makers). The X sperm are tougher and stronger and are thought to live longer. The Y sperm are lighter, faster swimmers. The theory is if you want a girl, you make sure the sperm has been waiting around in the vagina and uterus. If you want a boy, you make sure that the ova is ready and waiting for the winner of the race.

The main problem is that no one seems to agree how best to ensure the required outcome. In theory, though, the ideal method to ensure a girl is one that will deliver old sperm to the waiting ovum; so abstain for a few days, then make love before ovulation.

For a boy, you should deliver newly produced sperm to the waiting ovum. A combination of barrier methods of contraception, to ensure newly produced sperm (no hanging about in the vagina and uterus), and making love at ovulation without the barriers is probably best.

Whatever you decide, remember no one claims anything more than an 80 per cent success rate, and that in any event you have a 50 per cent chance of getting the sex you prefer. You can, therefore, do little better than marginally increase the odds. Never bank on the outcome, and don't take the matter too seriously.

104 The Q index

For most women to menstruate normally, about 25 per cent of their body weight needs to be fat. If you are underweight, you may be infertile, or if you do conceive, you may have a small baby. If you are overweight, there may also be problems. A man's weight also can influence his fertility. Check where you and your partner appear on the 'Q' index chart below; you should lie beween the two dotted lines.

$$\text{Q index} = \frac{\text{weight in kg}}{(\text{height in m}^2)}$$

A woman 1.62 m (5 ft 4 in) tall who weighs 58.5 kg (9 st 3 lb) would have a Q index of:

$$\frac{58.5}{1.62 \times 1.62} = 22.3$$

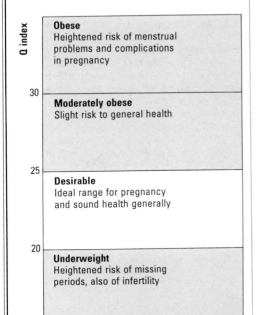

Q index

Obese
Heightened risk of menstrual problems and complications in pregnancy

30

Moderately obese
Slight risk to general health

25

Desirable
Ideal range for pregnancy and sound health generally

20

Underweight
Heightened risk of missing periods, also of infertility

105 The ovum

The egg, or ovum, which is released each month is special. All the other cells in a woman's body have 46 chromosomes – 23 pairs. The ovum has just 23 single chromosomes.

When the cells of the body multiply for growth, each cell makes a copy of itself: a little building brick with 46 chromosomes, in which each instruction is given in duplicate. The cell in an ovum has just half the genetic material: one set of instructions. So each ovum has only one instruction (on chromosome 11) for how to make insulin; one instruction for blue eyes, and so on. It also has one 'X', or sex, chromosome.

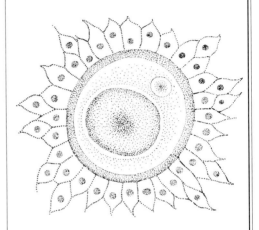

106 The sperm

Sperm are similar to ova, but smaller and more plentiful – about 300,000,000 are released each time a man ejaculates. Many are called, but only one is chosen. They are shaped like minute tadpoles, with pointed heads and long tails. They too have 23 chromosomes, 22 of them just like those in the ova, and the 23rd either X or Y. This is the duplicate set of instructions. When the sperm and ovum meet, they fuse to make the first building block of a new individual: an individual who will have 46 chromosomes, 23 pairs, with each instruction in duplicate.

There is just one way in which ova and sperm differ, one exception to this duplication of instructions. There is always an X sex chromosome in the ovum; sperm, by contrast, can carry either an X or a Y chromosome. The potential exists, therefore, for a female child to develop if an X sperm meets the ovum, or a male if a Y sperm meets the ovum.

X chromosomes are long, Y chromosomes are stunted and carry little genetic material, except initial instructions for forming the testes.

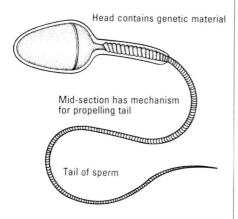

Head contains genetic material

Mid-section has mechanism for propelling tail

Tail of sperm

107 Determining sex organs

If an ovum and a Y sperm meet, then the baby will be a boy.

The ovum and sperm fuse together to make a cell with 23 pairs of chromosomes. Twenty-two will be identical, but one will be an X paired with a Y.

108 Genetic inheritance

Before reading on, see 43 for an explanation of genes and chromosomes; also 53.

109 Back to chromosomes

Twenty-three chromosomes come from the mother; 23 from the father. When the chromosomes are paired off, the gene from the mother which codes for eye colour will be opposite the gene for eye colour received from the father. (The same 'house' is always next to the 'pub'; see 43.)

This always happens with all the genes on all the chromosomes, except those genes on the sex chromosomes of boys; see 107. Anything that a boy inherits on the X chromosome, he receives from his mother. There cannot be a matching instruction from his father's Y chromosome: it is not long enough.

When it comes to giving instructions, some genes shout louder than others. Some are so quiet that their instructions are ignored if there are bigger voices around. These are called recessive genes; see also 71. Blue eye colour is like this.

Many people carry this gene without having eyes which are even remotely blue. To have blue eyes, both your eye-colour genes (the one from your mother and the one from your father) must be blue.

Sometimes a gene's voice is so loud that it overrules all the others (these are called dominant genes). Brown eye colour, for example, tends to dominate blue. Sometimes a gene's voice is on a par with others, so that both influence the offspring, and the child is 'in between' its parents.

Some inherited features are determined by a single gene, but most are determined by several; there are, for example, many genes that influence how tall a child grows. This is why human beings are infinitely varied.

110 Cultural inheritance

Now is perhaps the moment to step back and reflect on what may seem obvious: that a child's inheritance is governed not only by genes. For your baby will be conditioned by your attitudes from the moment she is born; attitudes you and your partner have in turn learned from others since childhood.

One attitude in particular will, I suspect, have a far-reaching effect on the future success of your relationship with your partner, and so on your child. It is whether you believe that the hard work and responsibility of childcare should rest mainly with the father, or with the mother, or whether it can be shared.

Society has, possibly, conditioned you from birth to accept that childcare is essentially a woman's work, although nowadays you are quite likely to be one of the generation of young people which, over the last fifteen years, has evolved a rather different set of expectations. Women, in particular, have come to question their role, and many relationships are now sharing ones, in which both partners work and both share household chores: at least before the children arrive.

You may expect that this arrangement will be easy to extend into your years of parenthood. Don't be too certain.

It is much more difficult to share childcare than many women think before they have children, and many find that men's attitudes, and society's as a whole, have moved more slowly in this respect than they had hoped. Someone recently went through everything ever written about fathers: it took 24 hours. Doing the

The female reproductive system

Outside the vagina are various protective flaps of skin – the labia. They are difficult to see without a mirror. Sit in front of a long mirror, legs apart, or hold a hand mirror between your legs. The clitoris is the only bit of the whole apparatus which has no other purpose but to increase pleasure. It has an obvious external tip, a thicker section just below the skin surface and two 'fingers' which extend along the pubic bone.

The uterus is connected to the vagina by the cervix; you can feel the cervix at the top of the vagina. If you do not know what it feels like, you can easily reach it with a finger: it seems close. When you are sexually excited, your vagina expands and the cervix moves back out of the way. The vagina lets penis and sperm get as close as possible to the ova. If you have not had a baby before, you will feel the ridged structure of the vaginal wall, less noticeable after your baby is born.

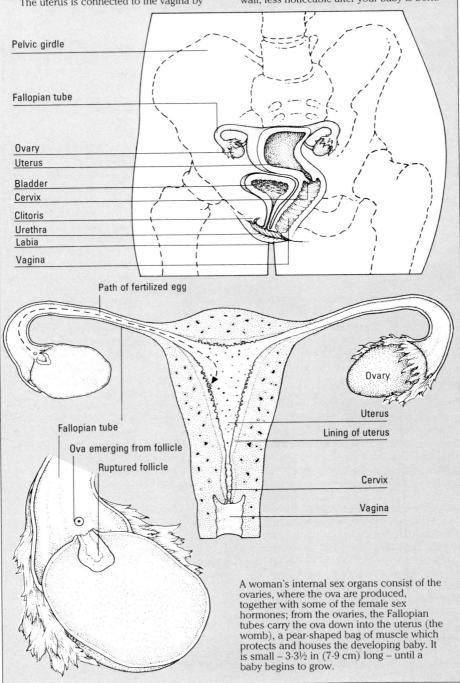

Pelvic girdle

Fallopian tube

Ovary

Uterus

Bladder

Cervix

Clitoris

Urethra

Labia

Vagina

Path of fertilized egg

Fallopian tube

Ova emerging from follicle

Ruptured follicle

Ovary

Uterus

Lining of uterus

Cervix

Vagina

A woman's internal sex organs consist of the ovaries, where the ova are produced, together with some of the female sex hormones; from the ovaries, the Fallopian tubes carry the ova down into the uterus (the womb), a pear-shaped bag of muscle which protects and houses the developing baby. It is small – 3-3½ in (7-9 cm) long – until a baby begins to grow.

The male reproductive system

The male sex organs are designed to deliver sperm, and to do so as close to the uterus as possible. Sperm are produced in the testes, which dangle outside the body in a bag called the scrotum or scrotal sac. This exposed position keeps the testes cool, necessary for normal sperm production. The testes also manufacture some sex hormones. From each testicle a tube, the *vas deferens*, takes the sperm by a circuitous route over the bladder to the base of the penis. Here the two tubes meet, and liquids from the prostate, seminal vesicles and another neighbouring gland are added to give nutrition to the sperm, and in which they can survive indefinitely. Then they pass on to meet the urethra near the point where it enters the penis.

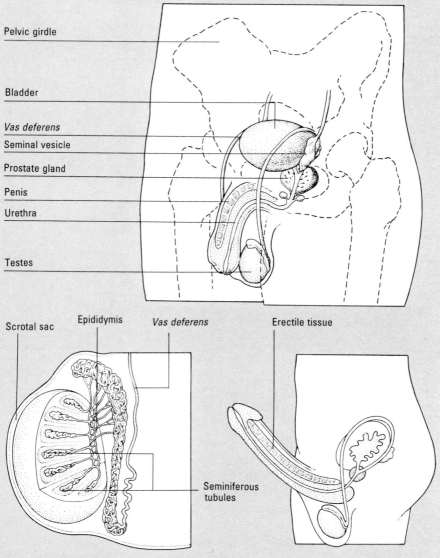

Pelvic girdle

Bladder

Vas deferens

Seminal vesicle

Prostate gland

Penis

Urethra

Testes

Scrotal sac   Epididymis   *Vas deferens*   Erectile tissue

Seminiferous tubules

Manufacture of sperm

The mature male's testes make sperm more or less continuously. Once produced, they travel along one of many channels (seminiferous tubules) within the testis to the epididymis. Here they stay for a period before continuing via the *vas deferens* to the seminal vesicles (see top illustration) for longer-term storage until ejaculation. Sperm may live as long as three months.

When sexually aroused, erectile tissue in the penis, containing many cavities, becomes engorged with blood, so that the penis becomes erect. (There is, incidentally, erectile tissue in the nipples and in the nose of both sexes.) At ejaculation, sperm and seminal fluid are deposited deep in the vagina.

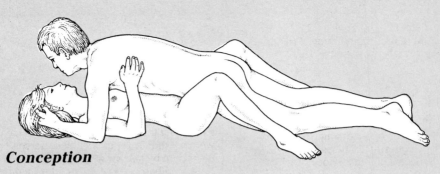

Conception

Only one sperm, of the many millions released when a man ejaculates, is required to fertilize the egg. What actually happens at the moment of conception is still only partially understood: it is thought that the sperm actually penetrates the ovum by swimming hard up against it. But it may be helped in this by the presence of other sperm secreting a substance which makes the egg

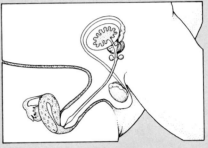

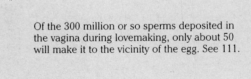

penetrable. As soon as penetration happens, the outer layer of the ovum seals itself so that no other sperm can enter. Only the head of the sperm penetrates – the tail is left outside. Once the head is inside, the genetic material it carries mingles with the mother's.

Of the 300 million or so sperms deposited in the vagina during lovemaking, only about 50 will make it to the vicinity of the egg. See 111.

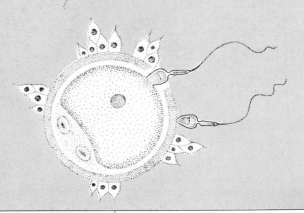

same for written material about motherhood would take weeks.

If you, as a mother-to-be, feel strongly that parenthood should be shared equally, you are setting yourself against a massive amount of pre-conditioning. Talk about this together now, and see 122.

111 Is it easy to become pregnant?

The chances of becoming pregnant are surprisingly small. The egg is only present for between 24 and 36 hours each month, and the sperm can survive for only about 24 hours. In addition, the sperm do not all race towards the egg; they simply swim about like tadpoles delighted with the new-found spaciousness of their surroundings. Of the 300 million or so deposited in the vagina, only about 50 will make it to the vicinity of the egg. And of the eggs that are fertilized, between a third and a half will be aborted (miscarried) in the first month or six weeks. It is something like an obstacle course; perhaps a necessary one, since in the production of so many sperm for each ejaculation, errors are made: sperms lack tails, have two tails, and genetic faults. The obstacle course probably ensures the survival, for the most part, of only the fit.

Typical faults in sperm

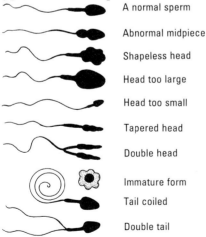

A normal sperm

Abnormal midpiece

Shapeless head

Head too large

Head too small

Tapered head

Double head

Immature form

Tail coiled

Double tail

112 Failure to conceive

In 100 couples not using contraceptives, 75 of the women will be pregnant within a year. Another five will become pregnant in the second year, and over their remaining child-bearing years, still more will conceive. But without treatment, ten will remain childless.

Wanting a child, waiting for pregnancy, can take over your life. From the period approaching menstruation (do I, don't I feel pre-menstrual?) to the disappointment of seeing the first menstrual blood, takes one week in every four. The disappointment of menstruation drags this sadness out to almost two weeks. Then follows a period of raised hope before the inevitable disappointment of the next month. Life becomes centered on something that does not happen. I know a woman who, at 78, can still find herself overtaken by sorrow as she looks at a new-born baby in a pram, and I remember my own five years of infertility as a time of growing obsession. A time when it was difficult to think of anything but that which I could not have.

113 When to ask for advice

If you have taken no steps to prevent pregnancy and have not conceived within a year, ask your doctor to refer you to a specialist.

Infertility has many causes, some of them more easiliy treated than others. A man is usually asked to give a sample of semen which will be examined to establish whether the sperm are sufficiently active and healthy. A post-coital test may also be done to check that enough healthy sperm are deposited in the vagina during love-making.

When there is difficulty conceiving, tests usually include:

● Keeping a temperature chart to check that ovulation is occurring. (Body temperature rises slightly at ovulation.)
● Estimating the levels of female sex hormones in the blood.
● A hystero-salpingogram, by which a dye is passed through the Fallopian tubes to check for blockages. This is usually done in conjunction with a laparoscopy in which a small optical instrument is passed into the abdomen to examine the uterus and tubes.
● A scraping is taken from the uterus, or a sample of vaginal mucus is taken, to investigate the response to female sex hormones.

Treatment will depend on what such tests show. Tests on women are more elaborate, since more can go wrong with them; but more can also be put right.

114 Male infertility

A man is considered to be fertile if, on ejaculating, he produces about 1.5ml of semen in which there are more than 75 million mainly healthy sperm that are still mobile four hours after ejaculation.

There are various reasons why sperm counts are sometimes low: hormone disorders, problems with the immune system and chromosome abnormalities, even trousers that are too tight.

Sometimes a varicose vein in the scrotum – called a variocele and usually on the left – blocks the passage of sperm. Sometimes there is an undescended testicle, infection or a disease of the prostrate or seminal vesicles. Other problems can be caused by congenital defects in the penis, too many hot baths, psychological impotence and hernia operations.

In the past, there has been an assumption that infertility was mainly a female problem. It is not. In 20 to 35 per cent of couples investigated, a poor sperm count or the complete absence of sperm in the semen are found to be the cause of infertility. I was investigated for four years before it was discovered that my partner had a variocele. It was not difficult to see. But since I had some hormonal abnormalities, no one bothered to look. I became pregnant within one month of the operation to correct the variocele.

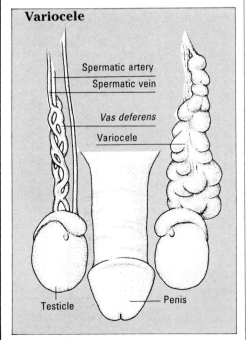

Variocele

Spermatic artery
Spermatic vein

Vas deferens

Variocele

Testicle

Penis

115 Female problems

There are three major reasons why women are infertile:

Blockage of the Fallopian tubes; disorders of ovulation, and a complex mix of problems including incompatability between the immune systems of the parents; thick, impenetrable mucus in the cervix, and involuntary movements or contractions of the Fallopian tubes which push out the sperm or block their entry.

Sometimes a woman does not conceive because the couple does not make love often enough, or at the right time. To be sure of conception, a couple needs to make love within a day of ovulation; see chart, page 22.

If love-making takes place only every two or three weeks, it is easy to miss this fertile period.

In many cases, both partners may be on the borderline; each could conceive with a more fertile partner.

116 Cures and treatments for infertility

Today many couples who would earlier have remained infertile can be succesfully treated. Drugs (so-called fertility drugs) can be used to induce ovulation. Blocked Fallopian tubes are a more difficult problem, but they can occasionally be repaired. If the tubes are irreparably blocked, a test tube baby' may be the only solution.

It is unlikely, however, that all infertile women wishing for this treatment will be able to receive it; nor does it always work. 'Test tube' fertilization involves taking ova from an ovary and mixing them with the partner's sperm outside the mother's body, then reintroducing the embryo into the womb where implantation can occur. Because implantation is problematic, a number of embryos is produced by stimulating multiple ovulation with drugs. All the ova are fertilized, and more than one embyro is returned to the mother for implantation. Sometimes more than one develops, in which instance there will be a multiple birth.

Male infertility is more difficult to treat. An operation may remove a variocele, and hormone treatment can sometimes improve sperm counts. Tight trousers and hot baths are also discouraged. Careful timing of love-making to coincide with ovulation, and choosing positions which deposit sperm as high up in the vagina as possible, may also help. It may also be worth trying to help the sperm on their

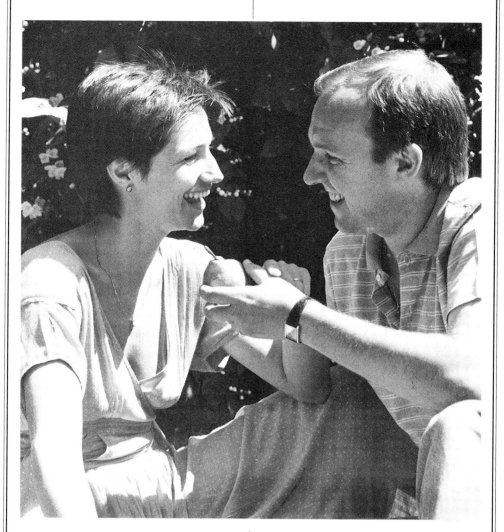

journey: you could simply lie on your back with your bottom raised on a pillow so that the sperm travel downhill, or certain lubricants may be suggested.

AIH (Artificial Insemination by Husband) may help: it is possible to collect a number of samples of semen from the man (freezing samples from earlier ejaculations) and insert them all beyond the cervix. Thus more semen is deposited closer to the goal.

AID involves inserting sperm from a donor – someone who is not the woman's partner. Sometimes the partner's sperm is mixed in with the donor's, so either man might be the father.

117 Forecasting ovulation

The easiest way to know if and when you have ovulated is to keep a chart of your temperature. It must be taken first thing

each morning before you get out of bed, and before you have anything to drink. Temperature rises by about one degree at the time of ovulation, and remains elevated until menstruation.

A second method is to examine your cervical mucus. Using a finger, take a small sample from high in the vagina and put it on to a mirror. You may find that the mucus is thick, cloudy, sticky and possibly a yellowish colour. It is like this when you are not ovulating. At other times, you will find that the mucus becomes quite runny: it is slippery and clear, rather like uncooked egg white. This is the mucus which is present at ovulation, you may even find it runs out of the vagina at this time. Obviously, semen and natural and artificial lubricants can confuse this picture; so can the fluid that some women secrete at orgasm. It is also difficult to read these changes if your normal vaginal discharge is excessive. See chart at 46.

Pregnancy
The First Trimester (First Three Months)

118 Signs of pregnancy

If your periods are regular, a missed period is probably the first clear sign. Some women have a very light, rather than a missed period, and for them the fact that they are pregnant may dawn slowly. Breasts which become slightly engorged before a period will remain full and tender, and this feeling will grow as the weeks pass. You may feel a tingling sensation and see a darkening of the tissue (the areola) around the nipple. A little later tiny swellings (Montgomery's tubercles) will appear. The nipple and areola will seem more prominent, and the breasts will seem fuller, much as when you are sexually excited.

Increased progesterone will now relax the bladder and the bowel (and many other body areas), so you will want to empty your bladder at frequent intervals. Your bowels will move more slowly than usual; you may find you are constipated. You may also have increased vaginal discharge.

You may also find that you have 'gone off' spicy food, or discover that tea smells sickly and oranges wonderful. It is these changes in smell and taste which make some foods seem repulsive, and others irresistible. You may experience a strange metallic taste in the mouth. See also 184.

The blood vessels may also relax, and the resulting drop in blood pressure may make you feel sick (often without actually being sick), not just in the morning, but throughout the day. And you will feel tired: unbelievably tired; a tiredness, which does not square with mere lack of sleep. See 191-192.

119 Pregnancy tests

Tests used to diagnose pregnancy are based on detecting the hormone human chorionic gonadotrophin (HCG) in a woman's blood or urine; see 120. It is not present unless you are pregnant. The most sophisticated (generally hospital-only) tests can confirm pregnancy within a week of conception. D.I.Y. tests, which are about 98 per cent accurate, can be carried out at home within a week of missing your period; some are easier to use than others. They will not, however, give results if carried out too early, or too late – check before purchasing.

You should use an early morning urine sample, which you have collected in a clean jar free from soap or detergent. Positive tests nearly always mean yes.

Taking up residence

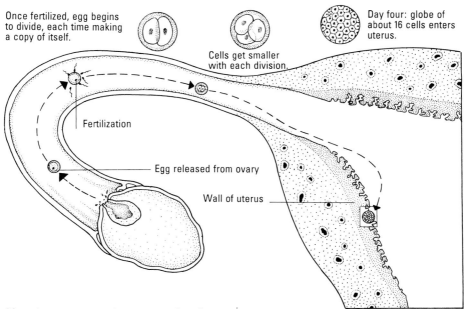

Once fertilized, egg begins to divide, each time making a copy of itself.

Cells get smaller with each division.

Day four: globe of about 16 cells enters uterus.

Fertilization

Egg released from ovary

Wall of uterus

Negative tests sometimes mean that the evidence is not yet clear. It is wise, in any event, to test more than once, especially if there are no other clear signs.

120 Taking up residence

The globe of cells that forms the embryo as it enters the womb have been wafted down the Fallopian tubes by little hair-like structures called cilia. The journey of 1-1½ in (3-4 cm) takes about a week. On about day seven the embryo comes to rest against the wall of the womb, and little tendrils reach out from the embryo feeling within the wall for the blood vessels beneath, much as a sea anemone searches for food. As it feels, the embryo slowly and gently embeds itself within the lining of the womb. Soon it is buried, leaving nothing but a little bump on the surface.

Now, the little tendrils, called chorionic villi, begin to produce a hormone, chorionic gonadotrophin (HCG). This tells the ovary to produce oestrogen and progesterone, preventing the next menstrual period. Without this instruction, the womb lining will be shed. See also 239.

The little tendrils are part of the embryo, and although they do not develop into the baby, they are made of the same cells and share the same set of genes. Samples taken from the tendrils will show the genetic composition of the baby, not that of the mother. If you are given a chorionic villi test to examine the genes of your baby, it is from these tendrils that a

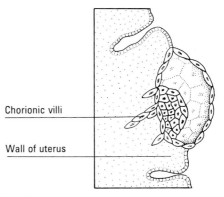

Chorionic villi

Wall of uterus

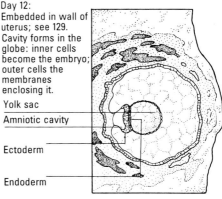

Day 12:
Embedded in wall of uterus; see 129. Cavity forms in the globe: inner cells become the embryo; outer cells the membranes enclosing it.

Yolk sac

Amniotic cavity

Ectoderm

Endoderm

sample is taken for examination. The advantage of this test over amniocentesis (see 232) is that it can be done much earlier in the pregnancy. Not all hospitals have facilities for carrying it out.

55

121 Minor problems

If your teeth and gums are not in sound condition, you may have a tendency to mouth infections during pregnancy. It used to be said that a mother loses one tooth for each baby. You need not; but you do need to take extra care.

You may find that your gums bleed; so may your nose. Neither is a sign of high blood pressure nor a cause for concern.

If a nostril starts to bleed, gently squeeze the tip of your nose between your fingers for about three minutes. This should stop mild bleeding. If the bleeding is persistent and heavy, you may .pa need to consult an ear, nose and throat specialist. The increased bleeding occurs because of the increased blood supply to this area.

Increased blood supply to the head can also cause headaches, even if you do not usually suffer from them. Take paracetamol rather than aspirin; see 59. If you get migraine, avoid preparations which include ergotamine. This may be the time to try bio-feedback technique for migraine. Ask your doctor if he can recommend a specialist, or consult one of the alternative health magazines.

122 Will you be a 'natural' mother?

See 110. According to the American sociologist Alice Rossi, one reason that women are predisposed to look after children is that they are made in such a way that child care is easier for them than it is for men.

This fitness is not just because they have breasts with which to feed babies, or wombs in which to carry them. They have, above all, skills which enable them to care for other people. Skills which men also possess, but for the most part to a lesser degree.

The skills Alice Rossi has in mind are responsiveness to people and to sounds; an edge over men in receiving, interpreting and responding to both spoken and unspoken messages. Women tend to be better communicators (look at any PR company and note the number of senior women executives). Men are better at fine discrimination of the physical world, spatial visualization and the physical manipulation of objects. Look at any design or engineering company and note how many senior people are men.

The combination of sensitivity to sound and face, and the rapid processing of peripheral information, makes it possible for women to judge emotional nuance better than men. These intuitive skills, plus an ability to communicate, mean that women are well fitted to talk about and express emotion and feelings. In caring for the non-verbal infant, or children who do not always express themselves well, women have a head start. They read the infant's face, the child's body language, and they can respond appropriately, harmoniously.

Male skills are, by contrast, with things that say what they mean.

Society builds on these natural tendencies, expecting women to be caring, thoughtful, emotional, intuitive, observant. Expecting men to be tough, not to show emotion, to care about possessions and inanimate things.

Parents encourage this in the toys they buy for their children: construction kits for boys, dolls for girls. The biological make-up of the sexes unfolds in a social setting in which these tendencies are exaggerated. That, at any rate, is one view. How true is it?

I think it is an open question. It is true that there are differences between men and women. The stereotypes reflect a reality. However, I think it is an exaggerated reality. Yes, women tend to have communication skills. But it is an average difference, not an absolute one, and the differences in ability are quite small. There is much more variation among women than between men and women.

Try thinking of it in the context of height. There is plenty of variation in the size of people, but that does not stop us saying that men tend to be bigger than women. Now suppose that instead of being 6 in (15 cm) bigger (on average) than women, men were actually only 1 in (2.5 cm) bigger. The average man would still be taller, but we would not think of it as crucial. We are, in fact, talking of differences in communication skills which are on a par with such a difference in height. They exist, but they are not that obvious to the naked eye.

They may contribute to a woman's tendency to mother, but they hardly explain it, nor make childcare an impossible job for a man. See 180.

123 The placenta

During the first week or so in which the tiny embryo lies buried in the wall of the

The developing placenta

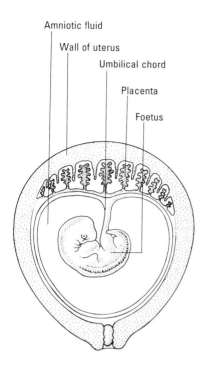

Amniotic fluid

Wall of uterus

Umbilical chord

Placenta

Foetus

womb (see 120), it is nourished by digesting the tissue around it. One might say, in fact, that it eats its way into position. But obviously, it cannot keep doing this. Later, all nutrition must pass to the developing baby via the mother's blood. The little fingers, or villi, that feel into the wall, searching for blood vessels, provide the early route for nutrients. Gradually the placenta develops from these villi, but it is difficult to say exactly when this happens. At five weeks, the villi are branched and blood vessels are developing; eventually the placenta will have 200 tiny blood vessels and be divided into 15-20 lobes, each made up of masses of these villi.

The blood vessels are rather special. They have very thin walls, which enable the nutrients to pass from the mother's blood stream into the baby's. However, the two blood supplies do not mix: the baby's stays inside the baby and the placenta, while the mother's stays inside her blood vessels.

The walls of arteries and veins are like fine sieves. Anything small can pass through, anything large cannot. Blood is made up of large cells which cannot pass through, but the nutrients and waste products are all small and can easily move

in and out. This is why it does not usually matter if your baby's blood group is different from yours. (But see 229.)

When the placenta is fully developed, it is a dark red disc weighing about 1 lb (500 g). It is about 1 in (20 cm) in diameter. The side facing the baby has a smooth surface, and the side attached to the womb is spongy. It looks like a lump of raw liver with a stalk on it. This stalk is the umbilical chord.

The placenta will usually attach itself to the top of the womb. If it attaches too low, this can create problems during birth.

124 Placental function

There are four. It supplies oxygen and nutrients to the foetus from the mother's blood. It takes waste products from the foetus back to the mother's blood. It forms a barrier to keep certain infections and drugs from the foetus, but it cannot block them all: aspirin, alchohol and many other substances can cross to the foetus. So, fortunately, can some antibodies, which can protect the baby from infection in the first weeks and months of life.

Lastly, the placenta secretes hormones, chief of which are progesterone, oestrogen and human gonadotrophin. These maintain the lining of the womb, the growth and development of the breasts and uterus and the pregnancy in general. Progesterone stops the womb from contracting and pushing out the baby. At birth, the progesterone level falls and labour begins.

Although the ovaries also produce oestrogen and progesterone, a pregnancy can be maintained after their removal.

125 The umbilical cord

It is bluish and shiny. If you look carefully, you can see one large vein and two arteries which wind around it. These are surrounded by a jelly-like substance called Wharton's jelly. The large vein carries nutrients to the developing baby; the arteries carry waste products away.

As the pregnancy progresses, the cord grows and twists upon itself. There are often up to 40 twists (and it may twist around the foetus too).

By the time the baby is born it may be up to 80 in (200 cm) long, although it is usually much shorter, and occasionally only about 3 in (7.5 cm). This can make conventional delivery through the vagina impossible. See 128.

126 How does the foetus breathe?

Although babies do make breathing movements, they do not actually breathe. Oxygen is diffused into the baby's blood from your own in exactly the same way as yours receives its oxygen from the lungs. It is then pumped around the baby's body by the baby's own heart.

Foetal circulation

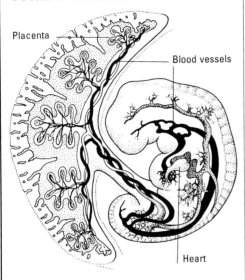

Placenta

Blood vessels

Heart

127 Length of pregnancy

Pregnancy is said to last for 40 weeks, but this calculation is based on the date of the last period, and conception will normally occur about two weeks after that. The figure of 40 weeks is, however, only an average: babies are usually born within two weeks of this date.

Some, of course, are born much earlier. These days it is possible for some babies to survive when they are born as early as 24 weeks after conception. But babies born earlier than 36 weeks after conception will need special care.

128 Day by day

The baby changes day by day. In the first three months it will develop from a single cell to a miniature baby who swims and kicks in your womb. Its little hands will clench, its heart will beat, and it will drink the amniotic fluid that protects it as it grows in the sac attached to your womb.

From three months, it will grow in size, the brain will continue to develop and the lungs will mature. It will slowly become capable of independent life over the following six months.

129 Days ten to 14

On the twelfth day, the tiny embryo (correctly called a blastocyst) is embedded in the wall of its mother's womb. It looks at this stage like a hollow blackberry, but it gradually forms into two layers which are known as the ectoderm (the outside skin) and the endoderm (inside skin). Think of them as the bread of a sandwich; the filling, the mesoderm, will develop later.

Forget the arms and legs and head for a moment and imagine the baby's body as a tube with the skin on the outside and the the gut surrounding a hollow tube on the inside. The cells that now make the ectoderm layer will divide and change and eventually form the child's skin and hair, and after folding inwards will form the nervous system and the brain. A thin layer of cells will move out from the main body of the blastocyst to form the bag that fills with water and protects the baby as it grows and develops within the womb. The endoderm cells give rise to the alimentary canal (stomach, intestine and so on) and all the internal structures that arise originally from the gut, such as the lungs and the liver. A yolk sac for early nutrition of the embryo develops on the inside, next to the endoderm.

130 Three to four weeks

During the third week the sandwich (see 129) begins to fill. It starts to fill at the back of the embryo and pushes forward in a thin line, called the primitive streak, like a thin layer of cheese squeezing between the bread and pushing slowly forwards. From this filling the Illustration. muscles and blood will develop. As the streak pushes forwards, part of the 'bread' curls over to make the notochord, a supporting structure which eventually forms the basis of the backbone. At the same time, the cells that form the sac which contains the baby move back, separating themselves from the exoderm except for a thin layer which attaches to the embryo (for that is what it is now properly called) to the edge of the sac. You are four weeks pregnant, and beginning to believe it.

131 Four weeks

At four weeks, the embryo starts to look like a small tadpole. A head can be made out at one end, and you can see where the eyes will be and the buds that form the arms. A primitive heart is developing and it will begin to pump blood almost at once. At this stage there is also a long tail.

There are other indications of our ancient history. Primitive forms of life, from which humans, like all creatures, have evolved, often display a segmented body form – indeed, fish still do. The human foetus now passes through this 'segmented' phase; indeed, by counting the segments, it is possible to tell the exact age of the embryo.

Now the nervous system begins to develop. Near the notochord the cells of the ectoderm start to move inwards, forming a long valley called the neural groove. It is as if someone has made a wheel mark in the snow. But the valley does not stay open for long. The 'tops' curve over, like trees arching over a sunken lane, to form the neural tube, a long strip rather like a piece of macaroni.

It is faults in the fusion of this arch which produce spina bifida.

132 Five weeks

From tip to tail, the embryo is now between ¼in (5 mm) and ½in (8mm) long: about the size of a baked bean. The early gut is developing, and by the end of the week there will be a mouth. There are a rudimentary brain and heart, arm and leg buds, and on the side of the head the beginnings of the eyes and on the side of the neck the beginnings of the ears. These will move into place next week.

133 Six weeks

Now the embryo is beginning to look like a baby. It is 1 in (2.5cm) long, the main internal organs are formed, the heart is pumping blood around the body. The head is large, and you can see that the eyes and the nostrils have moved from the side of the head to the front. The inner ear is growing, but the outer ear is not yet formed. The limbs are developing. See 135.

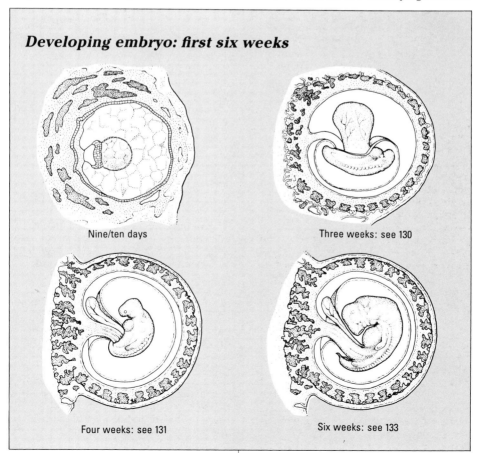

Developing embryo: first six weeks

Nine/ten days

Three weeks: see 130

Four weeks: see 131

Six weeks: see 133

134 Drugs

See also 120, 123 and 128-130. Watching how the blastocyst develops into an embryo, and later into a foetus, it is easy to see why drugs and diseases have different effects at different times. Cells move about in the embryo, things start to develop and change at different times. It is like a symphony or a ballet, a dance here, a dance there, the development of one theme and then another.

If damage is done at a very early stage, if, say, something stopped the blastocyst segregating into two layers, or the mesoderm did not develop, it is clear that death would occur. Without a mesoderm, there would be no muscles or blood: the embryo would reach a point beyond which it could develop no further and would die.

At a slightly later stage, things can go wrong which produce profound handicaps without killing the embryo. If the neural tube does not quite fuse, the baby can still develop, but it may never walk. If something goes wrong as the limbs bud, the baby may have abnormal arms or legs (as in children who received thalidomide at this stage in their development). The development of the eyes and ears can be disrupted by Rubella, but blindness or deafness is not fatal to the embryo or the child. A child whose eyes, ears or nostrils do not move into position may look stange, and its brain development may be abnormal, but it can live.

An embryo with some abnormalities of the gut or other internal organs may be viable while it is protected within the womb: while it receives its nutrition, and excretes waste, via the mother's body systems. Once outside the womb, it must use its own organs, and independent life may be impossible.

For most of us, these are the stuff of nightmares. The care required to reduce the risks to a minimum is well worth taking. Nothing can guarantee the health of your child, but everyone wants to say they did all they could to ensure it.

135 Genes at work

Each cell of the developing embryo has all the genetic instructions it needs to make the baby. The cells that form the eyes have all the instructions to form the liver, those of the liver the instructions to form the eye. The reason one becomes part of the eye and the other part of the liver is that they are told which genes to 'turn on'. By being part of the endoderm, and later part of the group of cells that becomes the liver, they are instructed to perform in certain ways. For example, at first they must take note only of the 'gut' instructions, and later follow only the 'liver' instructions. They must ignore all those which tell them how to become a bit of a bone, or a nerve cell in the brain.

Genes are, in fact, switched on and off as if controlled by a giant switchboard. As I sit at my phone, I have the possibility of calling millions of people all over the world, just as that first cell holds the possibility of becoming any part of the body. I dial 010, and immediately I cut out the possibility of dialling anyone in Britain. I add -1- and now cannot call anyone in France or Australia, only any number in the U.S.A. or Canada. In the same way, becoming part of the endoderm restricts the possibilities of those cells.

By dialling 212 next I can call anyone in Manhattan, but calls to Dallas or Miami are out. In the same way, our endoderm cell later is restricted to becoming part of the lungs. It can no longer be part of the liver. Dialling 960 will resrict me to an area of uptown Manhatten, as further development can restrict the developing lung cells to part of the spongy tissue or part of a small airway. The final four digits ensure that it is my friend's number I reach: just as in the end a cell will develop to be exactly right for the area surrounding it.

136 Who is the boss?

So, you have growing inside you a little scrap of tissue. How is it that something so small can alter you so? The old view of pregnancy was of a baby growing rather like a parasite in your womb: a scrap of a thing which you gave unwilling shelter. But this little scrap does not leave much to chance. It can, and does, control its environment – and that environment is you. It needs the womb walls to maintain their thick lining. It has to stop the womb from rejecting it. It wants the womb to grow, giving it plenty of space in which to move, and the mother's breasts to grow and develop in readiness to provide nourishment after birth. Ordering for now, investing for the future, it takes over a substantial part of your hormone production. And this can change the way you feel.

Few women are immune to the effects of hormones. They can undermine feelings of well-being, make us depressed, alter our sexual libido or, indeed, make us impossible to live with. Their action is not simple.

Suffering from P.M.T., a woman will turn on the nearest scapegoat unreasonably, or react out of all proportion to some minor offence. Few women feel as desperate as this *every* month, but few go through life without the occasional depressing day. Hormone action is quite unpredictable, and it makes women unpredictable.

It may be helpful to view adverse hormone action as something that makes it more difficult for a woman to snap out of moods. If the world seems to be against you, you find it hard to stand back and say, 'Look you are being stupid here, you are not important enough for everyone to gang up against you in this way'. If someone does us a wrong, P.M.T. makes it hard to control those initial feelings of anger and the desire to lash out.

The hormonal changes of early pregnancy and childbirth hit us in much the same way. We feel tired, we feel sick, we feel high, we feel low. But mainly we feel unpredictable. We feel unbelievably tired, yet can, on occasions, dance the night away. You have your longed-for pregnancy, yet feel strangely uncertain now it has happened. You may even find yourself blaming others for what you have, after all, planned and desired. This unpredictability can, in itself, make you feel worse. Especially if you are usually in control of yourself. 'This does not feel like me', is a common reaction to the first weeks of pregnancy. See 151.

137 But I still have my I.U.D.

No one quite knows how the interuterine device (I.U.D. or I.U.C.D.) works. But it usually does. There is, however, a failure rate of between four and six out of every 100 uses.

One likely explanation of the I.U.D.'s function is that it makes the Fallopian tubes beat more rapidly, speeding up the egg's passage down the tubes. The embryo, therefore, ends up in the uterus before it is ready (it needs to be six or seven days old) and thus naturally aborts. The I.U.D. also restricts the area to which the embryo can attach itself.

But some embryos overcome these obstacles. If you do conceive with an I.U.D. in place, there is no need to worry. You can have it removed if the thread is accessible, or it can be left in place. It cannot harm the baby, who is separate

from it in her own bag of water. Usually, the I.U.D. is compressed between the membranes and the uterine wall and can be seen pressed on to the side of the bag like a piece of abandoned chewing gum. Congenital damage to the baby is not a problem, either, but there is an increased probability that you will have an ectopic pregnancy. This can be dangerous. Make sure you are aware of the symptoms; see 167. There is also an increased probability that you will suffer from an early miscarriage.

138 Phantom pregnancy

Occasionally women who very much desire a baby, but cannot have one, develop a phantom pregnancy. They may have many of the symptoms of early pregnancy, but tests will show they are not pregnant. The reasons are almost certainly emotional and psychological but can also include hormonal disturbance. It is hard to convince women that they are not pregnant, and once the realization dawns, they need much psychological support.

139 G.P. visits

Once your pregnancy has been confirmed (or indeed, once it seems to you to be highly likely) you will need to visit your G.P. (family doctor) to arrange for antenatal care. The doctor will offer a pregnancy test, if this has not already been given, and will ask you about signs and symptoms. You may be given an internal examination and will almost certainly be told the expected birth date; see 140 and 213. Take this opportunity to ask about carrying on with work and about anything else which worries you. Ask about the antenatal care available, and let the doctor know your preferences for the birth; see 141. You could also ask about local antenatal classes.

140 What date

On average, 266 days from the day of conception: 40 per cent of women have their babies within seven days of this date.

141 Place of birth

In Britain and most other English-speaking countries, in the U.S.A., through western Europe, with the notable exception of

Holland, most babies are born in hospital. You can, depending on local legislation, have your baby at home, but in many areas this will be difficult. Many countries have an organization which supports home births: write to it if you are having difficulty arranging one. Hospital is the best place to be if anything goes wrong; home is probably the best place if everything is going right.

Unless you live a long way from a hospital, have had previous difficult births, or if complications are predicted or likely to occur, there is no overwhelming reason why you have to give birth in hospital. In Holland, where a large proportion of babies is born at home, the infant mortality rate is actually lower than it is in Britain. True, it is a smaller country, but there are areas of Britain which are as densely populated. See 323.

142 Private or public

If you subscribe to a private health plan, you will probably find that this does not include private antenatal care or cover the baby's birth. But you can often take out special cover to include birth, or pay directly for private care during pregnancy and/or birth. You can engage a private doctor, a private consultant, or even a private midwife to care for you in pregnancy and/or during delivery.

Depending upon your inclination, and your pocket, you can choose from several variations on the theme of private antenatal care by a midwife, doctor or consultant, and private birthing arrangements with either consultant or midwife. These can take place in a private hospital or clinic, or in a private bed in a state health service hospital. It is sometimes possible to buy a little extra privacy by paying for an amenity bed in a state health service hospital: the medical attention you will receive in this bed is the same as that for other patients and will be free. Remember, if you are opting for private treatment, that the bills can be unpredictable. An emergency Caesarian section can be costly: be sure you cover your 'worst case' scenario.

143 Hospital care

Hospital care throughout pregnancy and birth will certainly be advised if you have a history of miscarriage or if there are other potential problems. Obviously, the level of expertise at a hospital is high; the availability of special tests and the use of modern technology is usually impressive. But there are drawbacks. You are unlikely to see the same doctor or midwife on each visit; you may have a long journey to the hospital, and an indefinite wait when you arrive. It is in the nature of obstetrics that doctors get called away to emergencies at the most inconvenient times. Some women do need longer appointments than those given.

This said, I am not sure that the cattle market feeling instilled in me as I waited in these clinics was really necessary. Things may have changed since I had my last child, but I doubt it.

144 Consultants in the community

Some hospital doctors hold antenatal clinics at health centres or at family doctors' surgeries or offices. This makes available a high degree of expertise at the local level.

145 G.P. units

These are run by G.Ps (family doctors) together with local midwives. In some areas, they are run at a hospital, in others they take place at the health centre or at the doctor's surgery.

146 Shared care

Care which is shared between the hospital and the G.P: sometimes you will also see your midwife. This may mean alternate visits to the G.P. and the hospital, or that the hospital simply provides the back-up services such as ultra-sound scans.

147 What can I do?

Anything – except smoke too much, drink too much, or take in harmful drugs; see page 25. There is no need to give up travel or work, unless you work with dangerous chemicals. You may feel like resting, but you don't have to rest unless you feel the need. You do not have to give up sport.

148 Should I give up sex for a while?

Sex in pregnancy can be enjoyable, and safe – it is a mystery why so many books

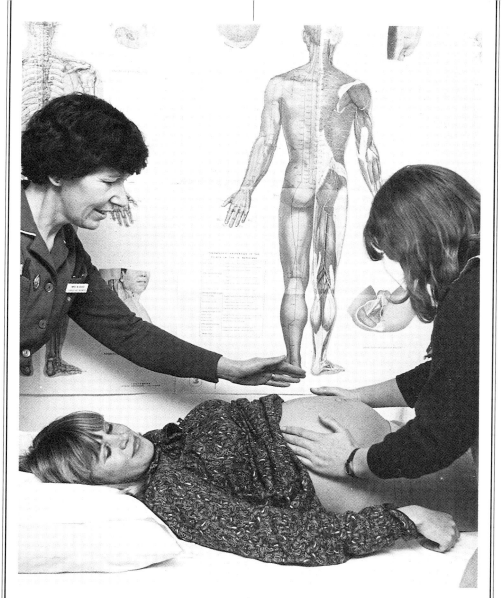

imply that the majority of women need holding and cuddling, rather than sexual excitement in pregnancy.

I do not know who these majority are; most of the women I have asked have found sex especially sweet at this time. Maybe some men find their pregnant wives less desirable than usual, or some women become inhibited by their own pregnant bodies. Certainly, some couples worry that they may harm the baby. They need not.

The womb, as always, lifts up out of the way when you become sexually excited. Unless you have had repeated miscarriages or vaginal bleeding, it is unnecessary to adjust your sexual behaviour.

Nevertheless, many couples still feel worried by the idea of deep penetration, almost as if it might intrude on the baby. Aggressive sex may seem to you somehow wrong or inappropriate during pregnancy, but however it feels, there is nothing to suggest that the deeper the penetration, the more likely a woman is to miscarry. The embryo is well and truly secured to the top of the uterus. Unless you have a history of early miscarriage (when you may be advised against any penetration), it is safe.

Still not convinced? Consider this. There are records of pregnancies surviving D. & C. (dilatation and curettage) operations in which the surgeon scrapes the inside of the womb with a metal spoon. It is unlikely that a penis (which may not even reach the cervix) could dislodge what a sharp spoon right inside the uterus can leave in place.

If your doctor does advise against intercourse, this will include anal intercourse which puts pressure on exactly the same areas. But as long as vaginal intercourse is possible, anal intercourse presents no problems.

Oral sex is also perfectly acceptable if that is your pleasure. But since semen contains one of the hormones which induce contractions (and this might be absorbed through the mouth and the gut) it is inadvisable to take semen into the mouth if you have had any vaginal bleeding with pain.

It is also dangerous for a woman to allow her partner to blow into her vagina: there is a possibility that this could cause a fatal air embolism. It would obviously be foolish, too, to engage in oral sex if the man has a cold sore on his lips (a condition allied to genital herpes), which could spread to the vagina. Primary herpes can be a serious illness for a tiny baby: it can be caught as the infant passes through the infected vagina at birth. If you have a vaginal infection at the time the baby is due, a Caesarian section would probably be given; see 429.

149 Can orgasm cause contractions?

Orgasm does induce vaginal contractions, and can, at term, provide an enjoyable start to labour. But your body will only go into labour if and when it is ready. In fact, the uterus practises contracting thoughout pregnancy; see 306.

150 Prostaglandins

Prostaglandins are found throughout the body but have a particularly high concentration in seminal fluid. Prostaglandin is used to soften and open the uterus before abortions, and it is thought to be involved at the onset of labour, since it can start contractions if present in the vagina. How then can sex be safe? The answer is that the uterus responds to small amounts of prostaglandin only when ready, and that although semen is a rich source, it is not rich enough to induce abortion. See 384 for inducing labour.

151 Togetherness

During pregnancy, especially the early months, a man can easily become an outsider as the woman communes with her growing baby. But he could, not unreasonably, see the baby as taking over a body and a person upon which he felt he had a major claim. She may be less attentive, he may feel jealous, and he may find it hard to feel close and involved with the child. Sex is something the three of you can share. You were there together at the beginning. It is right that you continue to be together throughout. See 189.

152 Old wives' tales

• If you carry a baby in front, you are having a boy.
• If you go off tea, you are having a boy.
• You can guess the sex of the baby from the heart beat.
• Don't stretch – the baby will be strangled by his cord.
• If you are frightened by a black animal, your baby will be covered with thick black hair.
• If you are frightened by a one-armed man, your baby will only have one arm.
• Don't eat strawberries – your baby will have a strawberry birthmark.

True or false? In fact, one is true. You can guess the baby's sex from the heart rate. Boys usually have heart rates below 140 per minute, girls above. If your baby's heart rate is monitored you may like to use it to try to predict the baby's sex.

153 Twins

There are two types of twins: identical and fraternal.

Identical twins develop from the same fertilized ovum. They share all the same genetic material and are, therefore, always of the same sex. They do not run in families as fraternal twins do. No one knows why this happens – it just does.

The fertilized egg begins to divide as it moves down the Fallopian tube to become embedded in the womb; at some very early stage in the process, the cells divide into two clusters and each cluster develops separately into a baby. Occasionally, when this division happens extremely early, the babies will have separate placentas; but usually they have the same placenta, growing, however, within their own amniotic sacs. The blood streams of the two babies mingle within the placenta. Very occasionally, the separation between identical twins is not complete, and so-called Siamese, or conjoined, twins develop. They can share not only one placenta but heads, legs, and body cavities. Fortunately, such twins are rare.

Fraternal twins develop in an entirely different way. They occur when two eggs are released at ovulation and both eggs are not only fertilized but continue to develop. Apart from the fact that they are developing in the same womb at the same time, these babies are no more alike than any other two siblings; indeed, they can even have different fathers. They have separate placentas, separate genetic endowment and may be of opposite sexes.

The tendency to produce fraternal twins (in spite of the name) is inherited from the female side of the family. If you are a twin yourself, you are twice as likely to be the mother of twins. It is often said that twins skip a generation, but there is no evidence for this.

How twins lie

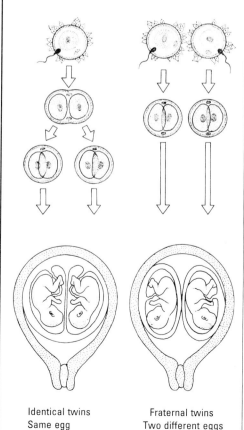

Identical twins
Same egg

Fraternal twins
Two different eggs

154 Blighted ovum

It is thought that as many as one in six miscarriages occurs because the embryo cannot develop beyond the earliest stages. The reasons may be genetic, or they may be due to high temperature, illness or harmful substances. The pregnancy begins normally, but thereafter only the 'supporting' pregnancy tissue develops. Bleeding is usually followed by miscarriage before the tenth week. Examination will usually show a small amniotic sac, but no foetus inside.

If this happens to you twice, your partner should ask to have his semen analysed. It is sometimes the result of an ovum being fertilized by an abnormal sperm.

155 Pyelitis

If you have a slight temperature, low back pain, and it hurts when you press the area of your kidneys, you probably have a kidney infection called pyelitis. You may also vomit. Seek medical help immediately: not only is it painful, but it can affect the functioning of the placenta. Antibiotics will clear it up, but until these take effect, drink plenty of fluids.

156 Cystitis

Cystitis is a recurring problem for many women, and especially during pregnancy. The best remedy is to drink: drink at least a pint of water when you get up in the morning, and another pint every time you pass urine. Ask the doctor for antibiotic treatment.

157 Yeast growth

Vaginal discharges increase in pregnancy, but if you become sore, red and itchy, you probably have thrush or *candida*. The acidity of the vaginal fluids changes during pregnancy, and this disturbs the bacteria in the vagina that usually keep thrush in check. (The contraceptive pill, or a course of antibiotics, can have the same effect.) The doctor will give you some pessaries to treat the complaint, but I find plain yoghurt works wonders, while others swear by vinegar in the bath water, or painting the whole area with gentian violet. If the problem persists, it is worth cutting sugar and white flour from your diet.

158 Varicose veins

Pregnancy is a time when many body tissues soften, and this can happen to the valves in the veins which carry the blood back to the heart. This impairs their function and results in a build-up of blood in the veins, especially of the lower limbs: the resulting distended, swollen blood vessels are varicose veins.

If you have a tendency to varicose veins, or if a close relative has them, avoid sitting in a position which allows the blood to pool in the legs. Keep your legs uncrossed, avoid sitting so that your thighs press hard on the edge of a chair, and exercise your feet and legs to keep the blood flowing. Wear support tights.

159 Vaginal varicose veins

These are just like those in the legs, but since the cervix often presses down on the swollen veins, they can be very painful. Ice, wrapped in a clean handkerchief and applied to the vaginal area, can relieve the pain.

160 Piles

The likelihood of internal haemorroids (piles) is increased in pregnancy because of extra pressure on the veins of the lower abdomen. Normally, the bowel is closed between passing stools by a mechanism consisting of three pads. If the pads hang down into the anus, haemorrhoids develop: the large veins inside the pads become prone to bleeding.

You may also suffer from external haemorrhoids: swellings at the external margins of the anus caused by blood clots in the veins.

Never be content with self-diagnosis of haemorrhoids: rectal bleeding is often due to piles, but it sometimes has other, potentially serious, causes. Always report it to a doctor.

> ### Preventing piles may be as easy as curing them:
>
> - Don't let yourself get constipated.
> - Sleep on your side.
> - Avoid long hours of standing.
> - Don't strain when passing stools.
> - Do pelvic floor exercises: follow the directions on page 39.
> - Eat plenty of natural fibre.

The simplest treatment is to sit in a bath of warm salty water two or three times a day. Dry yourself by dabbing with a towel and place a cotton wool pad over the anus. Keep yourself scrupulously clean. Soothing lotions or anaesthetic creams may also help, but don't use mineral oils.

161 Sinusitis

The hormones that soften up the vagina and cervix have much to answer for: here is yet another effect of their lack of precision. They often make the mucous membranes inside the nose and sinuses swell in pregnancy; it is rarely a serious problem, more of an irritation, particularly in the last weeks when it can seem as if you have a permanent cold. If it is a problem, a glass of water (or a small spray) by the side of your bed will counteract the dryness caused by breathing through the mouth.

162 Nose bleeds

Nose bleeds are yet another consequence of the softening effect of hormones. Blood vessels in the nose are especially delicate. Avoid blowing your nose (if you can) and blow gently if you must. Petroleum jelly is useful for stopping nose bleeds. Simply push some up the nostril.

163 Breast problems

Breasts become tender in the early weeks of pregnancy. A common enough statement, but you may feel that tender is not the right word. Acutely painful might be more appropriate. Pain is subjective, and some people are more sensitive to it than others: it is not that they are inclined to make a fuss. People vary, too, in the sensitivity of different body areas; that of breasts varies enormously.

If you find that your breasts are exceedingly tender, a supporting bra will help. So, if things get bad, will an ice compress and a warm bath. The problem should resolve itself by the middle trimester, but if it persists beyond this point, and particularly if the pain is localized, ask your doctor to check that you do not have a cyst.

Giving up coffee (you should be cutting down your caffeine intake anyway) may make a cyst disappear. Cutting alcohol and cigarettes, again advisable in pregnancy, should also help.

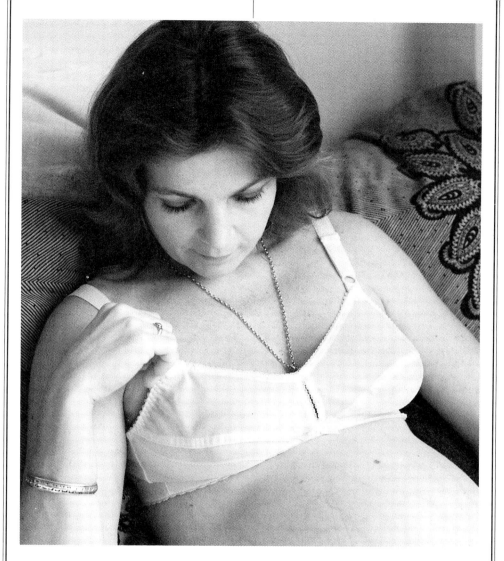

164 Brassières

Changes in the breasts are one of the earliest signs of pregnancy. Even if you do not normally wear a bra, you will find one necessary while you are pregnant and lactating. Heavy breasts allowed to hang freely will almost certainly develop stretch marks, which never disappear completely.

A bra to restrict the movement of your breasts is a great plus, particularly if they are tender and painful. You may find a light bra useful at night, especially if you are normally full-breasted.

165 Likeliest times for miscarriage

Pregnancy brings an end to periods for at least nine months, often much longer; but see 168. However, something of the rhythm remains. Miscarriages are most likely to occur at four weeks, eight weeks and 12 weeks after your last period. If you have any bleeding at these times, however slight, go to bed immediately. If it persists, call the doctor. See 166. It may be due to a polyp, or to erosion of the surface tissue of the cervix: in this case bleeding is usually slight and coloured dark brown. But it could be a threatened miscarriage, or the beginning of a true miscarriage.

Ask friends with children, and you will find pregnancy often fails to survive the first few weeks. Most women are able to conceive again and carry the child to term, since the fault is usually with the embryo, not the mother. If it happens to you, it is little comfort to know that the foetus was probably not viable and not developing correctly; see 170-179.

166 Bleeding

Any bleeding in pregnancy after your last period should be treated as abnormal, but it is not uncommon: as many as one in three women has some bleeding.

It is not safe to ignore it, even if the blood is dark brown and 'old'. Blood can stay in the upper vagina for a few hours without leaking out. If there is a small brown-coloured blood loss, it is probably safe to wait until morning before calling in the doctor. If you feel any pain, or there is more than a little spotting, call the doctor at once and lie down until he comes. If the spotting is accompanied by low abdominal cramping, dizziness or shoulder tip pain, it could be an ectopic (tubal) pregnancy. Contact your doctor without delay. These can be dangerous; see 167.

The commonest cause of bleeding is threatened miscarriage; see 182. It will help your doctor if you can describe the level of bleeding and the colour of the blood.

167 Ectopic pregnancy

Ectopic means out of place, and that is just what this is. It happens to about one in every 300 pregnancies, more in older women and in women who have an I.U.D. fitted. It is thought to occur when there is abnormal movement in the Fallopian tube. Normally, little hairs waft the egg down the tube at a steady rate. If this movement is too slow (perhaps because of infection), the fertilized ovum will develop to a later stage in the tube. About 90 per cent of ectopic pregnancies occur in the Fallopian tubes, but they can happen in the body cavity, they can embed in an ovary, or at the point where the Fallopian tubes join the womb.

The main symptom is pain and bleeding, and a distinctive feature for many women is shoulder pain. This happens because the pressure of internal bleeding on the abdominal cavity fools the body into thinking the shoulders are sore: this is known as referred pain, quite common in many medical conditions. If you have ever had an endoscopic examination of the abdominal cavity, you will recognize the pain.

Ectopic pregnancies cannot survive: the womb is specialized to support a baby, the Fallopian tube is not. An ectopic pregnancy always requires surgery. Sometimes a tube can be repaired, but

more often it has to be removed. But you do have two Fallopian tubes and even after the operation, you can conceive. The chance of having a second ectopic pregnancy is one in ten, nevertheless, even after two, you may still go on to conceive normally if one of your Fallopian tubes is functioning.

Ectopic pregnancies are dangerous. You can loose much blood. Do not delay treatment.

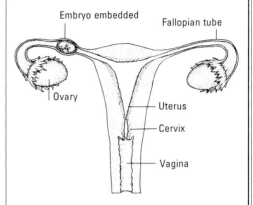

168 Periods in pregnancy

As many as a third of women will have periods in the early stages of pregnancy. Often the periods are more scant than normal, but they can be extensive enough for a woman not to suspect that she is pregnant. If there is a chance you could be pregnant, and your periods are slight, it is always wise to have a pregnancy test; see 119.

169 Are these periods dangerous?

Periods happen because the levels of progesterone (see page 42) are not high enough to suppress bleeding entirely. It may also happen as the placenta begins to take over the function from the *corpus luteum*; see 207. The bleeding is not from the embryo, but from the thickened walls of the womb, as it is in a normal period.

170 Miscarriage or 'abortion'

You probably call it a miscarriage: your doctor will call it an abortion. He is not implying that you intended to abort the foetus; this is simply the medical term for losing a baby before the 28th week.

The cause is not always known. Development may be abnormal, you may have kidney disease or high blood pressure. Even stress and emotional disturbance can contribute. The fictional scenario in which the heroine loses the baby under the stress of impending disaster is not entirely without foundation. Other factors include an abnormally shaped uterus, hormonal abnormalities, infections, the use of certain drugs (see page 25), fibroids, and cervical incompetence (see 247).

171 Consequences of miscarriage

Women do not die from miscarriages, nor do they bleed to death. You are simply expelling the uterine blood and tissue, which will come away in clots, like a heavy period.

There is nothing that can prevent an inevitable miscarriage.

Although it may seem a distasteful thing to do, save the tissue (the grey bits among the clots of blood). By examining them, the hospital may be able to tell why you have aborted, and help you next time around. *Do not use a tampon.*

172 Terminology

A threatened abortion is one that does not in the end occur.

A missed abortion is one in which the foetus dies, but does not abort. The pregnancy does not progress, and many of the signs of pregnancy disappear. Spontaneous abortion will occur eventually, but once a diagnosis has been made, a D. & C. will usually be given, or, if the pregnancy has reached a certain stage, labour will be induced.

Recurrent abortion (see 173) is the term used when abortion happens more than once.

A hydatidiform mole, a rare complication, happens when the chorionic villi (see 120) develop abnormally and grow a grape-like mass of cells filled with fluid. The foetus stops developing and usually aborts naturally. This condition always needs careful aftercare.

173 Recurrent abortion

If you have two or more abortions in successive pregnancies, you will almost certainly be referred to a specialist for tests.

The chances of aborting in a first

pregnancy are high (about 20 per cent). There is a small chance (less than two in 1,000) that a second abortion will happen randomly.

Most women go on to have perfectly normal pregnancies, but if you do miscarry two pregnancies, one after the other, there is probably a cause which needs investigating. Read on for the possible reasons for recurrent abortion.

174 Hormonal deficiency

In the first 12 to 14 weeks of pregnancy, before the placenta is working efficiently, the embryo is kept alive by a yellow yolk-like structure called the *corpus luteum*. If there is hormonal disturbance, this will not function correctly.

Your hormonal balance can be checked. You will be asked to keep temperature charts; samples of blood and of the womb lining will probably be taken. Your thyroid function will be checked (it has a minor role in hormone balance) and you will be checked for latent diabetes.

175 Infections

Recurrent abortion may also be caused by infectious organisms known as mycoplasma; 'T strain' is the culprit.

Mycoplasma are a cross between a virus and a bacteria, and live in the vagina or in a man's genital tract. They cause no symptoms.

The problem can, however, be identified, and treated. One month on antibiotics for both partners should clear it. If you are already pregnant, treatment with a safe antibiotic is usually advised.

The bacterium *Chlamydia* may also cause miscarriages; again this can be treated. Toxoplasmosis has also been implicated.

Virus infections cannot be treated. Some of them, such as *Herpes simplex*, are known to influence miscarriage.

176 Chromosomal factors

Most miscarriages are due to chromosomal abnormalities. If you have three miscarriages, you, and your partner, should ask for genetic counselling.

If you have a history of abortion due to chromosomal abnormalities, your doctor should offer you amniocentesis (see 232) or a chorionic vilus biopsy. If no one offers, ask for such a check. You are at increased risk, and these simple tests can tell you whether or not the foetus has chromosomal abnormalities. Not all such abnormalities are fatal, but all produce handicaps.

177 Coping with miscarriage

Miscarriage is difficult to accept, especially if you don't go on immediately to have a successful pregnancy. Every woman who has a miscarriage asks if there was anything she could have done to avoid it. The answer is usually no. You may feel that you should not have gone for that run, not stayed late at the party, taken more care on the stairs, or made love less vigorously. You may feel guilty, but you should not. You will be sad; don't think it unnatural to grieve. It was to be your baby: bottling up your emotions will not help. Don't rule out asking the hospital to let you see the baby: this may help you come to terms with what has happened. Not eveyone will find this an acceptable idea, but it may help some.

For a woman, the realization of pregnancy comes earlier than it does for a man. It is, after all her body. She can feel the changes long before he can see them. It is often difficult for a man to understand and share grief after an early miscarriage. You may find it helpful to talk to other women who have shared this experience.

178 Starting again

After the miscarriage, you may long for another baby. Take care. Be sure that your previous miscarriage is understood. Don't set up a situation in which you might have to cope with two miscarriages in rapid succesion.

Take care, too, that love-making does not just take on the role of baby-making. Love is to share, to enjoy and to give mutual pleasure. Don't let your pain make you forget this.

179 Reaction to a threatened miscarriage

If your pregnancy survives a threatened miscarriage, it is natural to worry that the baby may not be normal.

You may also feel something less than relief; wonder if, in fact, you really do want this baby after all. Again, this is quite normal. You have set yourself on a course which will make you totally responsible for another human being for about 18 years. Self-doubt is natural; reprieve from a miscarriage really opens up these doubts. It is as if you had been offered an escape and did not take it. Accept your doubts and uncertainty as a natural emotional reaction. Don't turn them into fear that the baby will not be 100 per cent healthy. It almost certainly will be: most babies are.

180 Why don't I feel maternal?

See 122. If it is your first pregnancy, you may find that you do not feel maternal.

The maternal instinct is a much over-rated emotion. If you suspect that it is as real as the average unicorn, you are probably right. Think of it as an emotion invented by men to keep women looking after the children. An over-statement? Of course, but no less true than the preconception that maternal instinct sweeps in with the seminal fluid, or overcomes us at the birth of a child. Most of have to learn to love our children, as we learned to love our partners. Love at first sight does exist, but it is not the only true love, or necessarily the best.

Not feeling maternal or emotional in these early weeks of pregnancy is normal. See 188.

181 Weight gain

Most women put on between 24 and 28 lb (11-12 kg) during pregnancy. As much as 3 lb (1.3 kg) of this can be extra blood, but some of it is also fat and due to fluid retention. You can gain weight quite quickly: don't panic. If you are not over-eating, the weight gain is probably not out of place. Chart weight gain.

182 Some views of pregnant women

Interviewer: *"Do you find Nancy just as desirable?"*

Norman: *"Well, I don't know. She looks pretty good in clothes, and in the dark you can't see, so it is not so bad."*

"People stare, unbelievably. Pregnant women must be most awkward-looking things to other people . . . I think to myself, my God, I must be a freak. And it's a little amusing, but it also angers me."

– From recent research papers.

If you have always flirted with men, you

may start to feel that in your present state this is not 'quite right'. If you don't feel it yourself, you may find others do.

On the whole, men don't flirt with obviously pregnant women. It is not necessarily that they find them unattractive; more the feeling that they 'belong' elsewhere. 'Belonging' in this sense may not be how you want to feel.

If you have depended upon casual flirting to reinforce your own feelings about your worth, you are bound to miss it, especially at a time when you have many doubts about yourself. It can easily undermine your feelings about the sort of woman you are, or want to be.

There is little you can do about it, except to re-value yourself for all your other attributes. Talk it over with your partner. If you and he have in the past played a double flirting game, it will be especially hard to see him succeeding while you fail.

183 Changes in taste and smell

Changes in smell and taste happen to nearly all women. See 118. They are probably changes in the blood supply to the linings of the nose and the tongue. And yes, some women do crave for things – such as coal – not normally considered food.

184 Skin changes

One of the pregnancy hormones tends to make skin cells containing dark pigments enlarge. Birthmarks, freckles and moles will darken, so will the nipples and the areas around them. Also any scar tissue. Some fair women develop chloasma, an area of dark skin, like a patchy suntan, on either side of the nose which extends across the cheeks. The upper lip may darken, also the nose and inner thighs. You may also notice a dark line going from the navel downwards: the *linea negra.*

Most of these changes start in the first half of pregnancy; all except the breast changes will disappear after the baby is born.

185 Feeling sick

'Morning sickness' (it starts when you wake, but only 10 per cent experience it just in the morning) can take you by surprise. The severity of the symptoms, and the wretched mental state that can accompany them, may seem inappropriate, even unnatural.

You may be able to put such reactions into perspective by reflecting on how differently you feel emotionally at different stages in your menstrual cycle; see 136.

186 Not hormones alone

But it is not so simple: neither premenstrual tension, nor sickness in early pregnancy, are an inevitable consequence of the hormonal trigger. If women who regularly suffer from premenstrual tension are asked just prior to their period how they feel, they are quite likely to answer 'Fine'. If the tension were just a function of the hormones, it would always be felt; it is not always felt, and it is not always with a woman in the days before her period. So mood is not simply switched on by hormones, however potent.

Up to 70 per cent of European and American women suffer from nausea in early pregnancy, but in other parts of the world it is virtually unknown. The most obvious hormonal explanation of nausea is the rise in H.C.G. (see 120), which occurs in early pregnancy and which declines after the first trimester. But all women, the world over, experience this rise in H.C.G., so it cannot be the only reason why some women feel so sick.

Diet may be a contributory factor: a woman whose diet is high in protein, and low in carbohydrates and vitamin B6, may suffer more sickness. This may in part explain why women in developed countries suffer more than their Third World sisters; but again, there is more to it than that.

187 Sickness: purely psychological?

It has been said that feeling sick is purely psychological: a woman's unconscious desire to be rid of the baby.

Just the sort of thing a psychologist *would* say? Not entirely. Few of us, after all, face pregnancy, especially for the first time, with no qualms at all. We may have a deep longing for a child and feel our lives empty without one, yet once pregnant, the nagging doubts begin. One minute you are filled with happiness, the next worried about the changes motherhood will bring.

One would be naïve, foolish, not to have such misgivings. There are, after all, questions impossible to answer until it is too late. Today, having a child is usually a conscious decision; naturally you worry that for you it may be the wrong one.

188 Feeling uncertain

There is some evidence that such ambiguous feelings contribute to the nausea (just as the excitement of a holiday, and worrying about travelling can also combine to make you feel queasy). A doctor studying pregnant women in France found ambivalence about pregnancy was common, and that ambivalent women were more likely to feel sick. Women who greeted pregnancy with unquestioning joy hardly ever vomited; those who totally recoiled from it were even less likely to do so. It was the ones who swung from joy to uncertainty, or who combined overall certainty with some nagging doubts, who suffered most from nausea.

There is a positive balance to these findings: studies of London women suffering badly from nausea in early pregnancy suggest that these same women become, as pregnancy progresses, more confident and happy in their pregnancy than those who get off lightly. Almost as if feeling ill to begin with helps one to come to terms with the change in lifestyle.

Of course, just because someone has shown in one study that nausea and ambivalence are linked, does not prove that it will be so for you. The figures say only that it is possible that if you are sick you are more likely to feel ambivalent, not that you are ambivalent.

189 Does he care?

It may be constructive to air ambivalent feelings about your pregnancy with your partner. Until a woman's belly truly begins to swell, nausea may be the only way of recognizing that her pregnancy really is happening. For a man, there is no such prompt – just a partner who is always sick and tired; someone who is now completely absorbed (151) in her own problems.

He may have his doubts, too. (Indeed, some fathers have morning sickness.) His doubts are, however, culturally more acceptable. Women are supposed to want children, and men are persuaded to have them. It is sometimes easier to accept this myth and accuse your partner of being unsure than to accept that you, too, share his doubts from time to time. See 203.

190 Combatting nausea

First, thinking again through the decision you made together (see 10-15) can be therapeutic. Bear in mind that one tends to feel what one expects to feel. In the West, we expect to feel sick in early pregnancy. In the early weeks of pregnancy your body gives out many new signals which you must learn to interpret; perhaps you interpret some of them as anticipated sickness.

Second, check your diet – see the box. There is also the old adage about plenty of exercise, fresh air and rest. All may help, probably none will cure.

Third, if things are very bad, talk to your doctor; he can prescribe certain safe medications provided there are no complicating factors.

Lastly, reflect that the nausea will probably soon diminish and, towards the end of the first three months, disappear; it rarely goes on for longer. You may reject this as poor consolation, but it is good medicine.

191 Feeling tired

The tiredness of early pregnancy, like the nausea, takes most of us by surprise, even if we have been warned. There is nothing quite like it. I remember sitting on a bench watching a traffic warden moving towards my car, knowing I would get a ticket unless I hurried, but without the energy to move. I felt faint when I got up, and had to sit down again. It cost me a fine.

Tiredness never seems to me to be quite the right word: overpowering fatigue is closer. If you are working, or looking after small children, this is a difficult time. You do not yet look pregnant, and are unlikely to arouse much sympathy. You may need that seat on the bus more than you will at eight months, but no one gives it to you now. Fortunately, this tiredness almost always passes. Like coming out of some long-term anaesthesia, it lifts in the third or fourth month to leave you, if you are lucky, with unbounded energy. My first two pregnancies followed this path, but my third did not. The tiredness lifted only at the moment my son was born.

192 Why the tiredness?

No one really knows. There are far-reaching metabolic and hormonal changes in the first weeks of pregnancy; it takes time to adapt. One possible culprit is the hormone detected by pregnancy tests, human chorionic gonadotrophin (HCG). The level of HCG rises sharply, reaching a peak at seven weeks, before dipping to less than 20 per cent of its top level by 20 weeks.

Another culprit, especially responsible for feelings of faintness and dizziness, is the alteration in the pattern of blood supply. The pelvic area, containing the womb, demands more blood to ensure a rich supply to the developing embryo. It takes time to adjust to this.

Finally, the increased level of progesterone causes a softening of the ligaments that support the joints. This has a slight weakening effort on the muscles. Everything feels more of an effort.

193 Becoming a father
See 190. There are formalities to show that a woman is pregnant: she feels sick; has a pregnancy test; visits the doctor, goes to the first antenatal clinic.

For a man the decision to have a child is no less momentous, but his commitment is not marked by any obvious event, exept the changes (often for the worse) that he sees in his partner. It is difficult to feel that the baby is real; easy to see what he is putting her through.

He may feel anxious, sick, moody, depressed. This is natural. While she has a reason for her feelings, he has none. His moods and anxieties can be condemned as unreasonable: a cry for attention; selfish, even childish. He, after all, is not pregnant; but of course he is.

There is no reason why he should feel any less anxious than she does, and if we accept that some of her 'symptoms' result from her anxiety and nervousness, it follows that he might share them.

194 But she is a mother
Incest is one of the strongest taboos in all human societies, and none stronger than that between a son and his mother. In the

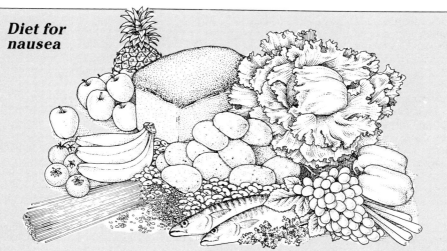

Diet for nausea

If you are suffering badly from nausea, it is doubly important to eat a balanced diet with plenty of unrefined carbohydrates and roughage:

- Wholemeal bread and pasta
- Potatoes with their skins.
- Vegetables and plenty of fresh fruit

Eat little and often.

Cut down on:
- Fatty foods, and those rich in protein, i.e. less red meat, butter, cream and cheese.

But maintain:
- Milk – you need the calcium it contains.

- Check the table on page 23 to ensure you are getting enough folic acid.

If this sounds like the diet you are always being told is best for you, you are right. Sensible eating is the same in and out of pregnancy.

Some women find a diet especially rich in vitamin B helps combat nausea: this means plenty of bananas, whole grains and yeast extract. Ask your doctor about taking a vitamin B supplement.

And some find a cup of sweetened tea (hardly any milk) with a dry biscuit or dry toast go down even when feeling sick; herb teas such as camomile, peppermint or lime may be palatable, too.

small nuclear families in which we live, a boy often has nowhere for his early sexual impulses to go but towards his mother. He loves her, he rubs against her, he may even masturbate next to her. Later, he must suppress all these impulses. Sexual feelings are not for mother.

Although women may 'mother' him, and indulge him, he separates them from the forbidden mother. He does not recognize their mothering as coming from a mother.

Now, suddenly, he finds that the woman he loves, his mistress, is to enter the class of forbidden women: mothers.

This *can* produce anxiety. It can also disrupt and undermine what was a mutually enjoyable sexual partnership. He may be 'turned off' (frightened off) by her pregnant shape; just as he once turned from his mother to other women, so he now turns from this new mother figure to another. It is not unusual for this to happen. Even if he does not consummate this relationship, it is not easy for a woman (or for the man himself) to be understanding and forgiving. It is, after all, asking a good deal.

195 An aside

Some books about pregnancy, written by women, suggest that sexual desire and pleasure are increased during pregnancy, especially in the middle months. "Never better", was how a friend put it, before correcting herself and saying, "never so consistently good". This is my own experience and that of almost all the women I have asked.

There are sound reasons why it should be so. A woman's sexual response depends upon an increased blood flow to the vaginal area (which is present at all times during pregnancy), is often accompanied by an increase in breast volume (present at all times in pregnancy), and is, for many women, increased just prior to menstruation when higher levels of progesterone are present. Progesterone levels are elevated in pregnancy. We might say that a pregnant women has many of the physical characteristics of a sexually aroused woman.

I have not seen a single book written by a man which suggests that women have heightened arousal in pregnancy. Most quote studies which show that the level of sexual activity is actually reduced.

Perhaps the causes of the fall in sexual activity are interesting here. Half the wives in one study said they were not attractive or sexy, while a quarter of the men agreed. A fifth of the men said that motherhood and sex conflicted, a few said that sex with a pregnant women was sacreligious. Half the women and a quarter of the men were afraid of harming the baby.

In another study, 27 per cent of couples feared they would injure the baby. A surprising 63 per cent found sex uncomfortable or awkward. But it takes little imagination to find a comfortable position. Perhaps the explanation is that successful sex takes two, and in relationships where the man has usually taken the sexual lead, there is a decline in activity.

196 He feels anxious

The financial responsibilities of a baby can be frightening. While two people are earning, chances can be taken, jobs can be changed. The financial responsibility for a family often still falls primarily on the man. It may seem like a trap – even if it is a trap he has chosen – and it may become an outlet for other anxieties.

A man is excluded by pregnancy. He is a postscript in the process, and let's face it, most men are not raised to feel like postscripts. Why should they be?

Moreover, he is asked to be supportive, stable, a tower of strength to his partner as she drags herself around. Yet this demand is made just as his own support is likely to have diminished or disappeared.

It should bring a man and a woman closer together, but it seems to be driving them apart. And he can be excluded not only by his partner but by the medical profession, her family and her girlfriends.

Will it go on like this? Will he be rejected from now on? The questions and anxieties are real.

197 Happy ever after?

So, it can be a touchy time. Together they face the biggest change in their lives since puberty. She feels sick, tired, emotional and anxious; he feels anxious, left out and a little guilty. It needs careful handling, especially in the early months.

The only way is to talk. Don't assume that your partner knows how you feel, or has no doubts. Discuss your sexual feelings and how the pregnancy affects them, especially the woman's worries about her attractiveness, and the possiblity of harming the baby. Sexual tension can only make a situation worse. Sexual pleasure shared can see you through a difficult patch. Tell each other that the difficult times inevitably pass. The middle trimester is much more fun.

198 How often to see a doctor

Once your pregnancy has been confirmed, your doctor will make arrangements for your antenatal care. You will probably see your doctor once a month until you are 28 weeks pregnant, then once a fortnight for the following eight weeks, and once a week for the last month. You may, in addition, see your midwife.

199 Eight weeks

She is 1½in (3.7 cm) long and has a large head and recognizable face. Through the paper-thin skull you can see blood vessels; the brain is developing in there. The tear ducts form this week, but the eyes do not yet open, although you can see them beneath the skin. The outer ear has formed and continues moving up from the neck into position at the side of the head.

The knees, elbows, ankles and wrists begin to form, and you can see the fingers and toes clearly. They are still webbed; sometimes they are webbed at birth. The baby is moving gently within the bag of water. You cannot feel this because the foetus is still so small.

You cannot yet see his or her sex, but the sex organs are beginning to develop about now; see 245.

Stroke the eyelids and they will squint; touch the foetus and it will move away. The heart beats, the blood flows around the body. The legs move in a gentle fashion.

200 Ten weeks

By now the foetus is 2¼in (5.5 cm) long. The head is more rounded, and the ears are now in place. The eyelids are formed. Finger nails appear, followed a little later by toe nails. They will grow out to the finger tips by the 32nd week. Next week it will be possible to determine the sex on an ultrasound scan. The foetus weighs about 1oz (28g).

She will close her fingers over anything she touches: not yet gripping, but holding in a rudimentary fashion. She can frown, and will turn her head away if you touch

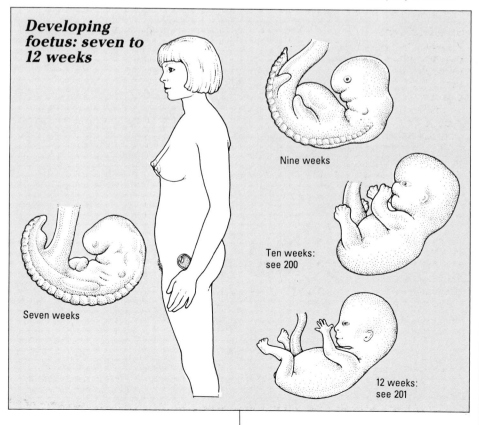

Developing foetus: seven to 12 weeks

Nine weeks

Ten weeks:
see 200

Seven weeks

12 weeks:
see 201

her forehead. She can curl her toes and lift her knees if you tickle her feet.

201 Twelve weeks

By the 12th week, the placenta is fully formed and operational. This is the end of the first trimester. All the foetal organs have developed, but the baby is still immature. She will not be able to survive outside the womb for at least another 12 weeks. From now on, the organs grow in size and capacity, fitting the foetus for independent life. The proportions are not quite right yet: the head is large, the limbs small and few of the muscles are working. The bones of the ribs and spine have yet to harden.

You still cannot feel the movements, but on a scan you can see her clench her fists, pucker her lips and kick her legs. She frowns, and twists and turns on the end of her umbilical cord. She can drink in the amniotic fluid and pass it out through her bladder. It is thought that the movement of fluid about the mouth helps the hard palate to form. In experiments, the tiny tongues of embryonic mice have been removed, and these tongueless mice are more likely than their litter mates to develop cleft palets.

202 Hang-over?

Movement is also essential for the developing limbs. One of the effects of alcohol on development is to put the foetus into an alcoholic stupor. Thus stupefied, it does not move and kick, or dance like a puppet on a string. As a result, the joints may be ossified at birth. So the kicks, twirls, twists and sucking movements have a purpose.

203 The growing womb

The womb is usually small, but throughout pregnancy it gradually stretches to hold, at term, a baby weighing in the region of 7-8 lb (3-3.5 kg), plus a sack of amniotic fluid and a placenta. At 12 weeks it has grown to about the size of a grapefruit: a little too large to remain hidden. You probably do not look pregnant – but you can feel the womb through the walls of your abdomen.

204 Bump

In a first pregnancy, or if you are exceptionally fit, you may not look pregnant until you are half way at 20 weeks. In subsequent pregnancies, it may be obvious by the time you are 14 weeks.

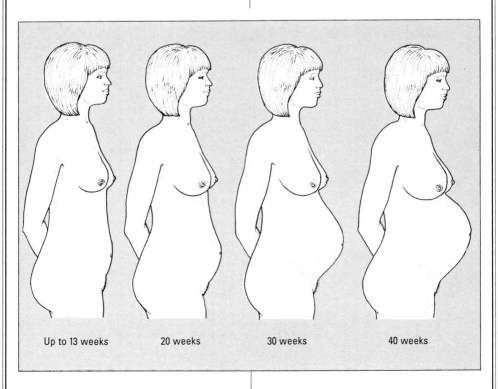

Up to 13 weeks   20 weeks   30 weeks   40 weeks

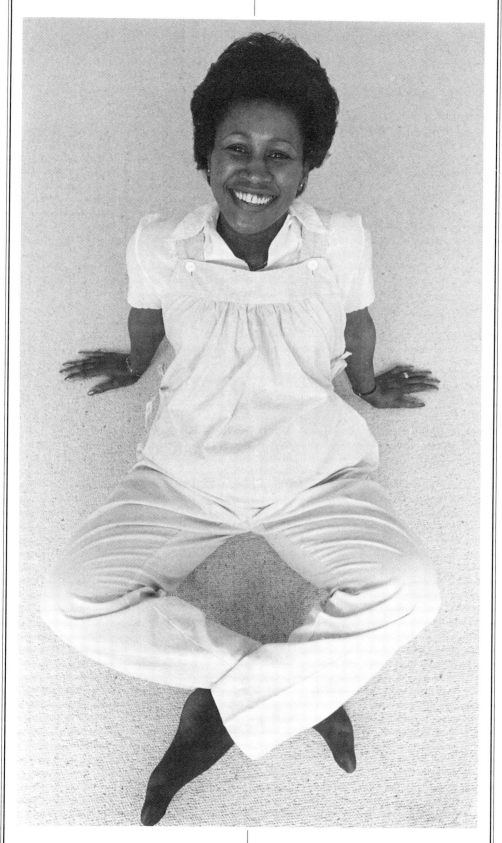

Pregnancy *The Second Trimester (Months Four, Five and Six)*

205 Feeling better

You may still feel tired (see 191-192) and sick (see 185-190), but over the next weeks these will (for most) be replaced by a feeling of great well-being.

Energy rushes back, life seems fun. The skin takes on a healthy glow (see also 260), your hair looks better (see also 261) than it ever has. You feel confident in your ability to handle the pregnancy and birth.

This confidence comes partly from the knowledge that miscarriage is now less likely, and that less can now adversely affect the baby's development.

206 Goodwill towards men . . .

Many women find the three middle months of pregnancy a time of great warmth, and of physical and emotional pleasure. Not only sexual enjoyment (with the return of your libido, sexual pleasure often reaches new peaks) but also the pleasure of physical and emotional involvement with others.

It is often a time when family ties are strengthened and a new closeness evolves with mothers and sisters. New friends are made. Suddenly the whole world begins to look pregnant.

207 Placenta power

At about ten to 12 weeks, the luteo-placental shift takes place: the baby's hormone support system is now managed by the placenta. Some women bleed slightly as this happens. The foetus is now recognizably a baby; it has only to grow, gain size, weight and maturity.

208 Signs of life

Sometime in the next few weeks you will become conscious of the baby moving within the amniotic sac. With a first baby it is difficult to be sure that the fluttering is the baby quickening, and it may be another two or three weeks before you are certain. But with a second baby you may recognize the feeling as early as 18 weeks; see also 248-249.

209 First hospital visit

If you are having your baby as a patient of the state health service, rather than privately, the first hospital visit could take about two hours. Two hours? Well, a great deal of that time will be spent hanging about. Waiting is the disease of state medicine the world over. 'Being seen' will probably take only about half an hour. But however awful the hospital may seem as you wait to be clothed, unclothed, then clothed again, labour and mother-and-baby wards are usually happy and caring places. It is not clear why they have to make you wait so long. There are staff shortages, doctors do get called away, but that hardly explains the situation; it is as if women have nothing better to do than just be pregnant.

The best defence is to treat it like a long train journey: take a book, letters to write, crosswords or a personal stereo. If you don't have to take small children, be thankful. You might even take a patient friend along.

210 Partner too

Your partner may want to share the experience. He is unlikely to be allowed much beyond the waiting area, although you could ask, politely. If the answer is no, ask again, explaining your reasons calmly and without aggressiveness. If your partner is still in the waiting room when you see the doctor, ask him or her directly if he could come in after you have been examined.

211 Baby clinic routines

You will hand over your urine sample (see 227) and change into a gown. You will be weighed, this weight being the base line against which weight gain will be monitored for the rest of your pregnancy.

On the first visit, a detailed medical and social history will usually be taken (218), which gives you a captive audience. Use it to ask any questions on your mind.

A doctor will then examine you. In some hospitals, particularly those used for midwife training, you may also be examined by a midwife, and by a trainee. There may be students present; they could be medical students, nursing students or trainee midwives.

You should be asked in advance whether you mind medical students sitting in, but in my experience this does not always happen.

It is easy in theory to say that you don't want to see students; difficult in practice.

They are the doctors, you are the patient; they know all about you, you know nothing about them. They are fully dressed; you have on a gown that ties at the back with two strings, one of which is broken. You walk into a room trying to hang on to some modesty by clutching the edges of the gown behind your back.

You are horrified to see them, but the consultant simply says, "This is an interesting case . . ."

Later you are angry, but at the time you are probably too embarrassed to complain. In a teaching hospital, students have to be taught, and you should not be surprised to be asked if they may sit in; but you should be given a genuine opportunity of saying no.

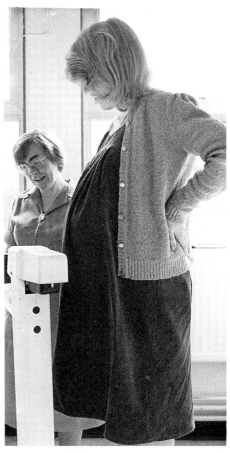

212 Initiative

I recommend taking the initiative by reminding yourself that they may there. Forewarned, it is harder to be patronized by insensitive medics. Even if you agree to have students sitting in, you need not agree to a student examining you.

But remember that students are often more forthcoming with answers to questions, reassurance and advice than are senior doctors.

213 LMP and EDD

The nurse who takes your medical history (218) will ask you the date of your last period (LMP), the number of days between your periods, and the regularity of your menstrual cycle. By adding nine months and seven days to the LMP she will get the estimated date of delivery (EDD), but if your cycle is not 28 days, or irregular, this estimate will not be particularly accurate. Nowadays, an ultrasound scan can be used to check the EDD.

214 Fiddling your dates

Don't be tempted to give the nurse a date earlier than the actual LMP. Wishing away the pregnancy will not make it go any faster, and you might later find yourself faced with an induced birth because you are considered overdue. More dangerously, the doctors may assume that early induction (as a cure for specific problems in the last months) is safe, when it is not. If you are unsure of the date of your last period, say so.

215 Contraceptives

They will probably ask what contraceptives you have been using. If an I.U.D. is still in place, say so. There is no danger, and it is possible to have the I.U.D. removed. You should also say if your periods have been very heavy (they often are when an I.U.D. is in place); you may need extra iron and folic acid.

A diaphragm or condom cannot affect a pregnancy, but if you were using a spermicide in conjunction with either, and became pregnant, you may be concerned about suggestions that spermicides can cause birth defects. Talk this over with the doctor.

216 Spermicides, the evidence

It is disputed. In one large study, there was no increase in the number of birth defects following contraceptive failures using spermicides.

In addition, spermicides have been used for years, and they have never been totally reliable so there must be countless perfectly normal people who were conceived accidently because spermicides failed.

217 Pregnant, despite the pill

If you became pregnant despite taking the pill, discuss this with your doctor. The synthetic hormones in the pill can produce serious congenital abnormalities, and if these are later proved to be present, you may wish to consider an abortion. There is no problem if you had stopped taking the pill before becoming pregnant.

When is the baby due?

Find the first day of your last period among the figures in **bold** type. Read off the figure immediately below in light type – it is your estimated date of delivery – EDD.

January	**1**	**2**	**3**	**4**	**5**	**6**	**7**	**8**	**9**	**10**	**11**	**12**	**13**	**14**	**15**	**16**	**17**	**18**	**19**	**20**	**21**	**22**	**23**	**24**	**25**	**26**	**27**	**28**	**29**	**30**	**31**
October	8	9	10	11	12	13	14	15	16	17	18	19	20	21	22	23	24	25	26	27	28	29	30	31	1	2	3	4	5	6	7
February	**1**	**2**	**3**	**4**	**5**	**6**	**7**	**8**	**9**	**10**	**11**	**12**	**13**	**14**	**15**	**16**	**17**	**18**	**19**	**20**	**21**	**22**	**23**	**24**	**25**	**26**	**27**	**28**	**29**		
November	8	9	10	11	12	13	14	15	16	17	18	19	20	21	22	23	24	25	26	27	28	29	30	1	2	3	4	5	6		
March	**1**	**2**	**3**	**4**	**5**	**6**	**7**	**8**	**9**	**10**	**11**	**12**	**13**	**14**	**15**	**16**	**17**	**18**	**19**	**20**	**21**	**22**	**23**	**24**	**25**	**26**	**27**	**28**	**29**	**30**	**31**
December	6	7	8	9	10	11	12	13	14	15	16	17	18	19	20	21	22	23	24	25	26	27	28	29	30	31	1	2	3	4	5
April	**1**	**2**	**3**	**4**	**5**	**6**	**7**	**8**	**9**	**10**	**11**	**12**	**13**	**14**	**15**	**16**	**17**	**18**	**19**	**20**	**21**	**22**	**23**	**24**	**25**	**26**	**27**	**28**	**29**	**30**	
January	6	7	8	9	10	11	12	13	14	15	16	17	18	19	20	21	22	23	24	25	26	27	28	29	30	31	1	2	3	4	
May	**1**	**2**	**3**	**4**	**5**	**6**	**7**	**8**	**9**	**10**	**11**	**12**	**13**	**14**	**15**	**16**	**17**	**18**	**19**	**20**	**21**	**22**	**23**	**24**	**25**	**26**	**27**	**28**	**29**	**30**	**31**
February	5	6	7	8	9	10	11	12	13	14	15	16	17	18	19	20	21	22	23	24	25	26	27	28	1	2	3	4	5	6	7
June	**1**	**2**	**3**	**4**	**5**	**6**	**7**	**8**	**9**	**10**	**11**	**12**	**13**	**14**	**15**	**16**	**17**	**18**	**19**	**20**	**21**	**22**	**23**	**24**	**25**	**26**	**27**	**28**	**29**	**30**	
March	8	9	10	11	12	13	14	15	16	17	18	19	20	21	22	23	24	25	26	27	28	29	30	31	1	2	3	4	5	6	
July	**1**	**2**	**3**	**4**	**5**	**6**	**7**	**8**	**9**	**10**	**11**	**12**	**13**	**14**	**15**	**16**	**17**	**18**	**19**	**20**	**21**	**22**	**23**	**24**	**25**	**26**	**27**	**28**	**29**	**30**	**31**
April	7	8	9	10	11	12	13	14	15	16	17	18	19	20	21	22	23	24	25	26	27	28	29	30	1	2	3	4	5	6	7
August	**1**	**2**	**3**	**4**	**5**	**6**	**7**	**8**	**9**	**10**	**11**	**12**	**13**	**14**	**15**	**16**	**17**	**18**	**19**	**20**	**21**	**22**	**23**	**24**	**25**	**26**	**27**	**28**	**29**	**30**	**31**
May	8	9	10	11	12	13	14	15	16	17	18	19	20	21	22	23	24	25	26	27	28	29	30	31	1	2	3	4	5	6	7
September	**1**	**2**	**3**	**4**	**5**	**6**	**7**	**8**	**9**	**10**	**11**	**12**	**13**	**14**	**15**	**16**	**17**	**18**	**19**	**20**	**21**	**22**	**23**	**24**	**25**	**26**	**27**	**28**	**29**	**30**	
June	8	9	10	11	12	13	14	15	16	17	18	19	20	21	22	23	24	25	26	27	28	29	30	1	2	3	4	5	6	7	
October	**1**	**2**	**3**	**4**	**5**	**6**	**7**	**8**	**9**	**10**	**11**	**12**	**13**	**14**	**15**	**16**	**17**	**18**	**19**	**20**	**21**	**22**	**23**	**24**	**25**	**26**	**27**	**28**	**29**	**30**	**31**
July	8	9	10	11	12	13	14	15	16	17	18	19	20	21	22	23	24	25	26	27	28	29	30	31	1	2	3	4	5	6	7
November	**1**	**2**	**3**	**4**	**5**	**6**	**7**	**8**	**9**	**10**	**11**	**12**	**13**	**14**	**15**	**16**	**17**	**18**	**19**	**20**	**21**	**22**	**23**	**24**	**25**	**26**	**27**	**28**	**29**	**30**	
August	8	9	10	11	12	13	14	15	16	17	18	19	20	21	22	23	24	25	26	27	28	29	30	31	1	2	3	4	5	6	
December	**1**	**2**	**3**	**4**	**5**	**6**	**7**	**8**	**9**	**10**	**11**	**12**	**13**	**14**	**15**	**16**	**17**	**18**	**19**	**20**	**21**	**22**	**233**	**24**	**25**	**26**	**27**	**28**	**29**	**30**	**31**
September	7	8	9	10	11	12	13	14	15	16	17	18	19	20	21	22	23	24	25	26	27	28	29	30	1	2	3	4	5	6	7

The pill can also influence the uptake of certain vitamins, and this slight deficiency can sometimes persist. You should be especially careful with diet if you have been on the pill for a long time.

If you did not have a period between your last pill cycle and becoming pregnant (discounting the period immediately after your last pill), let your doctor know. The EDD may well be inaccurate. Sometimes it takes two or three months for a women to start menstruating again after she stops taking the pill, and you may not have been pregnant at the first missed period.

Keep a note of the date of your pregnancy test and the time that the early signs of pregnancy (118) first appeared. It will be helpful in fixing the EDD accurately.

218 Previous medical problems

You will be asked about any operations and illnesses. Go armed with dates and details, especially of abdominal operations; the hospital may want to ask other hospitals for your case notes. You should also tell them about any blood transfusions you have had.

You will be asked if you have any heart problems, diabetes (see 222), or tuberculosis. You should mention any long-term illness, even if you think it is irrelevant.

Also check whether you have had *Rubella* (German measles). Don't worry if you are unsure; your blood sample will be checked for this. You will be asked about infections, such as cystitis and sexually transmitted diseases such as non-specific urethritis and thrush.

Make a note of any medicines you are taking and how much you smoke and drink. If you have a special diet, mention this.

219 Complications in previous pregnancies

Complications sometimes, alas, repeat themselves.

If you have had a Caesarian section, the hospital may suggest you have one again. You may wish to challenge this, but if you have a small pelvis, a Caesarian may be the only possibility.

If you have had a premature baby, there is an increased likelihood that this could happen again; you will need to rest in the second half of pregnancy.

You will also be asked about any previous miscarriages and about any induced abortions.

Between 15 and 20 per cent of women spontaneously abort their first baby. About 40 per cent of these abortions are inevitable, due to chromosomal abnormalities, and your next pregnancy will run exactly the same risk. Two miscarriages, following one after the other, are cause for reflection, since there is usually an underlying problem which needs investigating.

A late miscarriage – after three months – could be due to an incompetent cervix; see 247.

220 Previous abortions

Induced abortion is legal, but that does not stop a woman feeling guilty about it, and this is especially true if she has had more than one.

When she subsequently gets pregnant and wishes the pregnancy to go to term, this guilt can make her expect retribution. But it is very unlikely that a past abortion will affect a later pregnancy if the abortion was performed in a hospital by a qualified doctor. The expectation that things will go wrong is partly based on stories (sadly true) of back-street abortions.

221 Abortion by forcible dilation

If you have had a very late abortion (or more than one late abortion) which used forcible dilation of the cervix, there is a small possibility that you will miscarry in the middle trimester. The risk can, however, be controlled. The problem is that your cervix is more likely to be incompetent (see 247) because of the pelvic inflammation which sometimes follows this type of late abortion. Forcible dilation is, however, now rarely performed.

If your abortion occurred after 1975, and before you were nine or ten weeks pregnant, it is unlikely that it was performed in this way. Early abortions usually involve aspiration: the contents of the womb are sucked out.

Late abortions can be conducted without dilation if the cervix is softened with laminaria or prostaglandins. If you have had an abortion between 18 and 24 weeks, you probably aborted naturally. That is, labour was induced and you had a normal delivery. Again, this has no adverse effects on the outcome of subsequent pregnancies.

222 Pregnancy and diabetes

Pregnancy stretches your body in more ways than one. If you are at risk of becoming diabetic (and a family history of diabetes increases the likelihood), pregnancy could accelerate the problem.

Some women have diabetes only when pregnant. If this is diagnosed early, and your pregnancy is carefully monitored, there is only a tiny (2 per cent) risk of something going wrong. You will probably be treated by diet, but if this does not control your blood and urine sugars, you will be given insulin tablets or injections. The problem will probably disappear after the baby is born.

Mothers with diabetes are more likely to have premature, and large – over 10-lb (4.5-kg) – babies.

223 Already diabetic

Discuss pregnancy with your doctor before it happens. With care, there is no reason why pregnancy should not progress normally, or your baby turn out healthy.

Blood sugar can, nowadays, be monitored at home, and a hospital stay may be avoided if you are otherwise fit and well.

You may find that you accumulate amniotic fluid, and get rather large because of this; also that you are more susceptible to urinary tract infections. You also run a higher risk of developing pre-eclampsia (see 270-277), having the baby prematurely, and that the baby will be large.

Diabetics can sometimes have vaginal deliveries, but a Caesarian section may be needed.

224 Twins

You will be asked if there are twins in your family. Fraternal, (that is non-identical twins) run in families. They occur when two eggs are released. It is only your family, not your partner's, which is of interest.

At this first session you should also mention any genetic disorders which you know to be present in your family, such as haemophilia, cystic fibrosis, Huntingdon's chorea, phenylketonuria, or Duchenne's muscular dystrophy; for more details, see 71 and 72.

225 The examination

After checking your general health, the doctor will look at your abdomen. The height of the fundus can give a fairly accurate picture of how far the pregnancy has progressed. By comparing this estimate with your dates he can judge whether progress is normal. Later, he will be able to feel the baby and to judge how it is lying in your womb.

Next, he will conduct an internal examination. This makes many women tense; if so, it is worth learning to relax (see 303) and practising this during the examination.

You will be asked to lie on the couch with legs apart, knees bent and feet flat. The doctor will insert a metal or plastic instrument (a speculum) into the vagina. This keeps the walls of the vagina apart so the doctor can look at the cervix. The speculum is often cold, but it does not hurt, nor is it particularly uncomfortable.

The doctor will place two gloved fingers well up into the vagina and press on the abdomen wall with his other hand. This is to feel the uterus and the tissues around it. He or she will also take a cervical smear for later examination; note that the cervix is soft, due to the pregnancy; and that the size and position of the uterus are correct for this stage. The doctor will also feel for fibroids (local out-growths of the uterus) which can sometimes make vaginal delivery difficult.

Don't worry about the baby, there is no danger to it.

You will probably not need another internal examination until you are about 36 weeks pregnant.

226 How the baby lies

There is so much amniotic fluid in the sac (compared to the size of the baby) that the baby can swim up and down, twist and turn at will. Even if the doctor could easily feel how the baby is lying, at this stage it is immaterial. Later on, as the baby gets bigger, the way it lies becomes more important: from 24 weeks, the doctor will check this.

227 The urine test

Normally urine is clear yellow, with a typical smell. The sample you hand in will be checked for appearance and any indication of infection. It will also be tested for the presence of protein, sugar and

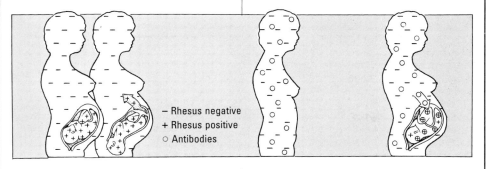

- Rhesus negative
+ Rhesus positive
○ Antibodies

ketones. You will probably see them doing these tests; ask if everthing is normal.

Protein in the urine may indicate kidney problems or infection, as may pus or blood. Later in pregnancy it may indicate pre-eclampsia; see 270-277.

Glucose may indicate diabetes. It could also be the result of hormonal change.

Ketones or acetone, present in the urine when the body is short of glucose, are a sign that the mother may not be getting enough food. This could be the case if she is extremely nauseous.

The urine will also be tested for the presence of any bacteria so that treatment can be given if infection is present. During pregnancy, the ureters (the ducts that pass urine from the kidneys) are compressed by the uterus as it lifts from the pelvis into the abdomen. Urine may not drain as readily as it should, which increases the likelihood of infections.

228 Blood tests

The blood sample taken at your first visit will reveal your blood group: occasionally women need an emergency transfusion following a haemorrage at birth.

The rhesus factor will also be tested; see 229. Tests for V.D., anaemia, and sometimes hepatitis will be carried out, too.

The blood will be tested for *Rubella* antibodies: if you are not immune to German measles, you will be offered vaccination soon after the birth so that you can protect subsequent pregnancies. If it is not offered automatically, it is well worth asking to be vaccinated. It is safe, even if you breast feed, but you must not become pregnant within three months of being vaccinated.

Your blood may also be tested for sickle cell disease and for thalassemia if you are likely to carry these; see 73. Finally you may be tested for spina bifida or some related disorder; see 231.

Since many of these tests are not automatic, do ask which are to be done. See also 256.

229 Rhesus factor

The red blood cells of most people (about 85 per cent of Caucasians) contain the rhesus factor. Such people are called rhesus+; if you do not have the factor, your blood group will be listed as A, B, AB, or O, rhesus-. It is only if you are rhesus- that you have potential problems. If you are rhesus- and your partner rhesus+, you could carry a rhesus+ baby, some of whose blood may seep across into yours. This is most likely to happen in late pregnancy or during delivery, but it can also do so if you have a spontaneous or induced abortion; during amniocentesis (232); or if you have an ectopic pregnancy; see 167. Once the blood has mixed with yours, you will react to the rhesus factor by producing antibodies, the usual defence to a foreign substance. The danger to your baby arises if some of these antibodies pass back into her bloodstream because they can destroy large numbers of her red blood cells.

230 Treatment of rhesus factor

If you know you are rhesus-, make sure you have your blood tested for antibodies at your first antenatal visit, and again at 28, 32 and 36 weeks.

At birth, blood will probably be taken from the cord for testing. If your baby is Rh+ and you have some antibodies, you will be given anti-D immunoglobulin injections. Given within 72 hours of birth, they can prevent the development of antibodies which could cause problems in subsequent pregnancies.

A fresh injection of anti-D immunoglobulin will be needed after each abortion or birth.

During a first pregnancy, there are rarely enough antibodies to harm a Rh+

baby. But with each subsequent pregnancy (unless the mother is treated, as above, within 72 hours), there is a growing possibility that there will be antibodies in the mother's blood that could pass to the baby.

It is possible to test whether or not the baby is affected by taking a small sample of amniotic fluid.

231 Alpha foetal protein tests

Alpha foetal protein, initially produced by the embryonic yolk sac and later by the baby's liver, passes to the mother's blood via the placenta. Monitoring of this protein (by testing the mother's blood) can give important clues to the baby's well-being.

A rise in AFP does not necessarily mean that anything is wrong; it does, however, indicate that further tests are necessary.

Very high levels of AFP frequently occur when the baby has spina bifida or amencephaly.

Increased levels of AFP can also occur when the baby has kidney or gastro-intestinal tract abnormalities, and if there is a threatened miscarriage.

But it may simply mean that you could be expecting more than one baby, (there is more AFP from two babies than one) or that you have your dates wrong since AFP levels double every five weeks in the fourth, fifth and sixth month of pregnancy.

An ultrasound scan (see 234) can test both these possibilities.

Low levels of AFP may also indicate that you have got your dates wrong – that your pregnancy is less, not more, advanced than you think. But it could also mean that the baby has Down's syndrome.

Again, ultrasound can check the age of the foetus, and if this is correct, then you will almost certainly be offered amniocentesis to find out if the baby has Down's syndrome.

If you have two elevated AFP tests, and there is no obvious explanation, you will also probably be offered amniocentesis as well. Together these tests detect about 85 per cent of babies with spina bifida.

Sometimes, neural tube defects can be seen on ultra-sound scans; certainly, with the increasing resolution of new machines, it is now possible to see the movement of the baby's pupils and eyelids in the third trimester.

If you undergo AFP testing, do remind yourself that AFP levels vary from woman to woman, and from foetus to foetus.

There are average levels which are typical of a pregnancy progressing normally, but AFP testing can never be a final answer: it is really a means of detecting those people who may benefit from further screening.

Of every ten British women with raised AFP levels between one and four will be carrying a child with neural tube defects. This is about four times the level of that found in the U.S.A., and higher than in most areas of Europe. The higher incidence occurs simply because Britons, an island race, are more inter-related than continentals. AFP scanning is often a routine procedure in Britain.

232 Amniocentesis

Amniocentesis is the process by which a small sample of amniotic fluid is removed with a needle from the sac surrounding the baby. For women in their middle and late thirties, this is a routine test, but it is not given to all mothers because it carries certain risks.

It can induce premature labour or miscarriage, and there is a small (less than 2 per cent) danger that the needle could damage the placenta or the foetus. This is reduced if an ultrasound scan is used to locate the baby before the test is done.

You will probably be given a local anaesthetic, then a long needle will be passed through the stomach wall into the uterus. You should not be aware of the needle passing through the stomach wall, but you will feel it passing into the womb. Most women do not find this is particularly painful, but sensitivity varies. So be prepared; it may hurt. It may also make you feel sick. It is sensible to go along for the test with a friend: although most women find the process relatively easy, some find it strangely upsetting.

The needle often leaves a painful bruise, especially if more than one insertion is necessary because there is not enough fluid, or if the sample taken contains blood.

The foetal cells contained in the amniotic fluid are grown in culture over three or four weeks, and examination of these can indicate chromosomal and certain genetic disorders. They will also show the sex of the baby. This may be important if you carry a sex-linked trait such as muscular dystrophy or haemophilia.

Occasionally, some of the mother's cells grow instead of the baby's, or there are not enough cells in the sample for analysis; however, 98 per cent of samples are successfully cultured.

Analysis of enzyme levels in the fluid can detect certain inherited metabolic disorders including cystic fibrosis. For rhesus babies monitoring of the fluid can indicate if treatment will be necessary; see 230. It can also indicate how mature the baby's lungs are, which could be important if a premature delivery is contemplated.

Since the test is examines the baby's chromosomes, and only the chromosomes, amniocentesis does not guarantee a healthy baby. It will tell you the baby does not have Down's syndrome; it will not tell you that the baby does not have another mental handicap.

It cannot test for heart disease, hare lip, club foot or intestinal disorders, but many of these can be seen on an ultrasound scan; see 234.

Neither can it test for beta thalassaemia or for sickle-cell anaemia, (see 71 and 73); these require a sample of the baby's blood or a skin biopsy.

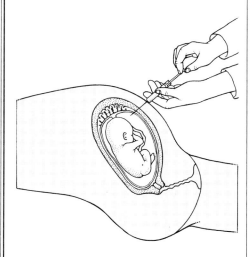

233 Risks in amniocentesis

The risk of inducing miscarriage is the one most often quoted: a figure of one or two miscarriages for every 100tests is usually given, but the figure is disputed. The problem is in finding the correct control group. Women having amniocentesis are usually older and have a history of complications; they are thus more likely to have miscarriages.

Recent studies suggest that when a woman having an amniocentesis is compared with a woman of similar age and similar history who does not, there is little evidence for an increase in the rate of abortion. Further study is needed.

234 Ultrasound scan

The technique was originally developed by industry to detect faults in metals. Adapted for use in medicine, it hasbeen around since the early 1960s.

Most hospitals scan routinely at 16 weeks, some offer a scan more frequently, some only when there is a potential problem.

A nurse will spread gel or oil on your abdomen to help conduct the sound beams, which are very high frequency, much too high for the human ear to detect.Each time the beams encounter a junction between two different substances – fluidand baby, foetal heart and baby's body cavity – some of the sound is reflected back.

Because a full bladder lifts the uterus, giving a better view, unblocked by the pelvis, you will probably be asked to drink large quantities of water as you wait for your test.

You can usually peep at the picture, (some hospitals will even give you a photograph of the scan). If you do not get an explanation of what you see, ask.

Although it is difficult for an untrained eye to interpret the picture, this first view of your baby can be very moving. It suddenly makes everything real; see also 250. Try to share it if you can: most hospitals will allow your partner to be with you, and his presence will almost certainly ensure that the picture is explained.

If you are lucky enough to have a real time scan, (a moving picture) itwill show the baby's heart beating and its hands clenching and unclenching.

235 What ultrasound can see

The amniotic sac at six weeks; the foetus at seven; multiple pregnancy; blighted ovum; fibroids; the point of placenta attachment; a number of foetal abnormalities, including heart defects, spina bifida, kidney and bowel disorders. Sometimes it is even possible to see the sex of the baby. Ask if you would like to know; some people say that this helps to make the pregnancy seem real.

236 Is ultrasound safe?

There have been studies suggesting that ultrasound increases the incidence of dyslexia and learning difficulties, but they are controversial. There is no evidence that ultrasound can produce chromosomal

Ultrasound test in progress

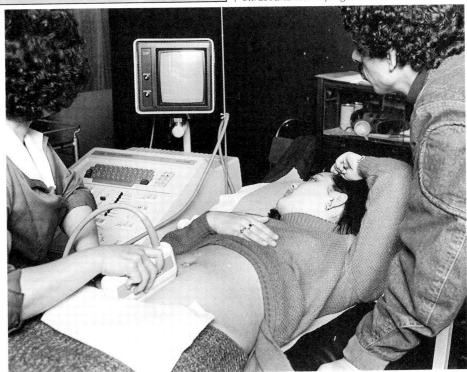

damage, cell damage, or induce miscarriage. It obviously needs further study but, since ultrasound is so widely used, it is unlikely that such studies will uncover any major dangers. You may, however, want to avoid routine ultrasound scans until the test has been given a completely clean bill of health.

237 A real baby, too soon?

After watching a tiny heart beating, and legs kicking, the 'thing' inside you becomes a baby. Bear this in mind if there is a possibility that something may be wrong. I know that when I had a real time ultrasound scan before my 16-week amniocentesis, I came away feeling unsure whether I could face an abortion. The waiting time between test and result was very difficult.

238 Facing an abortion

Many women report that they go into a state of shock when faced with the news that their baby has Down's syndrome or some other grave abnormality. They carry

on in an automatic fashion, making arrangements for the abortion, taking time off work, signing consent forms, acting as if they had always known of the problem. This shocked, unfeeling state may even last through to the abortion, for which you will not have to wait long – normally only a matter of days. See also 435.

At 20 weeks, the safest abortions are in fact induced labours. An intra-amniotic injection will normally be given which contains urea, prostaglandins and sometimes saline solution. You will go into labour and give birth. The labour will be painful and probably drawn-out – 12 to 24 hours. It will not be rapid just because the foetus is small: a lonely, painful time.

That this punishing outcome makes future conception more likely may seem an irrelevance, even an added cruelty at the time.

When you are delivering a live baby, any drugs you take must be strictly controlled because they pass across the placenta. But if your foetus is dead, you can take tranquillizers in order to soften the experience.

After the abortion, many women are further shocked to find themselves lactating; to be dripping with milk for a baby who will never be is unbearably sad. You may feel that it is as if your whole body mourns the loss. Strangely, this may help you to grieve. For grieve you will, and grieve you must.

Taking vitamin B6 in 200mg doses, and binding the breasts tightly, may help with the engorgement of milk. Kneeling in the bath with your breasts suspended in hot water will help them drain naturally and ice packs will ease the throbbing.

If you have to face a late abortion, you may find the experience difficult to share, even with loved ones. If so, you may find professional counselling a help and comfort.

Remember that the baby had a father too, and that he will feel the loss, and your pain. At 20 weeks the baby is less real to him than to you, his emotions are probably mixed, but that does not make the loss easy to bear. See also 436.

A woman may feel that the only way to fill the emptiness is to have another child as soon as possible; watching her pain and sorrow, her man may feel that he cannot let it happen again. Perhaps the best way out of the impasse is to accept that neither of you is in a position to make decisions now. There is no rush. Give yourselves time to grieve and to gather strength. A late abortion is unlikely to be necessary again, but remember that it could happen, and no one has unlimited resilience.

239 Chorionic villi tests

This can be carried out much earlier than amniocentesis. Samples of cells are taken under ultrasound guidance, from the villi (see 120) in the first trimester of pregnancy. The cells can be rapidly cultured and examined. If there are any genetic or chromosomal abnormalities, an early abortion can usually be carried out within the first 12 weeks of pregnancy using the aspiration method (221). At 12 weeks you will not lactate.

The test is relatively new and not available in all hospitals. No one is yet sure of the risks involved.

240 Placental function – biochemical tests

If at any stage in your pregnancy there is any indication that the baby is small for dates, you may be given one or more tests to examine how well the placenta is functioning. The most common of these is an assessment of oestriols, a group of

hormones made by the placenta, the mother and the foetus. Because substances pass between the blood of the foetus and the mother, these can be assessed by examining the mother's blood and urine.

241 Fetoscopy

To test if a baby has sickle cell anaemia or beta-thalassaemia it is necessary to take a blood sample from the foetus. The sample is taken from one of the blood vessels in the placenta. Put like that it sounds simple, but of course it is not. The first problem is finding the blood vessel.

A fetoscope is in fact a needle with a tiny fibre-optic telescope attached, which is inserted through your abdomen into the uterus. Looking down the tube, the operator can actually see into the womb and take tiny blood or tissue samples from suitable sites using special attachments.

A fetoscope can also look for cleft palate, limb abnormalities and other defects, and it can be used for surgery in-utero; see 242. It is a new technique which clearly requires skill and is unlikely ever to be routine.

242 In-utero surgery

The fetoscope (see 241) has made possible two types of operation on a baby still in the womb. One is a blood transfusion for a foetus made seriously anaemic by rhesus antibodies from the mother. The other is to help a baby with a blocked urinary tract, which can cause kidney damage. The blockage is detected on an ultrasound scan, but not all blockages can be helped by surgery.

243 New tests

Medicine is beginning to realize the ideal of examining the foetus without invading the womb.

Perhaps the most hopeful development is the ever-improving resolution of the ultrasound scan. There are already sophisticated ultrasound units which can look at the movements of the baby's eyelids and pupils in the middle trimester. It is not inconceivable that one day we will be able to watch all the minute details of the baby's development. Another new method of keeping a check on the baby involves taking a sample of the mother's blood and isolating the baby's blood cells from it. By reflecting light from the blood sample it is possible to see the chromosomes in the blood cells, and since the mother's cells and the baby's are very different, they can be separated. This tedious detective work is done by a computer. The cells can then be examined for abnormalities, but the major problem is that the foetal cells could be those of a previous pregnancy.

A more reliable sample can sometimes be taken from the small amounts of amniotic fluid that leak into the membranes.

244 Now can I smoke?

The organs are now all formed. The baby only has to grow. So is it safe to eat, drink and be merry?

The short answer is no. The longer answer is perhaps even more depressing: you should wait until you have weaned your baby.

Alcohol and cigarette smoke are not as dangerous now, but that does not make them harmless. Everything still passes to the baby. The brain is still developing, and will continue to do so for years, not months. The limbs need to stretch and move if they are to grow normally, and alchohol can leave your baby in a stupor which stops all movement. It can also make the brain develop abnormally (see below).

Smoking leaves the baby short of breath and caffeine makes its heart race.

In short, you should take just as much care of your body now as you did in the first three months of pregnancy.

245 Boy or girl: the crunch

The sex of a baby depends upon the genes: two Xs for a girl, one for a boy. Only a boy gets the Y; see 106-107.

But it is not quite as simple as that. The process is worth explaining in greater detail now because it gives an insight into how genes give instructions for growth. Each cell of the baby carries a complete set of genes. And since it has all of the genes, it has all of the instructions to make every part of the new human being. But it does not use them all at once. As cells divide and develop, the things they can become are more and more restricted. The first cell can become anything, later cells can become only one thing; see 135.

When the midwife says "It's a boy", she has not done a chromosome count, she has simply noted that the baby has a penis and a scrotum: the primary sexual characteristics.

There are other, secondary differences which we see at puberty (body hair, body shape, voice) and a different pattern of hormone release. Indeed, there are other less tangible differences in behaviour and perception. But most important of all, boys feel like boys, girls feel like girls. How does it happen? Science does not completely understand, but it does know what happens in the womb between six and 14 weeks after conception.

All babies, of whatever genetic sex, are programmed at conception to become girls, unless they are instructed otherwise. If the call does not come, nature makes a girl. A rudimentary tube in the foetus will grow and develop to become the Fallopian tubes, the uterus, cervix and vagina; so also will the slit-like external genitalia with a little bump (later the clitoris) at one end. If the instruction 'make a boy' is sent out, a different process goes into play. The female tubes are destroyed and another system develops into the internal male sex organs. The slit closes (you can see the line of closure quite clearly on the penis, it extends to the scrotum and looks like a weld-mark, which, in a way, it is). The little structure that forms the clitoris in women grows, in men, to form the penis. All this happens after the sixth week.

But what is the instruction? It is the male hormone testosterone. If the foetus receives testosterone, it makes a boy; if not, it makes a girl.

How is testosterone produced? The testes of the foetus have already grown, and are already making testosterone which is being pumped around the body in the foetal blood.

If there are no testes, the message is not given and a girl is made. In animal experiments, this has been shown to be true by removing the testes.

Occasionally, things do go wrong. At one time, a drug was used to stop miscarriage which, when it passed into the blood stream of the foetus, acted like testosterone. It gave genetic girls varying degrees of masculinity.

Testosterone also sets up the brain structures that organize a male pattern of hormone release.

No one knows whether behavioural differences are programmed at this early stage, or whether gender identity (the feeling 'I am a girl', 'I am a boy') is influenced by hormones.

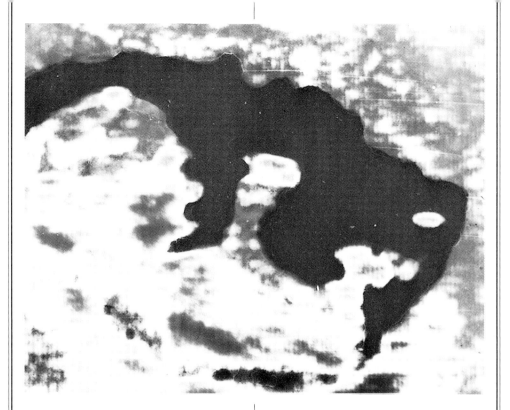

246 Blood pressure

If your heart pumps faster, or if the blood vessels narrow, or if your blood gets too thick, your blood pressure will rise. It is recorded by writing down two numbers, one above the other, like a numerical fraction. The top number is the systolic pressure: the pressure when the heart is pumping or beating. The bottom figure is the diastolic pressure: the pressure between beats. Think of the blood moving around the body in waves rather than simply flowing. Obviously, the top figure is higher than the bottom, but it is the bottom, resting, figure which is watched carefully in pregnancy.

Neither of the numbers should change much. Since there is much individual variation, it is impossible to say what is safe, high, or worrying, in anything but the most general way. But the resting figure should not vary by more than 15 to 20 points, nor should it go above 90.

If you start with a figure of 140 over 90, you will have 'essential high blood pressure' and your pregnancy will be carefully watched. If you have high blood pressure with protein in the urine, or a figure above 170 over 110, you will probably be admitted to hospital right away; see pre-eclampsia, 270-277.

247 Incompetent cervix

Some miscarriages are caused by an incompetent, or lax, cervix. Normally the cervix remains closed until labour begins, but sometimes the pressure of the growing baby makes it start to open. The membranes may bulge through, and this often leads to miscarriage.

If you have a history of spontaneous abortion after 16 weeks, the doctor will suspect incompetence. The treatment is to stitch up the neck of the cervix: stiches are inserted under anaesthetic at 14 weeks. (Non-absorbent tape may be used instead.) Stitches are usually removed a week or two before the baby is due, but if they are still in place when you go into labour, you will need to tell the doctor or nurse/midwife. Some women are born with a tendency to develop an incompetent cervix, in others it arises from injury.

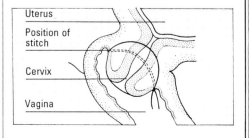

Uterus

Position of stitch

Cervix

Vagina

248 16 weeks

The foetus is about 6 in (15 cm) long, weighs about 5 oz (142 g), and is beginning to grow fine, downy hair, called lanugo. No one is sure why it grows, but it will disappear shortly before birth, or soon after.

A greasy white substance, known as vernix, covers the baby's face and scalp by week 18. Eventually it will cover the whole body; signs of it remain at birth, particulary if the baby is early. It probably serves to protect the skin, which is still very thin. The hand and foot prints are beginning to develop.

So, you have inside you a little, hairy, waxy baby with her lifeline already imprinted on her palms.

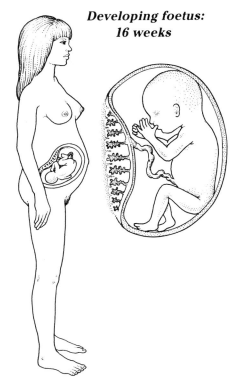

***Developing foetus:
16 weeks***

249 What can she do?

Move about with great vigor, twisting and turning in the amniotic fluid: it feels like butterfly wings deep inside you. If you could touch her, she would move towards you, not turn away. She grips with her hand more fully, but cannot yet hold tight. She would bend her knees and curl her toes if you stroked her feet. Her whole body is sensitive to stroking. She responds to sounds, and has her favourites: high-pitched sounds make her move more than low-pitched and set her heart racing.

Her world is dark, but not always pitch black. Her eyelids are still tightly closed, but the eyes respond to light. There is perhaps as much light in your womb as there is in the cinema: less when you have on your winter coat, more when you lie on the beach. She can probably taste the amniotic fluid she sucks in. Later she will drink huge amounts.

250 Reflections

It would be useful to stop for a moment and ask yourself what, apart from purely passing interest, is the purpose of these detailed weekly summaries of the development of the foetus?

Essentially, they can help you understand your pregnancy, prepare you for labour and birth by making it abundantly clear that the 'thing' inside you is not, in fact, a 'thing' – but a real, living being. That you are now a mother. It is fairly well established that women who are prepared for birth have easier and less complicated pregnancies. Their labour and delivery is shorter, and they have less pain. Their adjustment after birth is much better, and they are less likely to be depressed in the months following birth.

Starting to feel your child as someone to love, rather than a 'thing', is, after all, the most natural and easy way to prepare. Perceiving her as a person at this time gives everything that follows a happy, exciting focus: birth becomes less of a trial to be faced, more a time of meeting.

The bond between mother and baby can, and does, grow while the baby is still in the womb. Many parents – men and women – report that seeing the tiny embryo on the ultrasound scan made them suddenly feel she was 'real'; indeed, awakened a deep, instinctive sense of recognition if 'their child'. Others report that discovering the sex awakened the beginnings of love.

Bonding is just another word – over-worked at that – for a feeling of closeness to the child. Many ways have been suggested to promote this closeness; some even suggest that fathers should talk to their babies through tubes placed against the abdominal wall. You may think this sounds silly, but it could be that silliness shared with friends or lovers is one way of cementing the bond.

Of one thing I am sure: you cannot love anyone you do not see, or understand, at least in your mind's eye. See 419.

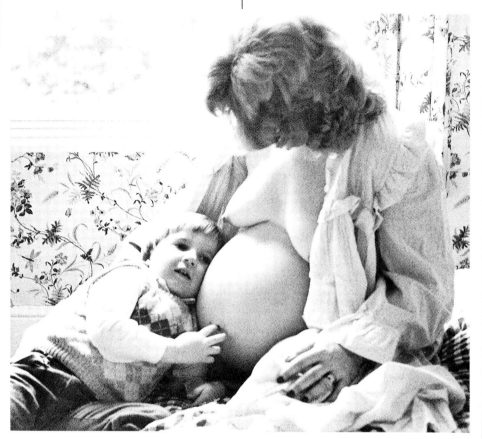

251 20 weeks

Half-way: she is half as long as she will be at birth, and weighs about 8oz (227g). You could hold her in the palm of your hand. The eyes are still firmly closed, the face rather gaunt, but hair is beginning to grow on her head.

By now you can almost certainly hear your baby's heart beating – use a glass tumbler. You may like to time the beats and guess the baby's sex: boys are usually under 140 beats per minute, girls usually above.

252 What can she do?

Try putting a glass of water on your tummy when she kicks: the movements will be amplified in the liquid: older brothers and sisters will be transfixed.

She can hear, too. A loud noise close to your tummy will probably make her move. She will also start to practise the muscle movements she will need for breathing. She will spend up to a third of her day practising these: that first breath which pulls her wet lungs apart after birth is hard to take.

253 Nothing fits

Sooner or later, and certainly by 20 weeks, you will start having clothes problems. The skirts with elasticated waists don't quite pull over the bump, the loose dress is no longer loose.

Clothes are a reflection of ourselves. We all dress (even if just in any old thing) to project an image. Feeling good about how we look often amounts to no more than feeling at ease with ourselves, but at other times dress is an important prop to a part we wish to play: to look young, to be pretty, to be intelligent, efficient, employable.

If we look right, we feel good. If we look wrong, we feel conspicuous in the worst possible way.

Maternity clothes only seem extravagant. They are four months' wear, but what wear. When did you last buy a dress that you wore every time you went out? When did you buy something smart for work that you wore every single day?

Trousers and boiler suits are especially comfortable in pregnancy, ideal if you are at home all day. They may be rather big at first. Get some braces to hold them up. You can also use braces to keep up

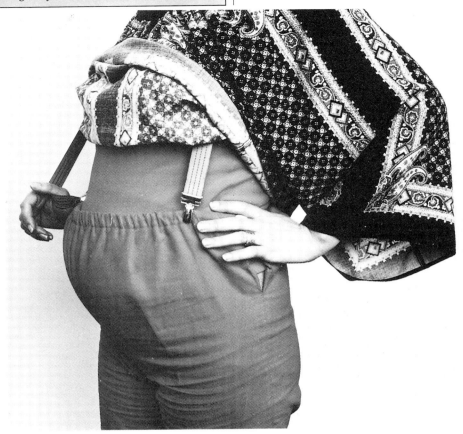

trousers and jeans from your pre-pregnant wardrobe, wearing them with the zips undone, the opening covered by a man's shirt or a long top.

Smarter dresses may be necessary if you are intending to work until late in pregnancy. You can wear fuller styles from the normal range, but do not imagine that you will wear them after the baby is born, by this time you will be heartily sick of them. If you do buy loose dresses, make sure there is some fullness in the back so that they do not hug your bottom. If you can afford it, one smart dress for outings will act as a confidence-booster in the last weeks. I found that up-market second-hand shops sometimes had a small range of high-quality maternity dresses at reasonable prices.

If you wear a sleeveless dress, or trousers with a bib front, you can make use of some of the blouses and sweaters from your pre-pregnant wardrobe. No one needs to know that the bottom buttons are undone. A dress may look smarter than trousers, or a sleeveless dress or pinafore, but these offer much greater variety.

254 Support

Second-hand clothes and old blouses semi-fastened: you can make do in many ways, but not with underwear. A proper supporting bra with wide straps is essential. I found the front-fastening type the easiest to put on, and the most flattering to wear. You should ask for the same size in a maternity bra that you usually wear.

Your feet also need support: they swell

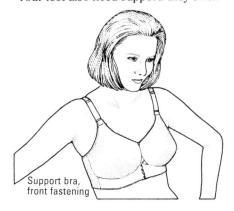

Support bra, front fastening

and flatten during pregnancy and you may now need a bigger size shoe.

255 Limits to activity

In the middle months of pregnancy, you may feel you can do anything. Often you can. Now is the time for travel, before sitting becomes too uncomfortable: a last trip before you have a baby in tow. Towards the end of pregnancy, most airlines will not let you travel, but before six months there is no problem. You will probably find that you are on top of your work and social life again.

Towards the six-month point, you may find yourself sleeping less, but this rarely bothers anyone. You could even regard it as practice for the sleepless nights.

Sex continues to be a pleasurable activity for most women; see 195.

256 Further hospital visits

These will settle into a routine: weight check, urine check and an assessment of the baby's growth. Later, the position will also be checked and recorded. You will ask be asked if you have felt any movements. If you keep a kick chart (290), you can tell the doctor about any changes in the pattern of movements.

257 Sweating

Something ladies used not to do. But because of dilated blood vessels under the skin, it now happens more than normally. You will probably find yourself taking extra baths and showers. Vaginal secretions may also increase: try to keep the genital area as dry as possible, and avoid using a great deal of soap. However troublesome the discharge gets, do not douch: this is dangerous during and just after pregnancy. Nor should you use vaginal sprays.

258 Breast care

The breasts change in pregnancy (see 118) and apart from support (see 254), need special attention. Make sure you don't use soap around the nipples. Later, you should roll the nipple between your fingers to draw it out, ready for breast feeding, and massage the breasts towards the nipple, squeezing the areola to express colostrum; see 469.

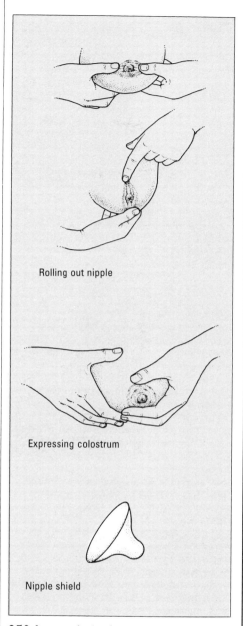

Rolling out nipple

Expressing colostrum

Nipple shield

259 Inverted nipples

If your nipples don't stand out, check with your doctor. You should try rolling the nipple area between your fingers to draw out the nipple, as in 258. Do this every time you have a bath. Sometimes you will be advised to try wearing nipple shields for short periods every day, starting at about the 16th week. Nipple shields are made of plastic or glass and are worn inside your bra. They gently draw out the nipple by suction. This does not hurt, but in hot weather they can irritate your skin. Wash carefully while you are wearing the shields and dust with talcum powder.

260 Skin changes

The middle months bring the bloom of pregnancy, literally: with extra blood being pumped to the skin, you take on a rosy glow. Dry skins become moister, oily skins less shiny. The high level of hormones in the blood plump out your skin, retain its moisture, and give it a smooth, velvety appearance. Your face becomes a little plumper, and this has the effect of smoothing any lines. Even if they call you an elderly mother at the clinic, you will probably not look it.

Use plenty of moisturizing cream, especially if you feel itchy over your bump and under your breasts. Try a body oil if the problem persists.

261 Hair

Sometimes the hair changes texture, becoming beautiful and shiny, or lank and lifeless.

Towards the end of pregnancy, most women's hair is oilier than before. The rate of hair loss is reduced, and hair growth is more vigorous. It rarely continues this way and most women lose hair for up to 18 months after giving birth. Your hair may become quite thin, but it will recover later on. Body hair will become more noticeable, especially if your body hair is darkened by pregnancy. Sometimes these changes are permanent.

262 Teeth

It is an old wives' tale that the baby steals calcium from your teeth, but the high levels of progesterone in your blood can make the gums soft and spongy, and this certainly makes infection more likely. Massaging of gums and regular brushing of teeth is essential.

263 Spider veins

These are broken blood vessels, often appearing on the cheeks, which are especially noticeable if you are fair. They will disappear soon after the baby is born.

264 Posture

Now, more than ever, avoid waddling like a duck. Lift your feet and don't shuffle.

265 Feet

Whenever you can, go about barefoot. Because of increased perspiration, tights will be uncomfortable in summer. In any event, make sure they are big and stretchy enough not to be constricting when they are pulled over the bump. Low-slung tights are possible, but not very comfortable. Avoid garters, stockings and knee-high socks: these, too, can constrict.

Low-heeled shoes of soft leather are best for winter, canvas shoes for summer. High heels may make correct posture difficult, causing both foot and back-ache, and they will be agony if your feet swell.

266 Father-to-be

With him now beginning to sense the baby's reality, if not regard her as actually real, it can be a good time for both of you, one of closeness and togetherness; but see 279.

267 Working mother

See 88. As the mid-point of pregnancy approaches, you may again be considering whether to become a full-time mother, or to continue in your job after the baby is born.

To help you make up your mind, it is worth taking certain facts into account. You might regard divorce as something that may happen to someone else, but there is, in fact, not far short of a 50 per cent chance that it will happen to you. Every woman is likely to be a widow for eight to ten years, and to lose her parenting role halfway through her life. Without education and employment skills, you could be high and dry.

It sounds depressing; it is depressing if you look at it this way. There is another way.

Your life is being re-structured. You do not have to keep working, or to stay in your present job. Many women take the opportunity offered by a period of full-time motherhood to re-think their careers. Once the children are at school, you can re-train, or re-educate yourself. You are entering a new phase in your life. Enjoy it. Life will still be there after the babies have grown. It is one of the positive aspects to being a woman today that women can, and do, change the course of their lives more than once. While those in continuous employment stick to the treadmill, women who take a break to have children often return with a new enthusiasm, more confident in their abilities, more sure of what they want.

268 Danger signs

In the second half of pregnancy, there are symptoms which require your immediate action: They are covered here, and in 269-278.

Bleeding is always a dangerous sign in pregnancy; in the second half it may indicate an incompetent cervix; see 247. You may miscarry without hospital care.

Late in pregnancy – from about six months – bleeding may also indicate that the placenta is becoming detached. This occurs because the lower part of the uterus grows and stretches in preparation for labour. But, unlike the uterus, the placenta does not stretch, so when the uterus begins to open out in preparation for birth, part of the placenta, failing to stretch, is torn away from the uterine wall. The danger for you, and the baby, is that as the placenta rips away blood vessels are broken, causing heavy bleeding and depleting the baby's oxygen supply.

Detachment, however, is rare, and occurs most commonly when the placenta is attached near the bottom of the uterus – the condition known as *placenta pravea*, which causes particularly heavy bleeding. But detachment can occur even when attachment is high in the uterus (high blood pressure may, in such cases, be implicated as a cause).

Sometimes blood is retained within the womb: you will feel a great deal of pain and go into shock. Such continuous pain, and a feeling of deep unease is *not* the start of labour, and you must get help quickly.

If the baby is mature enough, an emergency Caesarian may be performed. If a scan shows the baby's heart rate is normal, and if the bleeding is not severe, you will probably get away with enforced rest in hospital until the baby is induced.

Slight, continuous bleeding with no other symptoms is probably due to cervical erosion. It is not dangerous, but get it checked.

269 Premature rupture of membranes

Rupture can occur prematurely – usually in the form of a small tear. You will be watched carefully, but the baby will probably not be induced. The tear can mend, and the sac will then refill with amniotic fluid. See also 321.

270 Eclampsia

This is one of the few diseases that occur only in pregnancy. It is also one of the best examples of how well preventive medicine can work.

In the past, eclampsia killed many pregnant women, it still does in some parts of the world. It develops during the second half of pregnancy, starting with a slow build-up known as pre-eclampsia: for symptoms, see 273. If untreated, these can progress to blurred vision, bad headaches, irritability and severe abdominal pain. If these are neglected, full eclampsia can develop: a frightening condition, with fits, convulsions, coma and even death. Full eclampsia can occur before, during, or shortly after childbirth.

Pre-eclampsia is actually fairly common. Surveys in Britain suggest some degree of pre-eclampsia in as many as five in every 100 pregnancies. If untreated, about one in 20 women with pre-eclampsia will develop full eclampsia.

It is, however, almost wholly preventable through sound antenatal care.

271 Causes of eclampsia

In the past, a poison, or toxin, was thought to be the culprit. This is now disproved, but the precise causes are still not fully understood.

272 Susceptible to pre-eclampsia?

Pre-eclampsia (and in the past eclampsia) is commoner in the U.S.A. and Europe than in many other parts of the world.

Pre-eclampsia particularly affects:

- Undernourished women.
- Women under 5 ft 2 in (1.57 m) tall.
- Women having their first babies.
- Women under 20.
- Women over 40.
- Women with diabetes.
- Women with kidney disease.
- Women who suffer from migraine.
- Women who have had pre-eclampsia in a previous pregnancy.
- Women who suffer from hypertension, or who have a predisposition to hypertension, including family history.
- Women who are anxious.
- Women who feel ambivalent about the sexual and womanly aspects of their bodies; see 296.

273 Symptoms

> **The main symptoms of pre-eclampsia are:**
>
> ● Generalized oedema. This is swelling, caused by water retention. Puffy wrists, ankles and fingers may be the first signs.
> ● Sudden weight gain. This can be rapid, even overnight. It is sensible to keep a weekly check of your weight. We all know we can 'feel fat' and that this does not necessarily show on the scale.
> ● Protein in the urine.
> ● High blood pressure.

However, before you get really worried, consider the following:

Mild oedema is related to a normal, and necessary, increase in body fluids in pregnancy. Some swelling of the ankles and wrists occurs in 75 per cent of all pregnant women. It is particularly common in the evening and should disappear after a night's rest. If your hands and face become puffy, or if puffiness persists for 24 hours or more, then you should see your doctor. It may not be pre-eclampsia, but it could be. For treatment of oedema, see 276.

Some women gain excessive amounts of weight in pregnancy without having pre-eclampsia, and some were overweight before pregnancy began. A *sudden* increase, rather than simply being overweight, is the symptom to watch for. Although it is not wise to be overweight in pregnancy, it does not increase the risk of pre-eclampsia. Protein in the urine can, incidentally, be caused by many conditions.

If you have had high blood pressure throughout pregnancy, or indeed if you suffered from it before becoming pregnant, it will not necessarily develop into pre-eclampsia. But you are at risk.

It is the rapid onset, and the combination of these symptoms developing over a period of days, which are the true danger signs of pre-eclampsia; so it makes sense to be alert to any obvious changes in how you feel or look.

274 Dangers

Pre-eclampsia can lead to eclampsia, but even if it does not go that far, it carries risks and needs careful management.

The dangers to the mother are kidney failure and chronic hypertension. To the baby, they are separation of the placenta from the uterine wall and inefficient placental function. This will lead to poor growth, resulting in a baby who is probably small for dates and quite sick at birth.

275 Treatment of pre-eclampsia

The most important factor is rest, usually hospital bed rest, though if the condition is mild you may be able to rest at home.

If you have other small children, this is impossible, and it will be necessary to find someone to look after your children until the symptoms subside.

If you are hospitalized, you will almost certainly be released once the symptoms subside.

In hospital your condition will be carefully monitored, with blood pressure controlled by diet and drugs.

As with all poorly understood diseases, it is probably worth following any advice on diet which may be offered, as long as the diet is sufficient in nutrients.

276 Treating oedema

● Put your feet up.
● Wear sensible shoes.
● Don't wear stockings with elasticated tops.
● Try wearing tights with some support, and get them on *before* you get out of bed.
● Drink plenty of fluids.

277 Psychological factors in pre-eclampsia

As with morning sickness (187), there is some evidence that pre-eclampsia is associated with ambivalence, not so much about having a baby, but about womanly and sexual aspects of one's body. Women suffering from pre-eclampsia are also more likely to have P.M.T., sexual problems, pain and cramp during intercourse, and to fail to reach orgasm. They may also report that sex was a taboo subject in childhood.

A picture emerges of women who do not feel at home in their bodies, and who cannot readily accept the changes that pregnancy brings. They may, however, simply be women who are more than usually anxious.

278 Antibiotics

If you are ill late in pregnancy, you must be especially careful which antibiotics you take. It is always foolish to take anything you have around the house or which has been prescibed for someone else.

Some antibiotics can affect the development of the baby's teeth, and of the nerves associated with hearing.

> **Particularly risky antibiotics at this stage include:**
>
> ● Streptomycin and closely related drugs: there is a 10 to 15 per cent chance that they might damage the nerves associated with hearing, resulting in a partially deaf child.
> ● Kanamycin and gentamicin may also cause loss of hearing, but the evidence against them is not as strong.
> ● Tetracyclines given in the last six months of pregnancy can cause abnormalities in the development of the baby's teeth.
> ● New antibiotics should be prescribed with extreme caution, preferably not at all.

279 Marital power

See 197. Often in a marriage, one partner has most of the power. She is kingpin. He is kingpin. Two people may have evolved a stable balance, but adding a third can alter that. Her tendency to mother men may have been a major strength in their relationship, a hidden form of power. As the baby begins to move and seems daily more and more real, she may begin to switch her mothering from man to baby. Faced with a sudden loss of support, he may feel it necessary to reassert his power. Equally, he may find her mothering aversive: she is now a real mother, and mothers are sexually taboo.

On the other hand, the sickness and uncertainty of the early months may make her feel she needs more support: a father-figure to tell her it will be all right. He may not want this change of role. Try to be aware of these developments.

Talking it out is the only answer, but sometimes we are unaware of the games we play. Standing aside and deliberately reappraising your relationship may pay dividends. With the closeness many couples feel in these middle months, and with the increased sexual enjoyment of each other, this is the time to explore changes. The advent of children often gives a woman a more central and important role in the marriage. She can insist her partner comes home to see the children, when before she may have felt unable to insist he came home for supper. There is now an excuse to get what she always wanted.

Individuals within a family are constantly developing and adjusting their images of each other. This is what keeps relationships alive, but it also means the relationship is potentially unstable, even before a new member joins the family.

280 Looking forward

A woman's direct involvement with a child, which is, after all, exclusive throughout pregnancy, gives her a considerable power, but this can be a double-edged sword.

The mother's central role means that she emerges as the 'expert', while the father becomes her 'assistant'. She does all the essential and necessary parenting, while he helps with bits and pieces like bathing the baby and taking the children to the park. She will say to her friends, or her mother: "He helps, but can't really be trusted; he doesn't fully understand."

Once this pattern is established, it is difficult to reverse the roles. You may not feel it could happen to you, but it is in the middle months of pregnancy that many women make the beds on which they may later wish they did not have to lie. This debate is continued at 309, but you may find it interesting now to reflect on the fact that even if a man does genuinely feel he can share parenthood, society generally feels otherwise. In both the U.S.A. and the U.K., men have been refused social security payments which would have enabled them to look after their children after the death of their wives, or after they have left the family. In Britain, even poor-quality mothering is thought preferable to institutional care.

281 Antenatal care

Once the first antenatal visit has taken place (209), care takes on a typical pattern of monthly visits until six months, and fortnightly visits in months seven and eight. From then on, a weekly check is made until the baby is born.

At each visit, you will be weighed, have your blood pressure taken and receive a pelvic examination. You will give a urine sample, but a blood sample will not normally be taken at each visit, unless you are being specially monitored, nor is it likely that any further internal examinations will be made until the later stages of the pregnancy.

282 Faintness

Many of us have felt faint from time to time, especially when we get up rather too quickly, and this problem can be increased by pregnancy. The extra demand for blood by the uterus and foetus is the cause. It is worse when you keep still, so keep moving, even if only by tapping your toes. Get up carefully first thing in the morning, or after you have been sitting in one position for a while. If you do feel dizzy, sit down before you fall down. Breathe deeply for a few minutes, lowering your head towards your knees.

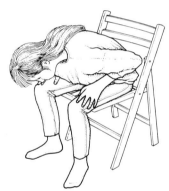

283 Flatulence and heartburn

As your baby gets bigger, the flatulence of early pregnancy may return. The movement of the gut is sluggish; and there is not enough room for wind to remain in the digestive system.

Heartburn is nothing to do with the heart (even if it does feel like a heart-attack), it is just another variety of indigestion. It occurs because of a tendency for the stomach contents to be forced back into the oesophagus (the tube connecting the mouth to the stomach). It increases towards the end of pregnancy because of the increased pressure of the uterus on the gut. Peppermint water may help, so may hot drinks. Avoid foods which cause flatulence – onions, beans, cucumber, fried foods, carbonated drinks – especially late at night. Little and often is the message, and keep drinking milk. If the heartburn becomes really painful, ask your doctor to recommend an antacid.

284 Oedema

Mild swellings of the ankles, feet, fingers or wrists can be expected – it happens because the body retains fluids. Rest is all the treatment you need for mild oedema; serious oedema always needs medical attention. Watching your weight gain may help. See 276 for treatment.

285 Rashes

Rashes may develop because you are overweight and sweat excessively, but sometimes there is no obvious reason. Calamine lotion is the best treatment, but check with your doctor that the rash is nothing serious. Bathing each morning and night may ease the problem.

286 Small for dates

If the placenta is not working efficiently, your baby will lack nutrition and oxygen. This can happen for various reasons, such as pre-eclampsia (270-275) or partial detachment (268) of the placenta. The outcome is usually a small-for-dates-baby, or, in extreme cases, the death of the baby in the womb. If the baby is thought to be at risk, a Caesarian section will be considered. In such cases, the health and safety of the baby are finely balanced during the last weeks of pregnancy. A premature, sick baby may be at greater risk than one which stays within the womb, even when conditions are less than ideal. Tests for placental function will be used in making this decision; see 240.

287 Taking care

All that extra blood being pumped around your body – there is 50 per cent more than there used to be – makes you look fit and well. But it is extra work for the lungs: another reason not to smoke.

Lungs at work need fresh air and exercise. A brisk walk every day will help them to cope with the extra workload.

Towards the end of the third trimester, when the baby is beginning to press against your diaphragm, you may begin to feel uncomfortably short of breath, particularly if you are expecting twins, carrying much fluid, or a big baby. You may need to take deep breaths, but be careful not to overdo it. Breathing too deeply for too long can make you feel dizzy.

Correct posture

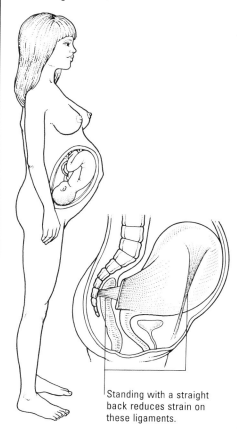

Standing with a straight back reduces strain on these ligaments.

If this happens, but you still need to breathe deeply, try this trick. Take a breath, put yout hand over your mouth, breathe out, and then in again. Remove the hand and start again. It works because you feel dizzy if you take in too much oxygen, and breathing in the air you have just expelled cuts the oxygen in the second breath. This is a useful technique to remember if you use breathing exercises during the birth, when the problem can arise again.

Standing or sitting up straight can also help you breathe more easily. You might even find it easier to sleep in a semi-vertical position. Experiment with cushions and pillows.

All that blood also puts pressure on the kidneys. They cope by working harder, filtering more efficiently, but also rather indiscriminately. They do not know which is waste and which is goodness. Vitamin C, being water soluble, is easily lost. Find extra sources in elderberries, fresh oregano, paprika, parsley, rose hips, blackcurrants, watercress, oranges and lemons. Folic acid is also lost, along with other minerals and trace elements. A

mineral and vitamin supplement is useful after the third month.

A well-balanced diet is now more important than at any other time, for you, and the baby.

Make sure that you take extra iron, with folic acid to help absorbtion. Explore alternative natural sources (see below) if you find iron pills upset you. You may be able to take fewer iron pills if your diet is already high in iron. Ask your doctor's advice or speak to the nutritionist at the hospital.

You will find iron in spinach, parsley, strawberry leaves (make them into tea), watercress and most green vegetables; apricots are another source. Meat, especially kidney and liver, contains a rich supply.

Calcium is needed for your baby's bones and teeth. Milk is the best source, together with milk products, such as cheese and yoghurt, but calcium can also be found in camomile, chives, dandelion root, nettles and sorrel.

As your stomach sticks out in front, your posture inevitably changes. Watch that you do not slouch or arch your back too much, it is easy to do and causes backache. Backache is a common enough problem once the baby grows, and sound posture now will minimize it.

Stand in front of a long mirror and make an honest assessment of how you are standing.

You should have your shoulders and knees relaxed. Never let them tense up; if you do, you will find that your whole posture is wrong. If your knees are relaxed (not sagging, just relaxed) your weight will automatically move on to the balls of your feet, rather than your heels. Get the feet and knees right, and your bump will fall into line. Be careful not to lean back. It is easily done, almost automatic, when you carry a weight out in front. Just watch what people do when they carry boxes out of the supermarket – this is a prime cause of backache.

The best way to maintain correct posture is to think of yourself as tall and stately, as a ship in full sail. Think of yourself as fat, and embarrassed about being fat, and you will automatically adopt the wrong position.

As you walk, keep your shoulders relaxed, weight evenly distributed; flow along, rather than shuffle. Lightness is the key, do not plant yourself with each step, nor drag yourself upstairs. Keep a lightness and a rhythm to your step. Feel good, and you will look good. See also 294.

A human baby is large, a human pelvis relativly small. How to get that big head out of a small hole is, essentially, an engineering problem. The solution is for the pelvis to open. The fibrous tissue surounding the joints softens, making the joints less rigid and more flexible.

Sometimes, the hormones that cause this softening are passed on to the baby. It hardly affects boys, but girls can have loose, clicking hips. It is the sacro-iliac joint of the lower back plus the joints of the pubic bone at the front which are mainly affected.

The loosening of your hips also alters the way that you walk, causing strange aches and pains from time to time.

Don't get over tired. If you are not sleeping well, try to go to bed early. Put your feet up whenever you can. Take a 15-minute recharge when you get in from work and in your lunch break. Try to relax completely, even if it is for a short period. See the relaxation technique described at 303. If you can rest for an hour or so at lunch time, or in the afternoon, that is ideal, but even ten minutes of total relaxation is worthwhile.

Because resistance is lowered in pregnancy, make and keep dental appointments throughout, and during the year after the baby is born.

288 Questions book

If something bothers you, or if you suddenly feel you are unsure about something, write it down in a notebook. This not only helps you remember to ask at your next antenatal visit, but forces you to define the problem clearly. Doctors are human – and busy – and respond best to helpfully expressed questions.

289 Complications

About 20 per cent of women have some complication during pregnancy. Many are minor, a few are serious; that is why it is important to keep all antenatal appointments. The simple tests performed will alert medical staff to potential problems.

290 Kick chart

A constructive way to monitor your baby's

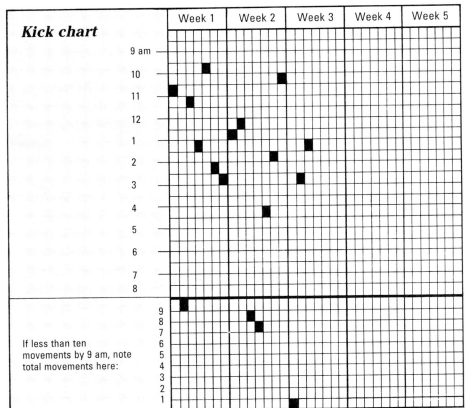

Kick chart

	Week 1	Week 2	Week 3	Week 4	Week 5

If less than ten movements by 9 am, note total movements here:

well-being – because it helps you to know her habits – is to record movement day by day. In the early months, at least, there will be somersaulting, arm-swinging, head-turning and leg-kicking, even hiccuping – so 'kick' is perhaps not the best description.

You will soon recognize your baby's habits. Many women find that their babies are awake when they rest in the evening; others when they bathe in the morning. Whenever it is, it is best to pick this time to start your daily observations.

Use squared paper: each square should represent half an hour. Starting at the same time each day, record the tenth movement the baby makes. Shade that square. You should find that the tenth movement is in the same square (give or take one or two) almost every day. As you approach labour, foetal movement may be reduced and the tenth movement may slip gradually into later and later squares.

If you feel no movements in a period of 12 hours, ring the hospital. The baby is almost certainly all right, but it is better to be safe than sorry. Nine times out of ten, there is no problem. But the baby might just be in distress.

If you feel that movements are reduced, try seeing how she responds to loud noises – for example a radio suddenly turned up to full volume, then down again. If the response is weak, it could be that she is short of oxygen. The hospital will do further tests.

Remember that babies do sleep. She will not 'kick' all the time. If you move, you rock her, and a rocked baby tends to sleep. In the last weeks, the baby will drop: the head becomes engaged and movement becomes much more resticted. She will often sleep for long periods.

291 Classes

These are usually attended during the last three months. There are normally several options, ranging from the expensive and fashionable through more reasonably priced courses run by organizations such as the British National Childbirth Trust, to discussion groups (often advertised in doctors' surgeries) and, indeed, classes run by the maternity departments of hospitals.

Consider also the possibility of learning relaxation and massage technique from a specialist group. The Alexander Technique is used by some people to prepare for birth, so is yoga and Shiatsu. Such classes

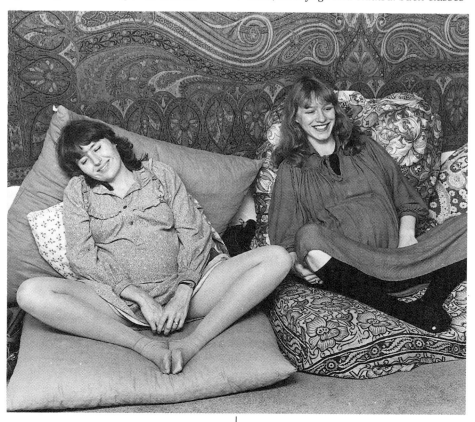

are often booked well in advance. Even if you opt for mainly private sessions, you may find the experience brings you together with similar couples who are learning from scratch.

There are classes about having a baby, *and also* on parentcraft, aimed at first-time mothers; these are often run by maternity hospitals.

If you intend to breast feed, you may like to contact a local breast-feeding support group. Ask your doctor.

292 Baby clothes

Once the baby starts too move, many mothers-to-be find their eyes turning towards the racks of baby clothes. Six months is a sensible enough time to start collecting. It makes the baby seem more real. It does not *have* to make you excited,

but it may. Baby clothes are a matter of taste, and self-indulgence. No one needs to pay a fortune for a baby suit, but many do because it gives them pleasure.

Winter babies obviously need more clothes than summer babies, who wear fewer, and those they have can be washed and dried more easily. Whether or not you opt for traditional or disposable nappies is to some extent a matter of lifestyle. The traditional ones do have some advantages, especially for night-time use.

293 Lifting

Because the ligaments of the back are softened during pregnancy, heavy lifting must be avoided. When you must lift, squat with your feet planted apart, lift the load close to your body, then stand. Use your legs to push, don't pull with your back. As you stand, your back must be

Clothes and equipment: first thoughts

Most modern babies wear stretch suits. You will need at least three. They are warm and cosy, easy to wash and require no ironing. The disadvantage? They don't provide loose material for the baby to touch and feel. An old-fashioned baby's 'dress' can be held in the hand and pulled over the face.

A compromise is to buy a couple of nightgowns. These usually fit new-born babies better than stretch suits, make nappy changing easier, and can be a source of stimulation in the second month.

Three cotton vests and three cardigans complete the basic summer wardrobe.

Winter babies will need warmer suits, leggings, mittens, hats and boots. Remember, there is a great deal of heat loss through the head, and a bonnet may be necessary even for spring and autumn babies if you live in a temperate, or in a cold climate.

Friends and relatives will surely give the baby presents, most of them first-size clothes. There is probably little point in expanding upon this basic wardrobe until after the birth.

Old-fashioned sprung prams look so comfortable, but they do not fit into many people's lives today.

At three months, a baby can be transferred to a push-chair for most outings, so few people get full use from a pram, and it is an expensive item. A carry cot on wheels, or a small, second-hand pram will probably be much more practical. Make sure both the wheels and the pram body can fit into the car. Check brakes and folding mechanism.

If you intend putting the baby out in the garden to sleep, buy a cat net to fit over pram, carry cot or Moses basket. Cats like to be comfortable, and lying on top of your baby is likely to be just that.

The fold-up stroller or 'buggy' has become more or less standard equipment. Well worth considering is the type with a removable seat. In its place you can attach to the frame a carrycot unit which converts the stroller to a pram, and which is more compact, and easier to stow in a car than a pram.

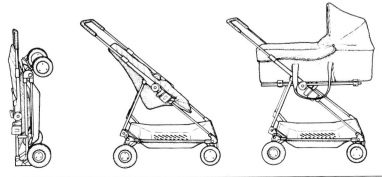

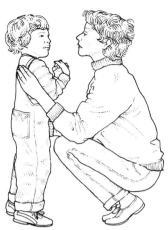

kept straight. Remember, toddlers are heavy: you should use this squatting technique whenever you pick one up.

294 Back pain

Posture changes, joints and ligaments loosen, and the weight up front can cause all sorts of aches and pains. Most of these can be overcome by good posture (287) and exercise, but some pains persist even when you walk tall, rest on the balls of your feet and concentrate on floating rather than shuffling along.

Low backache in late pregnancy is one such pain. This you can blame on the baby. Towards the end of pregnancy most babies come to rest head-down and bottom-over to your left (40 per cent) or right (25 per cent). About 13 per cent of babies come to rest head-down and facing slightly forward. Three per cent rest slightly left, 10 per cent slightly right. In this position, the baby's head presses against the base of the spine and can cause low back pain, especially when you lie or sit. You will get relief from kneeling on all fours and arching the back, or resting stomach-down on a pile of cushions.

Finding the most comfortable sleeping position can be difficult. I used to find it best to lie on my left side with my right knee tucked up and over my left leg. Soft cushions supporting the lower part of my stomach also helped.

Upper backache happens when you try constantly to 'lead off' with your bump; see 287. The best way to avoid this is to be conscious that you are doing so, and to roll forward on to the balls of your feet whenever you feel a twinge in the back.

Backache and the baby's position

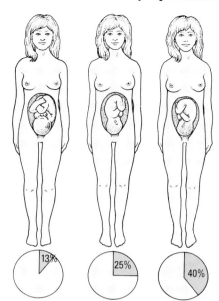

Rolling the shoulders backwards and forwards 20 times whenever you think about it will also help.

295 Miscellaneous aches and pains

Tingling and numbness in the hands is known as the carpal tunnel syndrome. It is caused by the pressures produced by the slight swelling of the hands and wrists and is most likely to happen first thing in the morning, because water builds up overnight. Stretching upwards, spreading the fingers and rolling the shoulders can help relieve the numbness.

Pain under the ribs is common. It is due to the large size of the baby and your small size. After 30 weeks, the fit is tight. A helpful exercise to relieve this is to hold your arms out to the side at shoulder height. Pass your left arm behind your head, reaching out along the right arm as far as you can. Then retreat back in little steps along the arm and across the shoulders.

Starting again, reach across the back to the back bone, and then down as far as you can. Push the elbow with your free hand. The effect is to lift the diaphragm off the uterus and the baby.

Pain in the groin is also common, and is caused by the softening of the pelvic joints described in 287. Avoid standing in one position for long periods, or standing at all if the pain is bad. The bottom exercises on page 39 will help.

Cramp, especially leg cramp, is

Relief from back pain

Try these as and when the problem occurs. It is worth experimenting with all of them to discover which helps you most.

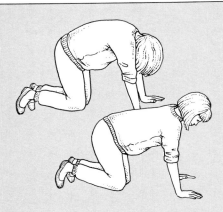

Right, arching and hollowing the back alternately a dozen times.

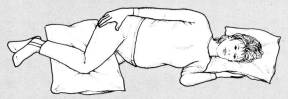

Above and **left**, lying with pillow or cushion support.

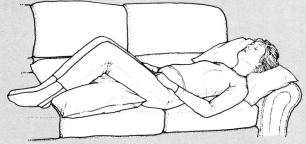

Below, using counter-pressure to ease cramp.

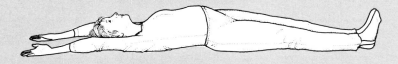

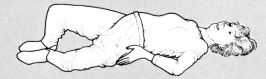

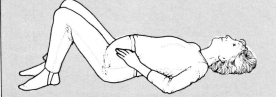

Left, pelvic roll: Begin by lying as shown below left. Relax. Then lift pelvis as shown above left. Repeat eight times to the left, eight to the right; then do four to each side; then two, repeating this four times; finally do one to each side, repeating eight times.

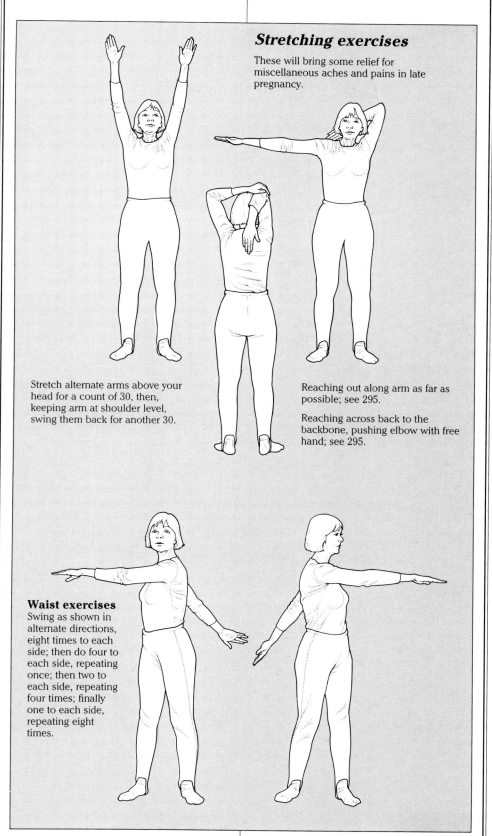

Stretching exercises

These will bring some relief for miscellaneous aches and pains in late pregnancy.

Stretch alternate arms above your head for a count of 30, then, keeping arm at shoulder level, swing them back for another 30.

Reaching out along arm as far as possible; see 295.

Reaching across back to the backbone, pushing elbow with free hand; see 295.

Waist exercises
Swing as shown in alternate directions, eight times to each side; then do four to each side, repeating once; then two to each side, repeating four times; finally one to each side, repeating eight times.

commonplace, especially at night. Try eating something salty before you go to bed. But if cramp persists, check that you have enough calcium in your diet. Adjust your diet (287) or try calcium tablets. Try to avoid curling your toes, and do some simple exercises before going to bed: lie on your back, knees pushed hard into the floor and push with the soles of your feet against a wall or solid object. This also helps relieve an attack of cramp. You can even do these exercises in bed: ask your partner to push against your foot and down on your knee at the same time.

Using a duvet or loosening the bedclothes can sometimes reduce cramp. It is also influenced by blood flow to the feet and legs. You can keep the blood flowing if you write your name with your foot, or circle each foot to the right ten times, then to the left ten times.

296 Your emotions: can they affect the baby?

If you are always tense, your whole body is affected. Your breathing changes, your level of adrenalin alters, and the fine tuning of your hormonal output can be disrupted. This can, of course, influence the baby's supply of oxygen and nutrients. But can your anxiety be passed on to the baby? Can you make her nervous?

Some people believe you can, and they could be right. Emotions are not just states of mind, they are states of body as well. It has been shown in animals that anxious mothers have offspring which grow up behaving differently from those of calmer mothers. But should you really bother about this? How good is the evidence?

At the very least, it gives food for thought. Women who feel positive about their babies have better births and their offspring have fewer mental and physical problems, but there are many reasons why this could be so. Groups of well-adjusted women have been shown to cope with most stressful experiences better than women who are anxious. This is probably as true for dental visits, or pap smears, as it is for giving birth.

Furthermore, the sample group of badly adjusted women in the experiment above almost certainly contained some with real mental problems, ones that preceded pregnancy, and continued beyond it. It probably also included women with problems such as pre-eclampsia and severe vomiting.

The children may have problems because they have disturbed mothers after, rather than before, birth, or because of poor conditions in the womb.

Nevertheless it will help to think as positively as you can.

297 Action of hormones

Progesterone is produced by the ovaries in early pregnancy, and by the placenta after 14 weeks. It relaxes smooth involuntary muscles, that is, all the muscles of the internal organs including the stomach and uterus. This allows the uterus to grow and stretch and allows more blood to be pumped around the body. We have seen the effects that this has on various bodily functions in 287.

Oestrogen is also produced by the ovaries, and later by the placenta. This aids the growth of the baby and placenta, as well as the development of the breasts preparing them for lactation. Oestrogen measurement is used to assess the health of the foetus and the functioning of the placenta.

HPL is another hormone produced by the placenta, (and is also used to check placental functioning). It is thought that the foetus uses it to signal its nutritional needs.

Prolactin is released by the pituitary gland, situated in the brain just above the roof of the mouth. The level of prolactin is high in early pregnancy and at birth. It falls after birth to a low resting level, but rises again every time the baby feeds.

Oxytocin, also produced by the pituitary, stimulates contractions, initiates the flow of breast milk and is released at orgasm: a confusing set of functions – no wonder mothering and loving get confused at times.

Once you have learned how the release of oxytocin makes you feel, you may experience something akin to sexual orgasm when giving birth, but I doubt this happens with a first child. You may also find (as I still do) that you sometimes feel something akin to milk let down (without the milk) long after you have stopped feeding babies; see also 468.

298 24 weeks

The top of your womb has risen to just above the navel. The baby is still growing, but the rate of growth is beginning to slow.

If you could see her inside the uterus, you would notice that she is beginning to

Hormone levels in pregnancy

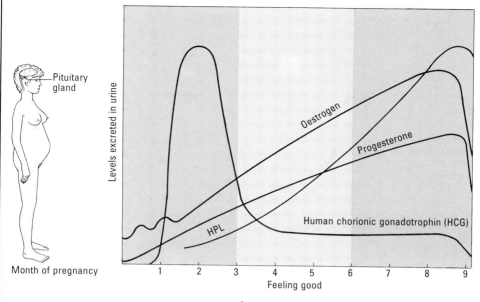

Pituitary gland

Levels excreted in urine

Oestrogen

Progesterone

HPL

Human chorionic gonadotrophin (HCG)

Month of pregnancy

1 2 3 4 5 6 7 8 9

Feeling good

look to the right. She is small, but in proportion, about 10 in (25 cm) long. She is active; you will definitely notice her movements. You may find that she is responsive to your voice or to music. What does she look like? Not quite as pretty as at birth: still covered in hair and vernix. Her skin is rather wrinkled; she is thin, scrawny. The features of her face look prominent because the fat pads which round out a face have not yet developed. In the next months she will become plumper and prettier.

Perhaps the major new development is that she would now have a small chance of survival if she were to be born. Her breathing is not yet stable enough to guarantee survival, and there is danger of brain haemorrage, but some babies have thrived when born at this stage.

299 28 weeks

Her birth from now on has to be registered, and death would be regarded as a still birth, not a miscarriage.

If born now, she has a 60-70 per cent chance of survival, even higher in a specialist unit.

Because she now almost fills her allotted space inside you, her movements are less free. Now she kicks; before she threw her whole body around. As she kicks, you can probably pick out parts of her body: a foot, her bottom, an arm.

Foot and knee movements are jerky, whole body movements smoother. It is now possible for your partner and children to watch and feel the baby move. They can even feel the movements under their hands if they touch your abdomen.

Developing foetus: 24-28 weeks

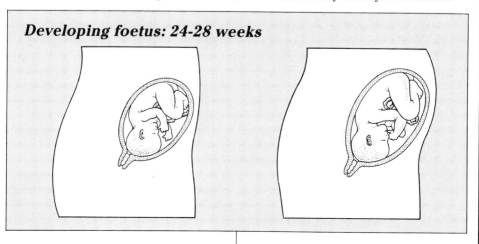

Pregnancy
The Third Trimester (Last Three Months)

300 Had enough?

Another month of pregnancy would be easy to bear, but thereafter, quite frankly, most women get weary of it. Uncomfortably large, stuck in maternity clothes, ready (but not ready), we wait. And wait: those last weeks can drag. It is an odd feeling to be living your life in the future. She could be born in two months, in one month, or tomorrow. By next week you could have a daughter. Your body does not let you forget what is about to happen.

You may now experience an odd fluttering feeling in the vagina. This is the baby lifting her head and lowering it against the pelvic floor muscles. You will see her make the same movements when you put her down on her tummy after birth.

Although you are becoming tired of pregnancy and want to get it over, perversely you are now used to it, and may be reluctant to let it go for the great unknown. Anxiety returns: there really is no going back. Can you cope?

Feeling low and depressed is common in the last weeks of pregnancy, and it is easy for these anxieties to get out of hand when you are suffering from lack of sleep. You are carrying extra weight, everything is more effort, and this in itself can make you feel low, especially if plodding along is not normally in your nature.

Muscle awareness

Unless you know which muscles are tense, it is difficult to relax them; there are several complex sets of muscles within the body of which you may not be aware. You can discover them by imagining you are doing something which involves one of these complex set of muscles:

- Chewing a piece of tough meat.
- Smelling a foul smell.
- Sucking a lemon.
- Feeling with the tip of your tongue, a piece of silver paper on the filling of a tooth.
- Watching an aeroplane flying overhead.
- Making a snowball.
- Pulling on a rope in a tug-of-war.
- Washing your hands.
- Walking on pebbles.
- Walking barefoot on hot sand.
- Sinking into mud.

Each has a characteristic pattern of muscle tension. Be aware of those tensions, and relax them. Breathe deeply, and relax.

301 Sleep

You need plenty of sleep, but needing is not getting. The physical discomfort of being large is not, however, the only reason for your sleeplessness. As the baby grows, the influence of her metabolism on yours increases. Waste products from her system have to be excreted from yours, and when she says 'Feed me', you cannot say 'No, I am too tired.' Your system tries to close down for the night, but hers goes on making demands.

These may help:

- A warm, milky drink at bed-time will relax you and reduce heartburn.
- A hot bath, followed by a gentle massage, will do the same.
- If your bed is small, consider sleeping apart from your partner in the last weeks. If you are conscious of keeping him awake, or of the ease with which he sleeps, you may find it harder to fall asleep yourself. Having room to spread and change position can often be an advantage.
- Go to bed early and relax. Take a book, or watch a video, play gentle music. Breathe deeply, and flop.
- If you wake in the night, get up and do something. Clean the stove, wash the fridge. Polish or dust. Use the time, and it will pass.

302 Massage

The massage sequences illustrated are especially designed for late pregnancy.

303 Relaxation sequence

If you cannot sleep at night, and even if you can, learn to relax by day. See the panel.

304 Sex

Even pregnant missionaries probably adapted their love-making late in pregnancy. Side by side, rear entry, or woman on top, are much more comfortable than the full-frontal 'missionary' position – not to mention more satisfying – in the later months.

All these positions give the woman more control over depth of penetration. Since she is the one likely to feel pain, or to be anxious about it, this can help her to relax and enjoy herself. Well-exercised pelvic floor and buttock muscles can be used to control how far the man enters, but it is much easier to suck in and push out if he enters from the rear. While on top, you do not have to work so hard either. Another advantage of the woman-on-top position, especially as birth draws near, is that your partner can prepare your breasts for

Relaxation sequence

- Arrange yourself comfortably in a warm place.
- Takle a deep breath, hold it, then slowly let it all out. Breathe in for a count of two, three, four, five; and out: two three, four.
- Repeat. Repeat.
- Now think of a beach, the sun and the waves. Watch the seagulls soaring on currents of air. Up and up. Watch the sailing boat coming slowly towards you, slowly, slowly.
- If a worry tries to intrude on this scene, say 'No'; stop yourself thinking about it by visualizing the seaside scene again.
- Become aware of how you are breathing. Think about it. Promote your breathing rhythm to the centre of your existence: make it your world.
- Say some soothing words to yourself: peace, calm, tranquility. Keep breathing rhythmically, and repeat the words.
- Now check that each muscle in your body is relaxed, starting with your scalp and working down to your feet.

You may find that tensing and relaxing muscles helps you to be sure of total relaxation. Start with your toes. Tense them, and relax. Make them feel heavy and warm. Then move to your feet: tense and relax; then ankles, calves, knees, thighs. You may find this easier if you roll your knees outwards, relaxing your bottom and pressing your back into the floor. Check the muscles in your bottom, one side at a time, release your abdomen and chest. Feel the relaxation flowing upwards and down each arm. Now consider your neck and face; make absolutely sure that your jaw, tongue and the area around your eyes is relaxed.

- As you relax, your breathing should automatically slow down. Slow it down deliberately if it does not.
- Lie like this for 20 minutes.
  Doing this twice a day can make up for lost sleep.

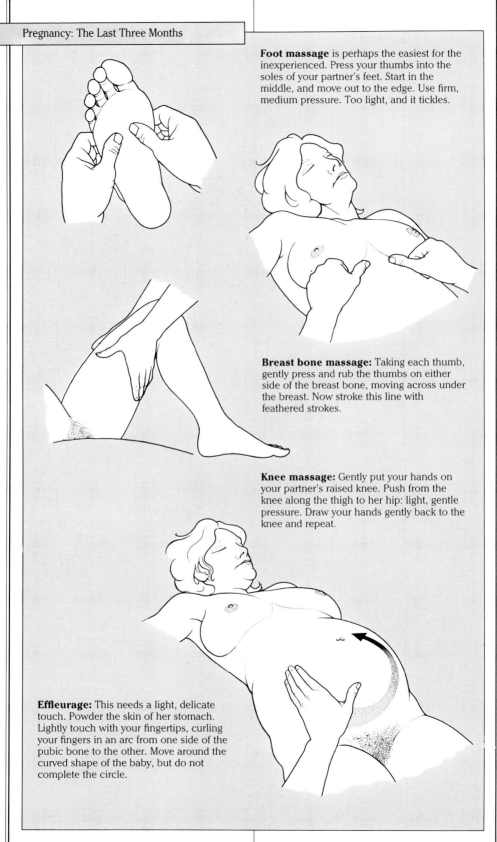

Foot massage is perhaps the easiest for the inexperienced. Press your thumbs into the soles of your partner's feet. Start in the middle, and move out to the edge. Use firm, medium pressure. Too light, and it tickles.

Breast bone massage: Taking each thumb, gently press and rub the thumbs on either side of the breast bone, moving across under the breast. Now stroke this line with feathered strokes.

Knee massage: Gently put your hands on your partner's raised knee. Push from the knee along the thigh to her hip: light, gentle pressure. Draw your hands gently back to the knee and repeat.

Effleurage: This needs a light, delicate touch. Powder the skin of her stomach. Lightly touch with your fingertips, curling your fingers in an arc from one side of the pubic bone to the other. Move around the curved shape of the baby, but do not complete the circle.

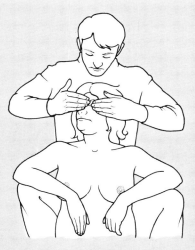

Brow massage: Let her lie between your legs, head resting on your shoulder and gently stroke her brow. Use your finger tips and a light feather touch. Stroke the eyelids and the hair line.

Gentle back massage: Turn over. Mark a line about one inch from the back bone on either side, paying special attention to the points nearest the shoulders. Gently apply pressure in different spots down to the small of the back, using the thumbs. Then, with feather strokes, touch this line. Move out another two inches and repeat.

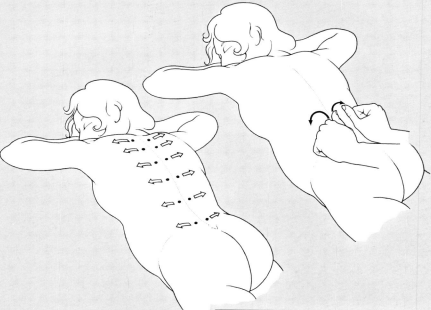

Stronger back massage: Knead the small of the back using a firmer pressure. Feel the base of the tail bone between the buttocks and press firmly with the heel of your hand. Make small circular kneading movements.

Touch relaxation
This is a combination of relaxation (303) and massage, and is especially good in the last stages of pregnancy. Start by getting yourself into a relaxed position, well propped up, with your arms and legs spread out. Now contract each muscle in turn as you did in 303. Get your partner to 'release' the tension by lightly touching each tightened muscle or group of muscles. Make sure his hands are warm.

feeding by gently sucking. Gentleness in this, as in all love-making, is the key.

By the end of pregnancy, some couples feel they do not want to make love. There is nothing odd about this. If you are tired, if it is painful, or if it makes you anxious, there is no point in trying to force it. Cuddling and caressing may be all you want or need. If this sometimes leads to a deeper sexual need for one or both of you, there is always masturbation or oral sex.

305 Sex and the baby

As you reach orgasm, your uterus begins to make small rhythmic contractions and these will continue for some time. The prostaglandins in your partner's semen have the same effect on your uterus. Could it bring on labour? Not unless you are ready. If, however, you have a history of premature births, you could be ready too soon. Ask advice.

306 Small contractions

It is normal to feel small contractions in the later stages of pregnancy. Indeed, they have been occurring throughout, but just as you did not feel the baby move until it had grown and filled the space in the womb, so it takes time to feel these movements known as Braxton Hicks contractions. They are probably beneficial: as the uterus contracts, it almost certainly squeezes extra uterine blood to the foetus.

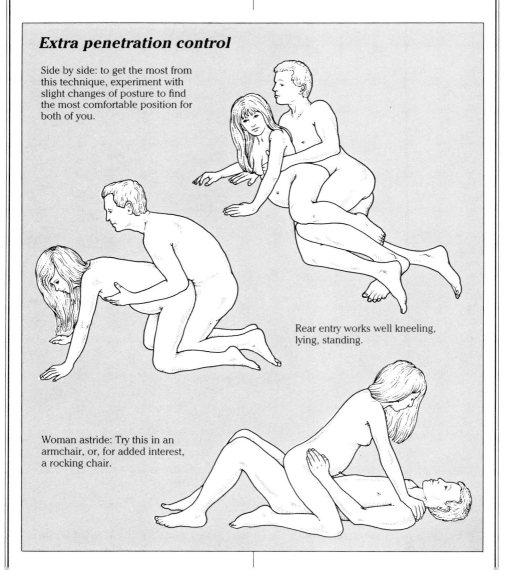

Extra penetration control

Side by side: to get the most from this technique, experiment with slight changes of posture to find the most comfortable position for both of you.

Rear entry works well kneeling, lying, standing.

Woman astride: Try this in an armchair, or, for added interest, a rocking chair.

307 More frequent checks

During the last months you will have to make antenatal visits at two-weekly, then at weekly, intervals. You will probably have at least one blood test. If you are rhesus negative, antibody tests will be carried out.

The doctor will monitor the position of the baby, and if she is presenting bottom-downwards (ie for a breech delivery) an attempt to turn her may be made at about 34 weeks.

308 Practicalities

If you are having the baby in hospital you will not have to stay there for long. If you come home soon after the birth, the community midwife – is in many countries, including the U.K. – legally obliged to visit you on several occasions during the first ten days. She will check your recovery, the baby's health, and will, in the early days at least, probably bath the baby for you. She will also be able to help you with any breast feeding problems and other worries.

In some areas, you can book into hospital for six hours, 24 hours or 48 hours. If you have other children, you may feel that just six hours in hospital makes the birth more of a family affair: you could be out of hospital before the rest of the family have time to miss you.

If there is a choice of hospital in your area, ask friends what they know of the birthing policies and facilities they offer. You could also ring the hospital to clear up any queries you may have.

309 Together

Learning parenthood is more difficult for a father than mother (280), and because learning is ultimately a voluntary activity, some men never learn. However, if a father does want to take an active role in his child's life, now is the easiest time to begin. Once he becomes involved in her life in the womb, and in birth, taking a role in the baby's development will follow naturally.

The golden rule for *both* partners is to be observant and involved in the other's needs. Sharing takes time, energy and hard work. Inter-dependence is never easy, especially if it is only just beginning. But it will be repaid a thousandfold, not just by the love of your child, but by the development of a deeper and more fulfilling friendship with your partner. The chance only comes perhaps twice in a lifetime.

There is no right way, no wrong way. With every new first child, parenthood must evolve naturally. Every family develops a unique identity, one that suits the character and mix of the individuals involved.

310 32 weeks

The baby is almost fully mature. She is practising breathing movements, and drinking large amounts of amniotic fluid; sometimes it gives her hiccups. The lungs may, however, still lack surfactant, the creamy fluid which prevents them from sticking together with the first breaths.

311 34 weeks

Almost ready for birth: about 17 in (42.5 cm) long, and about 5½ lb (2.5 kg) in weight. Her lungs are almost mature: if she were to be born now, she would have a 95 per cent chance of survival. In the last weeks, you will probably have felt that she is resting in one position: the feet pop out in the same place, the bottom on the same side. Her head may even be engaged in the pelvis in preparation for birth. For a first mother, 36 weeks is the most likely time for this to happen. It may be delayed for a week or two, but most women enter labour with the baby's head engaged. For .pasecond and subsequent births, the head may not become engaged until labour begins.

You will feel relief when the head does engage: pressure on the diaphragm is reduced, although pressure on the bladder may be increased; see also 346.

312 38 weeks

Your baby is now at full term. She is about 19 in (47.5 cm) long, and weighs about 7½ lb (3.4 kg). She looks good: plump, with blue eyes and, possibly, a mop of hair, though she may also be almost bald. The finger nails will be long enough to scratch you and the testes will have descended into the scrotum of a male baby.

313 Know the hospital

Make an appointment with your hospital to visit the labour wards and delivery rooms.

Developing foetus: 30-38 weeks

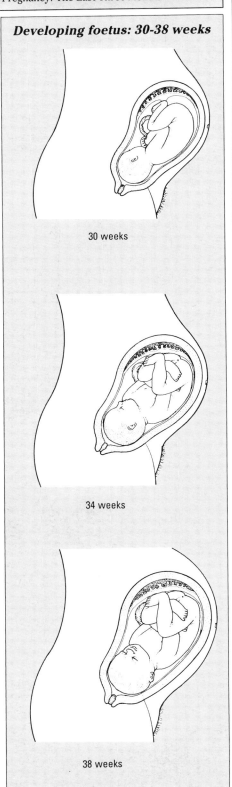

30 weeks

34 weeks

38 weeks

You need to know which door to use if you arrive at night, and where to park the car if you arrive at visiting time and find all the spaces full. These steps will make events simpler, less alien, as they unfold.

314 Labour pain

When you tighten your muscles, you automatically tend to catch your breath. When you relax, your breathing is also relaxed. Breathing techniques can help you both to relax and to stay in control during labour, which in turn can influence how much pain you feel. If you can expect less pain, you will probably feel less.

Pain is, in fact, difficult to understand. It is never simply an automatic response to tissue damage. Sometimes a person can break a leg and carry on running; some people are shot in battle without realizing it. If you imagine something will be painful, it usually turns out very painful indeed. See 365-367.

But be under no illusions: painless childbirth is a myth; childbirth with manageable pain a reality.

Natural childbirth is certainly not painless, but it does give you some means of coping with the pain, since the exhilaration of giving birth can counteract the negative aspects. Learning how to exercise and to use breathing techniques is immensely important.

315 Distraction

Distraction from pain is a difficult art. Try to choose a means of distraction which is at once mind-consuming and banal enough to be remembered at moments of stress. You could do worse than tap out the rhythmic line:

*There is a green-eyed yellow
statue to the north of Kathmandu.*

I chose it because I did not mind coming to hate the poem. The technique is to tap and sing, keeping the rhythm steady throughout the pain. You concentrate all your attention on doing this, watching your partner, doing it together. After the contraction subsides, you relax together until the next one comes. See also 369-370.

316 A little sister

Nine months is a long time for a child to

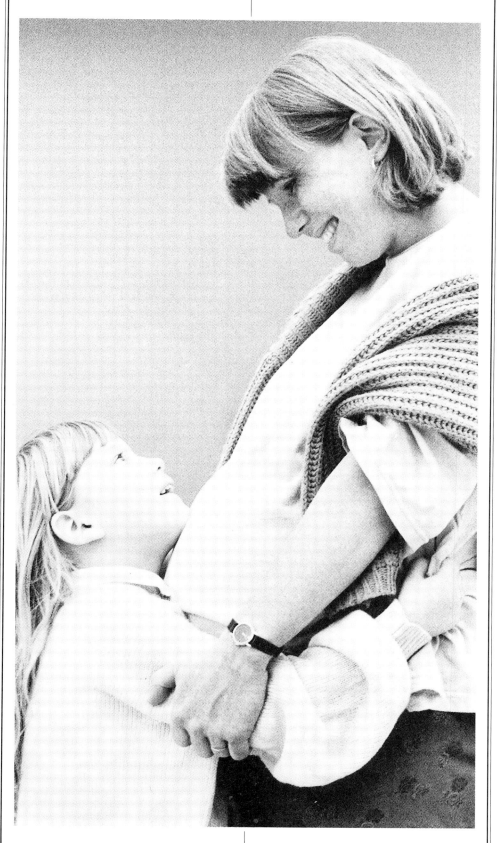

wait for the new arrival, and you may not want to break the news of your pregnancy to existing children in your family until some months have passed. But if everyone else is talking about the expected baby, they should be told too.

Time means little or nothing to young children, so try to find some marker that will make sense of the interlude before the birth: 'After all the leaves have fallen off the trees' or 'after we come home from holiday.'

Once the baby begins to move, a child may like to feel her kicking. Get out the snapshots of his baby years and some of his clothes if you still have them. As the birth approaches, prepare him for your hospital stay. Let him choose a present for the baby, and choose one for the baby to give him.

Involve him in preparing the baby's room. See also 506.

Some parents may want to consider allowing older children to watch the birth; of course, it will be necessary to contact the hospital in advance. Do examine your motives with total honesty, and discuss it openly with the children. You may want them to be there rather more than they wish to be present. They may find watching you in pain difficult and frightening. Once at the hospital it will be difficult for them to leave by themselves, and your husband may have to take them home when you most need his support.

317 Planning ahead

Just slipping out to the shops will be a major expedition after the baby is born. Fitting in the shopping between feeds is an art which also takes time to learn. If you have a freezer, you can prepare meals for a few weeks in advance, or buy them ready prepared. Consider doing a major non-perishable shop at least three weeks before the baby is due, and try to get on top of jobs such as cleaning the oven which will otherwise not get done for weeks.

318 Premature labour

There appears to be no reason for a normal pregnancy to end inpremature labour. Sometimes a woman will have two or three premature babies; sometimes just one.

Accidental early rupture of the membranes (269 and 321) can cause premature birth, so can multiple pregnancy, an excess of amniotic fluid or previous damage to the cervix. Occasionally, it will be brought on by shock.

If you think you are in labour, telephone the hospital, then lie down and rest while your husband fetches the car. If you have no car, call an ambulance. If you are under 30 weeks, you may be transferred to a hospital with special facilities for seriously premature babies.

The hospital will try to stop the labour and probably also give you steroids which help the baby's lungs to mature.

319 I can't wait

If you are overdue, there are ways in which you can speed things up:

• Castor oil. I don't recommend this but it *can* work. The old midwife's trick was to sit the mother in a hot bath and make her down half a cup of castor oil: unpleasant, and the effects upon your bowels can be dramatic. If it does not work, (and it will merely tip the scales) it can leave you feeling awful.
• Nipple stimulation is much pleasanter. Twist your nipples in your fingers. Douse your breasts in hot water, then stroke and massage them with warm oil. Best of all, get your partner to such them gently, since this releases oxytocin, the hormone that is involved in the birth process. Even if it does not work, this is an agreeable sensation with no unpleasant side-effects.
• Love-making works for the same reason. Orgasm releases oxytocin and starts contractions. Women are capable of multiple orgasms; just now, the more you can manage the better. Try to reach orgasm in any way you can: for each orgasm should initiate five to ten contractions. It is not necessary to have intercourse but the prostaglandins contained in semen, if this is released in the vagina, can help labour on its way; see 384.

None of these methods will work unless you are ready, and in any event, the hospital has more powerful means of inducing birth; see 384. In many hospitals, labour will automatically be induced if you go beyond ten to 14 days after the baby is due. There are sound reasons for this in most cases. The placenta does not always function efficiently so long beyond term, the baby is still growing, and birth could be difficult if she gets too big.

By 42 weeks, many women are only too pleased to get it over with and would drink whole bottles of caster oil, or readily accept induction. But if you have strong feelings against induction at 42 weeks, ask for a test of placental function. If the placenta is still working efficiently, it is safe to wait a few days.

320 Packing the bag

Have your bag packed at 36 weeks. The bag is really three bags: see box.

321 If the waters break now . . .

The phrase captures the essence of the problem rather better than 'rupturing the membranes'. Not all the waters are released, just the waters around the baby's head. Nor is it a flood: the baby is so big that the waters at this stage do not amount to much. For most women, labour is well under way before the waters break, but if you now start to leak, in a steady stream, or in a slightly faster rush, the membranes have ruptured.

I used to worry that I would not be able to tell the difference between the waters breaking and urinating. You will. It feels very different: much closer to the feeling of a heavy period starting, or the sensation of a tampon leaking. See also 361.

Another common worry is that the membranes will rupture in the supermarket or when you are out to dinner. I did hear once of someone whose waters broke on a train, but most women seem to be in bed or at home when it happens. Even if it should happen in public, you will probably be the only one who notices. Around term, labour usually follows quite soon after the waters break.

If you are more than 36 weeks pregnant, and labour does not now begin naturally, you will probably be given drugs to induce it. Don't try to induce it by love-making: the womb is now open to infection.

By 36 weeks, the baby's chances of survival are high, and the dangers of infection inside the womb are probably as great or greater than they are outside.

For labour, pack:

• One or two small, clean sponges for wiping your brow or sucking during contractions. You will not be allowed much fluid, and labour can last a long time.
• Massage cream and oil, to rub into your back and stomach.
• Talcum powder, a useful soothing agent.
• A sock with two tennis balls in it to ease back pain.
• Sweets or dextrose tablets to sustain energy.
• Chocolate bars, peanuts and biscuits to keep your partner going. It may be up to 12 hours before he can get anything to eat. You will not feel hungry during labour, he will. Make some sandwiches just before you leave home, and a flask of soup. You may be grateful for this after the baby is born.
• Lip salve for sore lips.
• A notebook or tape recorder for posterity.
• A camera and an ultra-fast film so you can take pictures without flash.
• Books, crosswords, cards, games. There can be ten minutes, or even half an hour, between contractions.
• A large-hand mirror to enable you to watch her head emerging.

For your stay you will need:

Nightdresses, dressing gown, slippers; a sanitary belt or pants.
• A wash bag with toothbrush, tooth paste, soap, two face cloths, creams and make-up. Also comb, hairbrush, shampoo and conditioner.
• You will need magazines, books, crosswords and perhaps a personal radio; pen, paper and envelopes.
• Hospitals have differing policies about baby clothes. They will tell you what to bring for the baby.

Finally the third bag, containing clothes for you and for the baby to go home in:

• A full set of baby clothes: vest, nappy, pants, stretch suit or nightie, cardigan. In winter you will need a bonnet and leggings; also a shawl or blanket in which to wrap her.
• Your clothes should be roomy. Don't be ambitious: you will probably still look at least six months pregnant. The morning after my daughter was born, I slipped next door to the shop to buy some tea. "Still about?" they said. No one noticed I had actually had the baby.

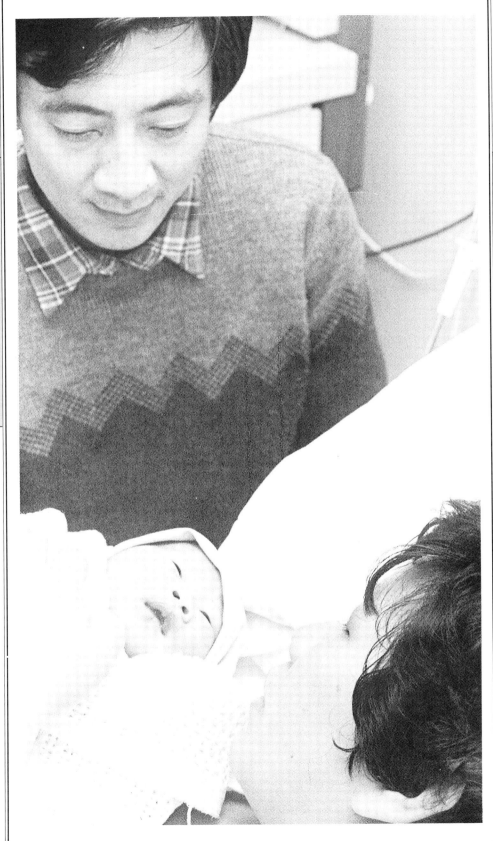

Birth

322-451

The Modern Birth

322 The day draws nearer

You can plan – but, of course, babies don't always arrive on the day they are due. You can expect your baby any time between the 38th and the 42nd week: today, tomorrow, this time next month. There is no perfect birth. What happens to you will not be 'right'; it will not be wrong either. It will be as it will be.

Don't imagine ecstasy and wonder when you find your baby in your arms. You may just feel tired and flat. Don't imagine you will cope efficiently, few do. Labour will take you by surprise; it will seem unbelievably long, and yet be over very soon.

It is birth, only birth. For all you have waited and looked forward to it, it is merely the means of getting the baby from inside your womb to the outside world. Learning to love her may take a few days longer. Birth is not the be-all and end-all, it is a passing phase. The point of your present condition is that you wanted a baby, to make a family, not to give birth. Sometimes, in your preparations for birth, it is easy to forget preparations for life. This is not just sophistry. Women who suffer from postnatal depression (almost two in every ten) often see a 'bad' birth as the focus of this depression. Looking beyond birth, thereby accepting it as it comes, could be the key to your future mental health.

323 Home birth: safety considerations

No analysis of perinatal mortality so far conducted supports the argument that all mothers should give birth in hospital.

Not a statement by a home birth fanatic, but by a British government minister in 1984.

In 1958, a survey carried out in Britain showed that perinatal mortality was almost twice as high in hospital as it was when birth took place at home. At that time, however, most births, except those with potential problems, first-time births and women in their fourth and subsequent labours, would have taken place at home. One would, therefore, expect the hospital mortality figures to have been the higher.

In 1970, when hospital birth was becoming popular among low-risk women, the perinatal mortality rate in British hospitals was 27.8 per 1,000 births. At the same time, it was 43 per 1,000 home births. Hospital appeared to be a safer place to give birth than home, but not twice as safe as it was in 1958.

In 1983, Britain and the U.S.A. both had higher rates of Caesarian section, induced labour and other obstetric intervention than almost any European country, but they did not have the lowest perinatal mortality rates. This honour rests with Holland and Sweden, whose rates are the lowest in the world. In Sweden virtually all babies are born in hospital, but in Holland 50 per cent are born at home.

324 Intervention

It is, perhaps, no coincidence that in Sweden and Holland midwives are in total charge of pregnancy and childbirth.

Doctors are trained to cure the sick, midwives to assist healthy women to give birth. The difference in their training and attitudes almost certainly influences the way women feel about giving birth: whether they consider it a natural process or an illness. It also influences how soon medical intervention (339) is considered.

325 In hospital . . .

- You may feel safer.
- You will meet other mothers.
- You have back-up facilities on call.
- You can be monitored.
- You can have an emergency Caesarian.
- Your labour can be speeded up.
- You can have epidural anaesthesia.
- You don't contemplate the washing up.
- You don't have your family telling you what to do.
- There is a special-care baby unit.

326 At home . . .

- You have family and friends around you.
- You are in a familiar place.
- Your family can share the birth.
- You do not have to leave older children.
- A single person will care for you.
- You will only hear one baby crying.
- There will be less medical intervention.
- Your baby can can stay with you at all times. (But this is not always unadulterated joy.)
- Your partner can stay with the baby too.
- No hospital infections.
- You will be less anxious, and probably give birth quicker.

327 Preparing for a home birth

- You will need a bed with a firm base to provide adequate counter-pressure when it comes to pushing. If your bed is soft, you could put a board under the mattress or perhaps consider using a large bean bag or a birthing stool instead. Consult your midwife before you buy. Not all midwives are happy about delivering in a squatting position. You will need to protect your bed, bag or stool from the amniotic fluid and blood which are by-products of birth.
- Make the bed up as usual, then put on the plastic sheet with an old sheet over the top. That way you can quickly strip off the damp sheet after the baby is born.
- Have other clean sheets to hand. If you intend to give birth on to the floor, you will need to spread one out. Or you could use newspapers. This may sound makeshift, but it is safe, and newspapers are especially practical for catching drips when you move between bed and bath.
- You will also need a spare clean nightdress, a sanitary pad and pants.
- Prepare the baby's bed and have a nappy and a nightdress or stretch suit ready.
- Prepare a table or clear a surface for the midwife's use.
- Move comfortable chairs into the birth room for the midwife and your partner.
- Clean the bath and be sure there is plenty of hot water for baths or showers.
- Wash well with antiseptic soap, paying particular attention to the vaginal area.

328 Birthing stools

These have been in use for many years. If you are contemplating a home birth, you may like to buy one. They look like small kidney-shaped tables and cost little more than a small coffee table. If this happens to appeal to your sense of humour, you could even use it as such between births.

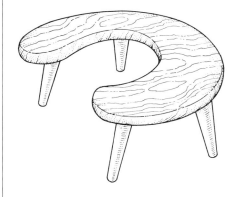

Equipment: the basics

- Wherever the newborn baby sleeps, your bedroom or her own, you will need the following:

- Moses basket: the almost universal choice for the first weeks: lighter and more portable than anything else.

- A crib or cot for when she outgrows the Moses basket.

- Sheets; blanket or duvet. Blankets are best for the first months because babies like to be wrapped up.

- Baby wipes and muslin nappies or squares, used for cleaning up the baby and to protect bedding and clothing if she is inclined to be sick.

- Nappies: see page 206.

- Baby clothes: see page 102.

- Plastic pants: the ones that tie are best for tiny bottoms.

- Changing mat: After your first baby you may well be able to change her on your knee, but few manage this with their first.

- Two or three new soft towels for drying the baby after baths.

- Natural sponge or soft face cloth.

- Cotton wool.

- Baby lotion, oil, petroleum jelly.

- Blunt-ended scissors for cutting nails.

- Cotton wool buds for wiping the creases of her ears and cleaning the edges of her nose.

- A bag or a box in which to keep everything together.
Feeding equipment if you are not planning to breast feed.

- Bouncing cradle chair.

- A baby bath is not essential. The kitchen sink makes an excellent substitute, provided the kitchen is warm enough. See 536.

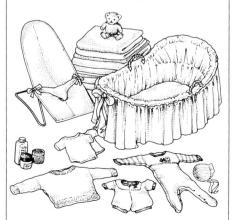

329 When home labour starts . . .

- Ring the midwife.
- Ring your partner.
- Contact whoever is to look after your children.
- Check that everything is ready.
- Have a hot drink, a snack and a warm bath.

330 Your choice

When I was giving birth I wanted my mother and my lover. I wanted loving familiar faces. Strangers and uniforms seemed grotesque accompaniments to the intimate rite of birth. We may be saving lives. . .but we may also be losing understanding of how life should be.
> – From Danae Brook's Nature Birth.

But home birth is not for everyone:

All that fulsome praise of Nature tends to infuriate the large minority whose babies, in Nature, would not have been a lot of fun getting out. Caesarian, drip induction, epidural anaesthetic and forceps victims have developed a tendency to complain bitterly about being 'cheated of the experience of birth'. . .like complaining about being cheated of the rack and thumbscrew.
> – From Libby Purves' How Not To Be a Perfect Mother.

331 Telling your children

Children, however small, should be prepared. They should know that the baby is coming and that you will need to go into hospital for the doctors 'to help her out'. Pregnancy and childbirth should be explained simply. Answer their questions honestly, using words and concepts they can understand.

If you are having your baby at home, make it as natural as possible. Banning a small child from the birth room throughout labour is not a good idea, but don't expect him or her to sit wide-eyed throughout, since boredom will quickly set in.

Hospital or home, you will need someone to care for your children if your partner is to be with you.

If a child is to be a birth companion or observer, you should give full warning of what he or she may witness – blood, grunts and all. You should also explain that for much of the time you will probably

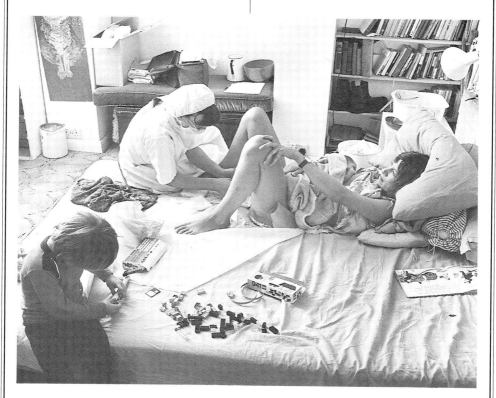

not be able to give attention, and that the midwife will be in charge – which means leaving the room if she asks.

332 Delivery rooms - what to expect

Labour and delivery rooms vary from hospital to hospital. Some are sterile, clinical and business-like, with delivery tables and machinery to the fore. Others are more comfortable and home-like. If you are lucky, you will find a hospital with birthing rooms designed to look something like bedrooms: there may be wallpaper, a television, curtains, even a rocking chair or bean bags. You will stay in this room throughout labour.

333 Such a squeeze

Human birth is difficult compared with that of most mammals. Why? Because of our big brains. Big brains need big heads, and a big head is difficult to pass through a small pelvis. In fact, so large have our brains become relative to our bodies that we need to give birth to our young long before brain growth is complete. Even at three years old, a child's brain is still growing; it has reached only 70 per cent of its final size. At birth, a baby's brain is a

mere 23 per cent of what it will eventually be when fully developed.

334 No boiling water?

Remember all that water boiling, and the constant demands for clean towels, in old films and books?

In the past, hot salt towels were applied to a woman's vagina. Alternating with olive oil massages, they helped enlarge the vaginal opening. Nowadays we snip instead; see 425.

335 Premature baby

A baby born too soon, very small for dates, or with medical problems, may go to the special care baby unit within moments of birth. A friend once described seeing the doctor tuck her tiny premature baby inside his white coat and run with him to the premature baby unit.

There, the baby will be nursed in an incubator, her temperature contolled, her heart and breathing monitored.

All the wires and tubes are essential, but they do distance parent and child. You may feel the baby is not yours. Time in the unit is a limbo between pregnancy and caring, an empty period before the baby comes home and belongs to her parents. See also 501-502.

While the baby is in an incubator, someone else does the caring, the parents sit and watch. You are not exactly a non-parent, but you are not a real one either. It could make you feel guilty, as if this had happened as a judgement on your inadequacies. Rest assured that any such feelings will vanish when your baby comes home.

336 More like home

Hospital maternity wards are undergoing gradual liberalization. Visiting hours are no longer restricted, and parents can come and go as they choose. Often, special gowns and masks (which can put a psychological barrier beween baby and parent) are worn only by staff, and efforts have been made to involve parents in the day-to-day care of babies in special care.

Unless the baby is too immature to suck, in which case she will be tube-fed, breast feeding is encouraged. Even when babies are tube-fed, mothers are encouraged to express milk, and both parents can fill the tubes; see also 440-449.

337 Short, sharp labour

Some labours last only one or two hours, but a short labour is not always as short as it seems. There may have been hours of painless labour before contractions are noticed, and the mother may be well into transition before the first contraction is felt. This slow build-up and quick resolution of labour places no extra strain on the baby.

Sometimes, though, the uterus may actually accomplish in minutes what takes hours in other labours. Here, the contractions are harder and faster, and for the baby this can mean stress. Her blood flow may be reduced by the pressure of contractions, and there will be less time between contractions for the baby's heart rate to recover; see 344. Despite this, such labours are not unnatural, and babies are rarely in danger.

338 Making it short

There are, these days, fewer prolonged labours – more than 24 hours – than there used to be. Better social conditions,

improved health, nutrition and antenatal care have probably contributed to this. So, too, has the increased tendency to perform Caesarians if complications seem likely, and to induce women whose labours are progressing slowly; see 384 and 429.

Making labour rooms more comfortable and familiar and keeping women active and upright in labour have also played their part. So have women themselves: mental preparation for birth almost certainly helps. In one study it was found that women who believed pregnancy was an illness had longer labours than women who believed it was a natural process. The women who believed it an illness had even longer labours when their doctors believed it was not.

339 Mechanized birth

If pregnancy and labour are uneventful, there is no medical reason why you should not have as natural a birth as you wish in hospital. Equally, there is no harm in mechanization – if the choice of epidural anaesthesia and foetal monitoring is yours. My ideal is that nothing should override this right to choose. The birth that causes you the least anxiety is likely to be the one that you find easiest.

It is bound to be different for different women. For some, an epidural or the foetal monitor can be a real source of stress; for others, not knowing whether the baby is safe is just as stressful, and being wired to a foetal heart monitor will do much to alleviate the anxiety. Against this one must, however, weigh the fact that the procedures can themselves increase risk to the baby.

340 Status symbols

Look around the hospital and you will soon notice the status that clothing confers. Consultants wear suits; young doctors wear white coats; nurses wear uniforms. For birth, a mother is dressed in a hospital gown. And father? In many hospitals, his lowly status is emphasized by full medical garb: overshoes, gown, hat, mask.

341 Fathers at birth

Nowadays, 70 per cent of fathers attend births. When asked what they consider the greatest benefit of fathers being present,

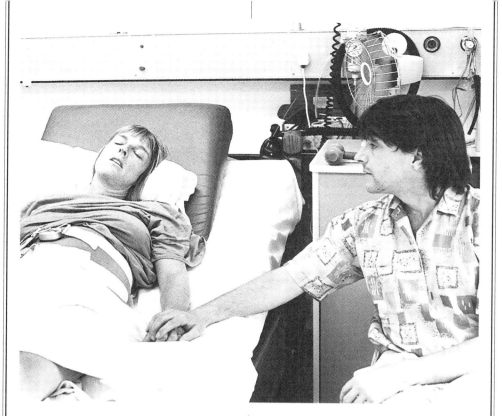

almost all women reply simply 'He was there.' I believe we should not underestimate the importance of his being there: above all, his presence demonstrates a commitment to family life.

But let us look at it coolly. In theory, both parents go to hospital to give birth. Put like that, it sounds like a joint experience, different but equal: it rarely is.

A man's primary role in labour is that of birth companion, a role without status and without any clearly defined activities. He is not naturally fitted for this kind of role, and it is asking a great deal of some men that they should suddenly assume it – especially the current generation of men experiencing feminist attitudes for the first time. They have not been brought up to be good birth companions; in addition, in the past, labour companions were women, often older women, with experience and expertise. A man generally has none of these, and in this sense he is an inferior companion.

He can, however, play a more active role as a birth coach. The sections that follow give suggestions as to how to coach a woman through labour. It is, nevertheless, not a role all men will want to play, nor will all women want a coach; some women may see it as demeaning – it is a matter for each couple to decide for themselves. The role of coach does not entirely supercede the role of companion, but it does enable a man to participate more fully.

The father can also, of course, act as a paramedic: psychotherapist, masseur, acupressurist, conveyor of complaints.

The committed father will want to play a parent role, too, but he cannot really do so until the baby's head becomes visible in the birth channel; then you can both share the role.

This still leaves unanswered the question of whether a mother-to-be should *expect* her partner to be present. He is in no strong position to argue; but beware of emotional blackmail – it can cause more long-term resentment than short-term gain. Just because most fathers are present at the birth does not mean they must be there. A man should have a choice, too. You may, out of vanity, not wish women friends to pity you, or think ill of your partner, because he does not want to be present. But those are poor reasons for insisting he comes.

Finally, it is worth remembering that, for a few men, seeing their wife giving birth takes the romance out of their relationship. The memory of the cursing, grunting, bleeding woman clouds their view of her ever after. See also 398.

The Last Few Days

342 As birth approaches

You will almost certainly feel a decline in foetal activity. At 30 weeks, babies make, on average, between 25 and 40 movements an hour; at term this drops to 18 to 28. It is not a sudden dip, rather a gradual decline in activity over the last few weeks.

The reasons? First, there is simply no room in there for gymnastics. Second, if the head has engaged, this will stabilize the baby. Third, there is now little fluid in which the baby can swim around. Finally, the baby is more mature: body, arms and legs will tend to move in a co-ordinated sequence so that you feel a single movement where before you felt many different movements as she exercised arms and legs at random.

The decline is not always obvious, and, unless you have been monitoring foetal movement, you may not be aware that it has happened. Nor is it inevitable. Some babies are born even though still active; others will arrive a week or two after they have quietened down.

343 Movements suddenly stop

Movements should be felt every day. If they become weak or stop suddenly, tell your doctor at once. The baby may be in distress; see 344.

If you are worried, test how the baby responds to a loud noise such as the radio being turned up to full volume. If the response is extremely weak, call the hospital, where they can test whether the baby is in distress. These tests may well be given routinely if you are overdue; see 344.

344 Foetal monitoring and oxytocin challenge test

Foetal monitoring, sometimes called a non-stress test (or NST), involves hooking the mother up to a machine which can detect the baby's heart beat. Normally, when the baby moves, her heart beat increases immediately. An NST looks for the acceleration of heart rate, following foetal movement, over a set period.

The oxytocin challenge test is more complex and time-consuming than an NST. Sometimes called a stress test, it assesses whether or not the baby can safely withstand labour. If the baby is stressed by the contractions of the womb, a normal vaginal birth would clearly put it at risk.

The test examines the baby's heart rate in respnse to uterine contractions and will normally be administered in conjunction with monitoring oestriols; see 240.

If the foetus is in distress, and responds poorly to this test, a Caesarian section will be considered.

345 Hyperactive?

As you try to get to know your baby in the tantalizing days before you can hold her, you have only feelings to quide you. If she squirms and wriggles a great deal, it is natural to wonder whether this will continue. Will she be a hyperactive, wakeful child? Be reassured: there is no evidence that this is so.

Babies do not squirm in the womb because they are restless, they do it to keep their joints free and their muscles exercised. Those who do not move in this way, perhaps because their mothers are alcoholic, spend their days in an alcoholic stupor, and may be born with ossified joints.

346 Lightening

If this is your first baby, she will probably descend into the pelvic cavity two or three weeks before birth. There is little mistaking it when it happens. You can even see that your bump is lower and tipped slightly forward. You will feel less

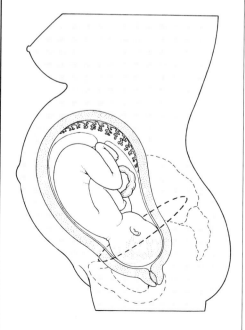

short of breath as the pressure of the baby on the diaphragm is reduced, and less bloated as the pressure on the stomach decreases.

Although you feel lighter at the top end, you will feel pressure lower down. The baby is, after all, still as big. You may feel pressure in the small of the back, the pelvis and the bladder. As the head presses on the pelvic floor, you may feel odd fluttering movements in the vagina, almost as though you were being tickled.

Because your centre of gravity has changed, you may also feel off-balance and clumsy. The loosening of your pelvis in readiness for birth can heighten this clumsiness; see 287.

If this is not your first baby, lightening may well be a positive sign that birth is about to take place. In subsequent pregnancies, lightening rarely occurs before labour is under way.

347 Bleeding and spotting

In the weeks approaching birth, many women notice a slight brown or pinkish spotting, especially after intercourse or following an internal examination. It is nothing to worry about. Bright red blood is another matter and should be reported immediately to the hospital or doctor. So should any spotting (whatever the colour) that occurs every day; see 268.

348 Will you know?

Everyone knows when they go into labour – or so they say. But how will you know?

The truth is that you will probably realize it, but not necessarily at once. Most women get to hospital in time, but that does not mean they suddenly know 'this is it'.

We expect a 'this is it' feeling because the only people we ever see going into labour are in films or on TV. What film wastes half an hour with the heroine uncertain of her condition?

So how do you tell the difference between Braxton Hicks contractions (306) and the real thing?

The first-time mother usually expects the contractions of real labour to be like Braxton Hicks contractions, but more so: more intense, more definite and more painful. That is a fairly accurate assessment, since in most cases, the contractions of real labour will be felt as pain. Even so, at the beginning of labour it is not always clear that they have started.

Three days before my daughter was born, I packed my son off to the friend who was to look after him. I was certain that 'this was it': I made some soup, had a bath, walked around. The contractions subsided. Nothing happened.

Three days later, I arrived at the hospital, totally certain, already pushing, just ten minutes before my daughter was born. "Well, you made it with time to get your boots off," the midwife commented as I gave birth on a trolley in a waiting room. This, I should add, was not my first labour, but my third.

349 Presentation

The technical definition of the baby being engaged is when the broadest part of the baby's head reaches the upper part of your pelvis. This is often indicated as a zero point. Movement during labour past this point is measured as 'plus' with a numeral from one to five; position prior to the head reaching this point is defined as minus with a numeral, also one to five. Examination will tell where the baby sits, but movement can be very gradual in the early stages, and the baby can move downwards without your feeling labour has begun.

350 Will anyone else know?

Doctors and midwives see countless mothers every year but still cannot predict when labour will begin. There are signs (351) that it is due, but no sign, or combination of signs, that provides an infallible guide.

Sometimes labour can last days, sometimes minutes, and the early movement of the baby into the birth channel can be equally variable. So can the early thinning of the cervix (effacement) and its early opening (dilation), both of which can occur hours, indeed weeks, before birth.

351 The signs

- Lightening (346), evident up to four weeks prior to labour.
- Increasing pressure in the pelvis and rectum as the baby drops into the birth channel. If the early stages of labour progress without clear signs of contractions, this feeling of pressure is a true indicator that labour has begun.
- If the baby is presenting in a posterior position, persistent backache.
- Weight loss: some women lose up to two or three pounds as labour approaches.
- Nest building: many women will tell you they scrubbed the kitchen floor, cleaned the stove or made 20 pounds of stew for the freezer the day before they went into labour. It does not always happen, but feeling energetic is quite a reliable sign.
- Vaginal discharge often increases; usually it also thickens. Up to three weeks before labour starts, you may notice that the mucus plug blocking the opening of the cervix has been dislodged.

As the cervix opens, small blood vessels are broken, and these can give rise to slight bleeding which is quite normal. (Heavy bleeding is abnormal at any stage.)

This light bleeding is, in fact, the 'show' which in some women is an almost certain sign that labour is about to start. But even this is not infallible; it can happen several days before labour begins.

- Diarrhoea often occurs just prior to labour.
- Braxton Hicks contractions (306 and 348) become more frequent and more painful for many women just before the on-set of labour.

352 Probabilities

Labour has probably not begun if:

- Contractions are not regular.
- Contractions do not increase in severity and frequency.
- Pain is felt in the lower abdomen rather than the back.
- Contractions die down if you walk around.
- Contractions ease if you have an alcoholic drink.
- The show (351) was brown.
- Foetal movements increase with each contraction.

Labour has probably begun if:

- Contractions are becoming more and more regular.
- Contractions are becoming stronger.
- Contractions intensify as you move around.
- Contractions do not feel any different, however you sit or stand.
- You feel them in the lower back and they spread to the lower abdomen.

- You have a pinkish show.
- The membranes rupture; see 361.

353 A time of transition

Think of your baby now in that watery world. Safe, enclosed, subdued. Moving her body easily and freely in her secure bag. Think of what she sees and hears: light and shadow, possibly red-tinged, the muffled, constant sound of two hearts beating separate rhythms. She thinks this is how it will always be – part of you, but separate. Soon she will be much more part of her father's life. You are giving up your exclusive care. Bringing her out into the world for others to share. My child, our child, their child; in time someone else's lover, someone else's parent. Maybe you should savour this moment of still-exclusive care. Like many women, you may find yourself holding too tightly to it after she is born.

Think of how she has listened to your voice, muffled by that watery world, and her father's, more distant, deeper tones. Think of the journey she now has to take from her world to yours. Try to vizualize it. Try to visualize her. Reflect on what it means to be born; see 385.

354 Assertiveness

Some people seem to be born with the confidence to say "That is how I want it to be", and without bullying, manipulating or grovelling, they make requests which seem so reasonable that they often get their way. But many women find it hard to be assertive. They often find themselves being dragged along by the force of others' views because they feel their opinions are less important.

As we approach the birth of a baby we are faced with two counteracting forces which may make it particularly difficult for us to assert our wishes.

On one hand there is the possibility that the medical profession will take over the birth. Doctors do not have a good press when it comes to telling patients what is happening to them, or to asking for patients' opinions.

Conflicting with this is the fear, deep inside you, of pain; you long for a labour free of it. You don't feel at all brave.

Deep down, you may wonder how something which is controlled by the muscles of the womb without any conscious input from the mind could ever be a mind-expanding experience, as liberated women sometimes describe their natural births.

Well – it seems like a conflict. But it need not be. To be liberated is to be assertive. To be assertive is to select *realistically* what is right for you. It may be a drug-free, natural birth; it may not.

What is right, in this more than anything else, is what *you* want.

355 Inhibitions

The key to coping with birth is to greet it willingly.

Relax for a moment. Think about each breath you take; feel yourself relax. Consider what lies ahead.

Think of that first breath, the breath you took at birth, the breath your baby will shortly take. Your breath now, hers then. Then, as you relax, think of the time in between. There is no point in being anxious about it: simply accept it. It is inevitable.

Think about sounds, of the sounds you make in loving, and the sounds you make in happiness. Then think of the sounds you make as you work, push, heave and strain. Think of the powerful forces that will pass through your body in the coming hours, and the sounds of those forces. Be ready to release them without restraint. You *can* cry out; you *can* moan; you *can* yell; you *can* swear. There will be pain, there will be stress; there need not be inhibition. Birth, and the earthy instincts that go with it, are among the most natural things in the world.

356 Self-esteem

- Write down four things that you do better than most people.
- Write down three things that you have done in your life which make you proud.

Many women can think of things that they do worse than others, and of things of which they are ashamed, but when faced with these questions, they find themselves looking at a blank page. They could fill the page if they were to write about friends or lovers; but not for themselves.

You are about to change your life. For better or worse, you must now renegotiate your relationship with your partner, as later you must form a relationship with your child. No woman who undervalues herself can achieve her true goal and develop her own style as a wife and mother.

357 How it should be

Everyone has a right to assert themselves, provided this does not infringe the rights of others.

In matters relating to the birth you have the right to:

- Ask for what you want.
- Express your opinion, feelings and emotions.
- Make mistakes.
- Say what you think, even if it is not logical and well thought out.
- Decide for yourself.
- Change your mind.
- Be told about things that concern you.
- Remain in ignorance if that suits you.
- Do it alone.
- Want to succeed.

These are, of course, difficult ideals in your present condition. You are caretaker of a child who is as much your partner's as yours. But as long as you are not putting that child in danger, you should feel free to say what you want for the birth.

358 Backache

A baby presenting in a posterior position (see diagram) will exert pressure on the mother's sacrum. The resulting backache has a habit of not letting up between contractions, and the contractions themselves can produce excruciating back pain. It will be a difficult labour. The following techniques may help.

- Stay off your back. If you lie down, the baby's weight will be pressing on your back. Keep upright and moving for as long as possible. While you are upright, gravity will force the baby downwards. Crouching, leaning forward against your partner or a wall, kneeling on all fours, squatting or lying on your side with your back well rounded will all relieve pressure.
- Heat applied to the back is a comforting counter-irritant. A hot bath or shower is best, but a hot-water bottle, warm compresses or a heated pad can help. A warm sponge alternated with a bag of ice (or even frozen peas) can sometimes soothe.
- Counter-pressure can be applied to the point where your pelvis joins the spine.

Ask your partner to experiment. Try applying different degrees of pressure to the point of pain and to adjacent areas. Intense counter-pressure normally brings the greatest relief. Ask your partner to use a heel, or the palm of his hand, with the other resting over it – or to try the same technique using his knuckles. You can also place your own knuckles just under your bottom as you sit in a warm bath. Two tennis balls in an old sock can work wonders: press them well into your back on either side of the spine.

- Another useful technique is acupressure: pressure applied externally to the points used in acupuncture. The point you need for back pain in labour is just below the centre of the ball of the foot. Apply light to strong counter-pressure with a finger to each foot – you will know when you have the right spot.

Pressure at this point can help relieve the pain from contractions, too. See also 380.

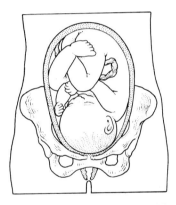

359 When to call the hospital

When in doubt, call. No one is going to think you foolish. The hospital will ask you a number of questions and tell you when to come in. Many women do not want to spend any more time than necessary in hospital, but if you are nervous, you are better sitting in a hospital waiting room than panicking at home.

However, most first labours are long, likely to take 12 to 24 hours, so there is normally no need to rush into hospital.

Many women, perhaps most women, go into labour during the night. The midwife and the hospital are well aware of this. If labour is progressing rather quickly, you don't have to wait until morning. If you feel ready to go, you *are* ready to go. Ring and let them know you are on your way.

Before ringing, time your contractions. Take the time from the begining of one to the beginning of the next. You will also be asked how long each contraction lasts, and how regular they are (360). Your partner can help with the timing, but it is better if you make the phone call. The hospital will ask other questions, and it is easier if you answer them directly.

360 Are the contractions regular?

Most descriptions of labour suggest that contractions gradually build up as labour progresses, and for most women having their first baby this will be the case. Contractions start rather irregularly, before settling into a pattern in which they become longer, stronger and more frequent.

But you may not be average. Progress is not always by the book. With some women, contractions do not settle into a rhythm until labour is well advanced; with some they never do.

It is perhaps safest to be guided by your strongest contractions. Labour is said to be established when contractions are fairly close together and lasting for 40 seconds or more. If your contractions are longer than this, labour is probably well established, even if the contractions are less frequent. It may also be well established if you have frequent short contractions.

361 Have the membranes really ruptured?

See also 321. Urine has a familiar smell, while amniotic fluid smells sweet. Urine is passed then the desire to urinate is over. Amniotic fluid goes on trickling, even if it starts with a rush. The baby's head acts like a cork to stop up the cervix; the cork is more effective when you sit, so if you leak while standing and stop when sitting, it is not urine but the waters breaking. See also 391.

362 Waters break: then?

Sometimes, after a show or the waters breaking, you will go into labour quite quickly. Sometimes you just wait – and wait. When this happens, the hospital will probably suggest induction if you have reached term but not gone into labour after 24 hours.

If the membranes have ruptured, keep the vaginal area as clean as possible. Wipe front to back when you go to the lavatory; don't make love.

Unless labour has started, don't have a bath, although you may have a shower. If labour is delayed, there is a small danger that an infection, particularly a lung infeciton, could enter the amniotic fluid, which the baby drinks, indeed breathes in.

However, if you are definitely in labour (see 352), this is not a serious problem. You can have a bath if you want to, but make sure the bath is clean by wiping it out with disinfectant.

363 Darkened amniotic fluid

If your amniotic fluid is stained with meconium, a greenish-brown substance from the baby's bowels, ring the hospital immediately. Meconium staining often occurs in post-mature babies, but it also occurs when the foetus is under stress. It is not a sure sign of stress, so don't panic, but it is a hint which should not be ignored.

364 How do contractions feel?

Contractions have been described as feeling as though a tight elastic belt, slung under your bump, is being gradually tightened. The closest comparable sensation is probably stomach cramps. Contractions are like the stomach cramps of a bad period, but more regular. They start in the lower back and move forward around the abdomen.

In fact, they feel as you might expect them to if you consider what is happening. Your cervix, which is normally a long canal hanging down from your uterus into the vagina, first becomes soft and stretchy – it is said to 'ripen'. Then contractions draw it up bit by bit until it is just a cuff at the base of the uterus.

It is through this cuff that the baby must pass. As the cervix is drawn up, it also draws apart so that the tiny gap at the centre of the cervical tube gradually widens (dilates) until it is possible for the baby's head to pass through into the vagina. You are considered to have entered labour when this gap is about 3 cm.

Think of the cervix being pulled up, stage by stage, in the same way that a boat is slowly dragged up a beach: it has to be done as heave, pause, heave, pause. The pull is starting at the back and moving around to the front, but low down, under your bump. It is, after all, here that the womb is opening up, here that the baby will pass.

Pain and Pain Control

365 But does it hurt?

Pain: a word always associated with childbirth. But to understand the question fully, we need to consider how pain is felt, and why we feel it.

There is one word for 'pain', but many feelings; it is rather like having the one word 'colour' to describe the great variation of different hues in nature. Pain can be sharp, nagging, dull. It can flicker and stab, pulse and throb.

To understand why we feel pain, consider what happens to those rare individuals who don't feel it. If you feel no pain you do not withdraw your hand from the hot plate, or stop chopping when you cut your finger. Your bones and joints could deteriorate from arthritis, but you would continue to go jogging until one day you irreparably damaged yourself. Pain, then, enables us unconsciously to monitor our bodies, but, at the same time, the perception of pain can break through into consciousness, either as a 'take care' signal (as, for instance when you jump and land heavily) or as a true danger signal.

366 The gate theory

The level at which these unconscious warning signals become pain has been examined in many groups of people. It was found, for example, that a stimulus most northern Europeans call 'warm' was called pain by people from farther south in Europe; that levels of shock which were intolerable to Italian women were easily acceptable to Jewish and Anglo-Saxon women.

To explain these observations, the researchers Melzak and Torgerson developed the gate theory of pain. They suggest that the points at which we set our 'take care' and 'danger' levels depend upon the context in which we perceive. As, for instance, with our perception of a pink flower: against a white sheet it looks decidedly pink; against a blue wall, it can look quite white.

Imagine now that the signals from your womb are a football crowd rushing to leave a stadium through a single gate. From inside the gate, you can see the crowd. You could say 'Look at all those signals, this will be excruciatingly painful.'

But imagine you are outside the stadium, watching the crowd come through. the gate is open wide, many signals pass through, and you say 'Ooh that hurts'. But if the gate is almost shut, you see only a few signals getting through.

You do not know how big a crowd is on the other side.

The brain, Melzak and Torgerson would say, is seated outside the stadium. It sees only what passes through the gate. How wide we open the gate we can, to some extent, decide for ourselves. For childbirth that is the good news. But there is bad news, too.

As you might expect, it is almost impossible to keep the gate (366) only slightly ajar all the time; the signals keep running through a little too fast for us to control. Even the bad news can help, since it means that the rush of signals will not be entirely unexpected: for if they do take you by surprise, you can lose control of the gate entirely.

The woman who taught the childbirth class I attended had experienced one painless birth, her first, but this was followed by two births with pain. I know of no other person who has given birth without pain at least at some stage of the process. But I know of many who found the pain manageable without drugs.

367 The knowledge of pain

There is little point in trying to pretend to Western women that labour is not painful. But I suspect that received knowledge from the older generation can make young women expect it to be more painful than it is – can make them automatically leave that gate wide open.

Until the 1930s, most women embarking on pregnancy knew they were putting their lives in danger; and 1930 is not so long ago. Death in childbirth is reportedly linked with great pain; but I think this may be misleading.

Of course there *was* pain. But anxiety and fear, when childbirth was a killer, must surely have contributed to our grandmothers' experience of pain. Death in childbirth was, in fact, most commonly death *after* childbirth from 'childbed fever', caused by the organism haemolytic streptococcus.

Eclampsia (270-275) was another killer: the dramatic death frequently described in literature. Before 1948 it was seen in one in 400 births in Sydney, Australia; after the introduction of strict monitoring of weight and blood pressure, it fell to one in 15,000 births.

Mothers also died from severe haemorrage and from the sort of obstructive labour which today would be safely and simply managed with a Caesarian section.

368 At one

Think of these women (367) as you enter labour, and be grateful for how different it is today. Think of how frightened they must have been, how you have nothing to fear, although you may still share some of the same uncertainty. Then think of all the other women all over the world who are going into labour, as you are now; who will soon hold their child, as you will.

369 Psychoprophylactics

Pain, fear and ignorance are the trinity which makes us open the gate; see 366. If fear and ignorance could be removed, much of the pain would also go. Psychoprophylactic methods (PPM) offer a way of reducing the pain we perceive, of pushing the gate a little nearer the latch.

Relaxation, feed-back relaxation (in which a test shows you how relaxed you are), and focussing your attention (on, say, a silly rhyme) are the basic PPM techniques.

When women who had been taught these techniques were experimentally compared to women who had not, it was shown that PPM reduced the perception of pain and increased tolerance. The women had to keep their hands in ice cold water for four minutes, take them out, warm them to blood heat and then put them back in the bucket of iced water.

Women who had been taught PPM were able to keep their hands in the bucket for longer and showed a gradual increase in tolerance over time. Those without training were less tolerant, and their tolerance lessened over time.

370 Breathing exercises

Many women are taught to control their breathing during labour as a technique for producing distraction and maintaining relaxation.

Be sure that your partner knows the breathing routine and can talk you through it. His instructions can form part of the whole pattern of relaxation and distraction. But if, on the day, you find you cannot get the breathing right, try other means of distraction and relaxation: look at the door handle, make rhythmic sounds, or recite a poem.

There is, however, an alternative approach. You can accept the power of contractions and go along with them. Accept that you are, for now, being

133

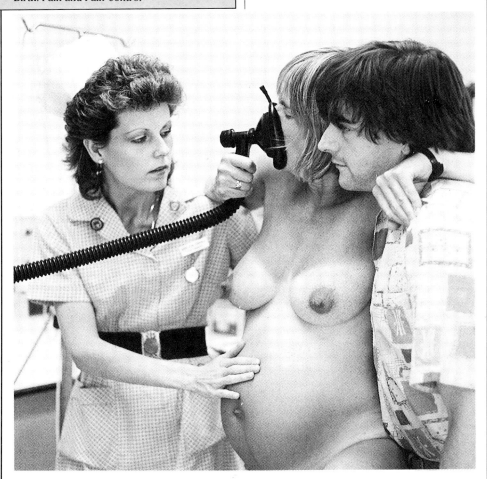

controlled by your body, not your head, and simply let go. Imagine that the contractions are waves in a great sea, and that you would do better to become liquid and move with the flow, rather than to stand firm and face it.

The key to 'becoming liquid' is to open yourself up to the experience by relaxation. Unless you have been trained in breathing relaxation, it is easiest if you breath naturally. Concentrate on each breath, not as a pattern or level, but as a breath; and let go all feelings of control. Some women find it easier to do this if they allow themselves to moan or sigh, even to shout.

371 But if you fail

It is easy to say 'I will not lose my temper, I will not give in, I will not let him/her/them do that to me again.' And we all know that in an emotional state, good

intentions can evaporate. You can use the emotion of giving birth in a positive way, as the books say, but you can also lose control. Birth *is* overwhelming. It *is* new, and however much you have prepared for it, cannot know how it will feel until you experience it. It can be scarey, just as all deep emotional feelings are. The regular pounding of contractions hour in, hour out, takes over. You feel as if you are no longer in charge.

Being out of control is, in this sense, right. In birth, our bodies take over; we don't control labour with our minds. The fight for control is doomed to failure.

For those of us who pride ourselves on how well we control our lives, accepting this can be especially difficult. It brings anxiety, and guilt. We want the birth to go as planned. We are upset when it goes wrong. Once you have lost command of the situation, it is difficult to get things back on an even keel. It can happen to all of us. It certainly happened to me. It is human. Maybe you will succeed next time, maybe not.

The important thing at the end of the day is not giving birth, but what is born. Not being a super birthing machine, but being a complete woman, a good mother.

Don't be afraid to take what help you can. It is *not* weakness to accept pain relief in labour. Nor to shout out, if that helps. You can be sure that anything you shout will have been heard before.

372 Pain relief

In 1847, James Young Simpson splashed some chloroform on to a handkerchief and held it over the face of a woman in labour; she became the first women to deliver under anaesthetic. This revolution in obstetrics was greeted with horror by the Roman Catholic Church, which saw the pain of childbirth as punishment for Eve's eating the forbidden fruit.

I will greatly multiply thy sorrow and thy conception; in sorrow thou shalt bring forth children; (Genesis 3:16).

Needless to say, the high clergy who reacted in this way were all men.

Similar criticism from the Anglican Church subsided when Queen Victoria agreed to use chloroform for the birth of her seventh child. It was not until 1950 that a papal decree accepted painless childbirth as consistent with the teachings of the Roman Catholic Church.

But it was not just the churches, or men, who opposed giving pain-relieving drugs in labour. The distinguished psychoanalyst Helen Deutsch said in 1942 that the pain of childbirth was essential for bonding.

Keep this in mind. Although there is a general acceptance of pain relief in childbirth, there is still, in some quarters, a feeling that it is not good. That you should grin and bear it, take it like a woman. That if you accept the pethidine, you will be a bad mother.

It is nonsense. Pain reduces bonding, by all accounts. And bonding is, in any event, an over-used concept. Loving your children, not sticking yourself to them with superglue, should be your aim.

Pain relief is an important aspect of any woman's labour, and prudent use of medication is often essential. Drug-free childbirth may remain the ideal, but it is probably an ideal to which most women do not subscribe. What they want are the pleasures, the emotion, the loving aspects of giving birth: wanting their cake, and eating it, perhaps. But to some extent we *can* eat cake. Maybe it is the guilt of eating, when we should be suffering for Eve, that makes many of us believe drug-free labour is ideal.

Although most women accept drugs for a difficult, prolonged, or breech delivery, or if forceps are needed, many feel guilty if they accept drugs for a 'normal delivery'. Be guided by your own feelings; accepting help is not an admission of failure: you do not feel a failure when you take an aspirin for a headache, or a drink for Dutch courage.

373 Drugs in labour

The medical aim of giving drugs in childbirth is not to eliminate pain but to reduce it. And since two of you are involved (often with conflicting interests) the aim is also to administer drugs in such a way that the needs of the mother and child are balanced.

Analgesics (374) are pain relievers; anaesthetics (377) produce loss of sensation; tranquillizers (375) you will sometimes hear described as ataraxics. Which you are given will depend on the situation, the way it can be given and the obstetrician's or anaesthetist's preference.

374 Analgesics

Pethidine is perhaps the most frequently used, although many new drugs are appearing. You will be given an injection into muscle, usually in your bottom or a thigh. Ask what dose you are getting. In the U.S.A., doses are often considerably smaller than those routinely used in Britain. The 100-200 mg dose normally given in the U.K. will almost certainly make your baby drowsy.

It is far from certain that large doses are more effective than smaller ones. Indeed, many doubt they have much effect at all. Pethidine is normally given when labour is well under way and is usually avoided in the later stages. Its side-effects vary widely. Some people like the drowsiness it produces, others feel it makes them lose control. It can make you feel sick and depressed (but this does not happen to everyone). In a study carried out by the British National Childbirth Trust, 70 per cent of women found it an ineffective pain reliever.

The new analgesics being tried in many hospitals are less likely to make babies drowsy. Whether they work any better than pethidine remains to be established.

375 Tranquillizers

Tranquillizers are not in themselves painkillers. You are likely to be offered Phenergan (chemical name promethazine) or Valium (chemical name diazepam), which make you feel calm and relax your muscles. If you are anxious, they will help you to participate more fully in the birth.

Again, reactions vary. Some women like the feeling, others think they lose control. It is, perhaps, worth trying relaxation techniques before you accept tranquillizers, since the general effects are similar.

376 Inhalants

Entenox (gas and air – a mixture of nitrous oxide and oxygen) is widely used in Britain. It is breathed in through a mask at each contraction and can reduce the sensation at its peak. Some women find the slight wooziness pleasant, some that they get a slight 'high'; others find that the main benefit is having something to think about and do.

It has the advantage of being quickly eliminated from the body, but it can encourage hyperventilation; see 402.

377 Epidurals and other nerve blocks

Anaesthetics injected along the course of a nerve are called regional nerve blocks and are used to deaden the sensation in a specific region. An epidural, the most effective form of pain relief in labour, completely numbs the area from the waist down. Other blocks may totally or partially numb a smaller area. The most frequently used blocks are pudendal, epidural, spinal, caudal and paracervical.

• A pudendal block is inserted into the perineal or vaginal area and reduces pain in this region. It is used in forceps deliveries and sometimes during stitching.
• An epidural block is administered through a fine tube into the epidural space which lies between the spinal cord and the outer membrane. It is used in both conventional labours and in many Caesarian sections. It can make blood pressure drop suddenly, so there will be frequent checks. Epidurals are unlikely to be used if you have had pre-eclampsia or blood pressure problems during pregnancy, or if your labour has been

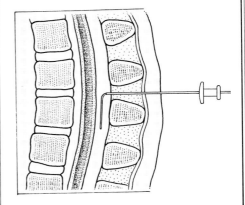

complicated by excessive bleeding.

More than 80 per cent of women say epidurals work, and although a few report a feeling of missing out, this happens to less than three per cent.

When an epidural works properly, it can be wonderful; but women are unpredictable. Some studies suggest that women who have drug-free labours are more satisfied than those who have epidurals. Don't agonize over this. If an epidural is your choice, remember that drug-free labours are chosen. It may be that women are most likely to be satisfied with the labour *they* choose.

There are reports of backache and headaches following epidurals, and a persistence of some numbness and tingling in the limbs. How common such findings are is not known. There are also reports that babies may be a little less visually alert after birth.

This may depend upon which anaesthetic you receive. (An epidural is a technique for administering anaesthetic, not a type of anaesthetic.) Bupivacaine is most commonly used, but many others are being tried.

One might also be concerned that some doctors are tempted to drive labour at speed by giving oxytocin IV as a drip to women who have epidurals. The thinking is that if a woman cannot feel pain, it may be sensible to get labour over as quickly as possible. But no one has assessed the effects of such violent labours upon the child.

A spinal block, for a Caesarian section, and the low spinal block (for vaginal delivery) are rarely used. After a spinal block the mother must lie flat on her back for eight hours, and may suffer from headaches. The anaesthetic is injected into the fluid surrounding the spinal cord.

• A caudal block is similar to an epidural, except that it blocks sensation in a more limited area. It tends to inhibit labour and for this reason is now rarely used.

• The paracervical block, also rarely used, reduces the pain of labour but not delivery. There is some danger to the foetus, and for this reason is a last resort.

General anaesthesia used to be common in delivery, but is now rare except in Caesarian sections. Today many of these operations are done using epidural nerve blocking.

378 Hypnosis

In qualified hands, this can produce impressive pain relief in some people. Some even go through painless Caesarian sections under hypnosis.

That hypnosis reduces pain may seem amazing, but it is not a mystical process, in fact it is essentially the same process as PPM; see 369.

If you want hypnosis, you will need to begin preparation at least six weeks before delivery. Choose a qualified practitioner.

379 Acupuncture

This has been used in China for 4,000 years to relieve pain, produce relaxation and restore energy. Certain acupuncture points on the body can be used alone to relieve pain, but it is better to have an overall treatment. Not all hospitals encourage acupuncture.

380 Acupressure

This does not need a qualified practitioner, just a partner with the know-how. Like Shiatsu, a similar Japanese massage technique, it can be used to relieve symptoms or as a means of strengthening and balancing your body's energies.

It is not known how these techniques work, but for some they are certainly effective. Both rely on nothing more than varying pressures applied by the fingers to different parts of the body. The massage itself is comforting, even if it does not relieve the pain.

381 TENS

Transcutaneous Electrical Nerve Stimulation is a big name for a little box about the size of a calculator, which passes electric current to four pads attached to the mother's back at the point where nerve fibres from the uterus enter the spinal cord. The principle is that the current, controlled by the mother, and applied through the skin to these fibres, can block the gateway through which pain sensations pass. It is also thought that the stimulation causes the body to produce its own painkiller, endorphin.

How does TENS feel? First like butterfly wings, then like birds' wings flapping. Pain is not exactly eliminated, it is broken up into a dull ache.

Increasing numbers of hospitals are now offering TENS to women during childbirth. In trials at a London hospital, 80 per cent of mothers reported that it brought relief.

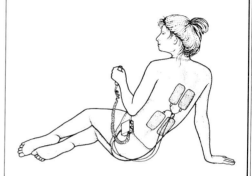

382 Which to chose?

Be flexible. Find out what is available at your hospital. Look into the various choices and discuss the possibilities with doctors, your partner and friends. Make a decision in principle, one which you could change later if necessary.

If you decide upon no drugs, or minimal interference, and find that you cannot live with that decision, be prepared to take any help that is offered. Labour is not the punishment of Eve nor a trial of endurance.

383 Warm baths

Women who had experienced several labours were asked what they thought was the most effective form of pain relief. All said that a warm bath or shower was more effective than drugs: this, however, did not include anaesthetics. Other methods suggested were:
• Keeping upright.
• Keeping moving.
• Massage.
• Warm compresses.

The Last Few Hours

384 Induced labour

Induction has a bad name, for a sound reason. In the past, babies were induced to suit the convenience of the hospital. But just because a technique has been abused does not mean that it is not sometimes necessary. And it is no use saying it was not used in the past, so why use it now? In the past many mothers and babies died.

Induction is advisable:

• If there is foetal distress.
• If the membranes have ruptured, and labour has not started within 24 hours. Twenty-four hours is a rule of thumb: you could ask to wait a little longer.
• If the baby is post-mature – say two weeks later than expected – you could ask to have an NST test or foetal monitoring (see 344) to establish the baby's well-being.
• If there is no progress with the labour; see 430.
• In maternal diabetes, the placenta often fails prematurely. You will probably be given tests for placental function at regular intervals.
• If there is concurrent illness in the mother.
• If there is severe rhesus disease.
A World Health Organization report on obstetric procedures suggests that no more than 10 per cent of labours should be induced in any geographical area. Before accepting induction, you should ask why it is being done. You may also want to know the incidence of induction at your hospital.

Induced labour is often rapid. Your membranes will probably be artificially ruptured, and this in itself may induce labour. You will probably be given oxytocin or prostaglandin to stimulate contractions.

Oxytocin is a hormone naturally produced by the body throughout pregnancy; see 297. As labour approaches, the uterus becomes more and more sensitive to its action, until finally the balance is tipped and you begin labour. In fact, as the baby approaches term, her pituitary gland also begins to release oxytocin, which passes into the mother's blood stream enhancing her own level of oxytocin, which in turn stimulates labour.

So, induction means by-passing the baby's ability to produce oxytocin, and giving enough directly to the mother for labour to start. It may be given as an injection into the bottom, as a pill placed under the tongue, or it may be sniffed. Most commonly, however, it is given as an intravenous drip, since this is the easiest way to contol the rate of uptake. Everyone responds differently to this hormone, and the dose may need adjusting to suit you: too much oxytocin can send you into rapid, prolonged contractions.

A sudden catapulting into advanced labour can be unpleasant, especially if you are unprepared: if this is the beginning, you may wonder how it is to be endured. Of course, it is not how labour really begins; you are starting somewhere in the middle. There are many advantages to a slow build-up, not least the time to practise PPM (369) of pain control. My middle child, although not induced, was born following a rapid, precipitous labour. When I say 55 minutes from start to finish, people always say You lucky thing. But it was, in fact, by far my most difficult labour. The 12-hour labour of my last child by far the easiest.

Labour is labour. If you are ready to go for it, go for it: you can do this even when dumped in at the deep end. Try to relax, practise breathing and distraction before the drip is in place. Hold your partner and face that first contraction knowing you are now in business.

385 The Leboyer method

Frederick Leboyer, the French obstetrician, believes that babies should come gently into this world. Birth is a trauma for the baby, a trauma we can minimize. In a Leboyer-style delivery room, the lights will be dim, voices soft and hushed. The new-born baby will be lifted immediately on to the mother's abdomen and gently massaged as she begins to perceive the world around her. Overhead heating or a soft blanket will be used to keep her warm. The umbilical cord is clamped and cut only when it has stopped pulsating, by which time the baby will have been breathing independently for some time. Once the cord is cut, the baby may be lowered gently into a warm bath where she can move freely.

Modified Leboyer birthing is offered by many hospitals around the world. No one really knows whether the approach really is best for babies. It is, however, almost certainly good for mothers. The less clinical the birth, the happier both parents feel about it. Women who give birth in comfortable, relaxed surroundings are far less likely to report pain and discomfort.

386 The Odent method

Michel Odent, another French obstetrician, believes that a woman's instinctive ability to give birth has been undermined by modern obstetric practice, which, in his opinion, can prolong labour. In this he is almost certainly right.

His delivery rooms contain no machines or medical equipment. They are gently lit and comfortable. There is no bed, but a platform on the floor and piles of cushions. Women are encouraged to remain upright throughout labour, and there are bars set into the walls to hold during contractions. He believes in using the force of gravity: that when a woman stands during a contraction, the weight of the baby on the cervix will accelerate its opening.

There is often a bath of warm water in the room, since bathing relaxes the muscles, and the baby can even be born in the water. This is, perhaps, the part of the Odent method we know best.

Few hospitals can offer full Odent facilities, but we can use many of the techniques to help labour along. Most hospitals will encourage you to stay as upright as possible during labour and birth. Some are expanding facilities for showers and baths during labour.

387 Staying upright

Most obstetricians now agree that remaining active and upright is best, and they also recommend warm baths for pain relief. In fact, one distinguished obstetrician is on record as claiming that there is only one delivery position worse than lying on one's back: hanging by the heels from a chandelier.

In fact, few women nowadays are delivered lying completely flat on their backs. It was never a natural position.

388 Am I missing out?

A sensitive birth need not depend on following Odet or Leboyer to the letter. In most hospitals you can, if you wish, stay upright; the baby is delivered on to the stomach, and few inflict bright lights or harsh voices on the newborn.

Taking a squatting position is no longer seen as odd. If you feel it is best for you, ask.

Women who have used the Leboyer method are probably not a cross section of the population, and neither are their children. The methods have not been scientifically tested, and no one has shown that these children are better adjusted than their brothers and sisters who entered it in the conventional, rough manner.

But why not make birth as happy, as gentle and as comforting an experience as you can? This certainly can do no harm – if back-up facilities are available.

389 Irregular contractions

No two labours are the same, even for the same woman. The picture of labour you gain from reading this, or any other book, will be an average. Just as many babies are not textbook babies, so not all contractions are regularly spaced, gradually getting longer and stronger, and building up slowly.

If you are having long, strong and frequent contractions which are, although irregular, sometimes less than five minutes apart, do not wait for them to become regular; they may never do so.

390 Shaving the pubic hair

This is a matter of fashion, and fortunately it is going out of fashion. It is unnecessary, and it can cause infection.

391 Rupturing the membranes

A World Health Organization conference on appropriate technology for birth came to the conclusion, after studying the evidence, that there was no justification for this becoming a routine practice. It suggested that the normal balance of pressures on the baby, placenta and cord during a contraction could be disturbed, producing an uneven pressure on the baby's head, and on the cord.

Obviously, if you or the baby is in real distress, these are minor worries. But it seems pointless to put the baby at unnecessary risk by using the procedure routinely.

Rupturing the membranes sounds awful, but it does not hurt: the membranes contain no pain sensors.

392 Your way

At the end of the day, the most positive

thing you can say is that you did it your way. The baby can come out head first, bottom first, facing up or down. You have no say. She can come out after 55 minutes of intense labour, or after 48 hours of drawn-out stopping and starting. Nothing you have done (or can do) will influence how the labour turns out.

You can, however, influence how you will feel, when it happens and after it is over. It is important to recognize this and not to feel it is your fault if things do not go according to plan.

Preparation really can influence the perception of how good or bad you feel the labour to be; how you perceive the contractions, and how easily you accept what is happening. Understanding, relaxing, breathing and distracting yourself from the intensity of the later contractions can make it an experience you will remember with emotion. Fear and ignorance are likely to make it an experience you dread and one you will want to forget.

Bear this in mind, and you are less likely to set yourself an unattainable goal.

Relaxing genuinely helps: you have to accept what is happening to you in order to achieve relaxation. Accept things as they are in your real labour, not your dream labour. Accept yourself, coping or not coping, and you are more likely to come through in a positive way; to look back and say: 'Not perfect, but mine.'

393 Admission to hospital

Read 359 before you read this. Ringing the hospital before you leave home enables them to prepare for your arrival, to get your notes and prepare a room.

When you arrive, you will normally be seen by a midwife who will prepare you for the birth. She will ask you about labour so far, how it started, if your waters have broken, and the frequency and nature of your contractions. She will also ask if you have had any bleeding, and if you have moved your bowels recently.

She will then examine you internally to see how far your cervix has dilated. She will listen for the baby's heart beat and palpate your abdomen to discover the baby's position. She will also take your temperature, pulse and blood pressure, and ask for a urine sample.

You are unlikely to be shaved (390) but you may be given an enema or a suppository if you have not emptied your bowels recently. Many feel this to be unnecessary. Labour usually ensures a bowel movement without the help of soapy water. If you do not wish to have one, say so.

You may then be told to have a shower or a bath and shown either to your birthing room, or to a labour room in which you will stay for the first stage of your labour.

Your partner, and any other companions may join you now.

Emergency delivery

1 Call 999 for an ambulance.
2 Ask the mother to pant to keep from bearing down.
3 Offer comfort, reassurance, the odd joke.
4 If there is time, wash your hands, and her vaginal area, with soap and place the cleanest fabric you can find under her bottom.
5 Delivery is best in a fairly upright position. Lying flat on her back can compress the large blood vessels and reduce oxygen to the baby. Probably the best position is for the mother to sit on the floor with her back agaist a wall. Place a folded coat or cushion in the small of her back, and raise her bottom slightly off the floor. Lying full length on a sofa with her back against one arm is another sensible position.
6 A shower curtain or bin bags will protect the delivery surface. Or use newspapers or towels.
7 As the top of the baby's head begins to appear, tell the mother to pant and apply gentle counter pressure to the head. It should not pop out suddenly, but emerge slowly. *Never* pull the head.
8 If the cord is around the neck, don't panic. It often happens. Ask the mother to pant, hook a finger under the cord and gradually work it over the head. If the mother tries to push, tell her to puff and blow and keep one hand gently pressing against the head until the cord is free. Babies can tolerate shortage of oxygen to some extent, so don't worry if the cord tightens for a second or two.

When the head has been delivered, stroke the nose downwards, and the neck and chin upwards, to express mucus.
9 Take the head gently in both hands and press it down slightly, asking the mother to push at the same time. This will deliver the shoulder. As the top of the arm appears, carefully manipulate the head to free the other shoulder. The rest of the baby will follow.
10 Lift the baby gently on to the mother's abdomen. Keeping it warm is essential. Wrap it in a clean towel, a blanket, coat or even in newspaper if nothing else is at hand. Remember to cover the head, too. Be careful not to tug the cord.
11 If the baby is pink, moving and crying, just keep it warm and wait for the placenta to be delivered. Don't tug or pull the cord. If the placenta arrives before the ambulance, wrap it in paper. The hospital will want to see it. Don't try to cut or clamp the cord. Keep the placenta level, or higher than the baby, so that blood does not flow from the baby into

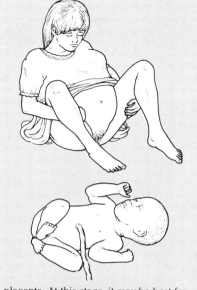

the placenta. At this stage, it may be best for the mother to lie flat. If there is much bleeding, she should keep her abdomen higher than her head.
12 If the baby is not breathing at birth, is blue or limp, try to stimulate breathing. Crying will make the baby breathe, so pinch, slap or rub the skin roughly with a towel or cloth.
13 If the airways seem blocked, place your mouth over the baby's nose and suck *very, very* gently.
14 If the baby still does not breathe, try gentle artificial respiration. Place your mouth over her nose and blow very softly. She needs little air to fill her lungs. Puff, pause, puff: just as you would breathe yourself.
15 Heart massage can also be given. At birth, a baby's heart beats at about 140 pulses per minute; 120 is two per second and easier to time. Using your fingers, tap the chest above the baby's heart, using a regular beat of 120 pulses per minute. The taps should be firm but not hard enough to break a rib.
16 Keep mother and baby warm until help arrives.
17 If the mother is bleeding, she should lie flat with her head lower than her bottom. This will help to stem the flow of blood.

In the car
Pull over, try to signal help. Keep the engine running and the heater on if it is cold. Sit the mother in the back seat with her back against the window then proceed as in **Emergency delivery**.

Labour

394 Definitions

Labour is traditionally divided into three stages.

The first is what we often think of as labour. It begins with the onset of contractions and lasts until the cervix is fully dilated. In most labours it is by far the longest stage. It can usually be subdivided into an early, middle and transitional phase.

The second stage is the delivery of the baby.

The third is the delivery of the placenta.

395 Stage one

It is a long, but not particularly intense, period during which the cervix dilates (opens) to 3 cm. See the illustration.

The gradual opening up of the cervix can in fact occur over days or weeks in which you may notice nothing more than the odd twinge or strong Braxton Hicks contraction; or, as described here, over a period of two to six hours during which you are unmistakably in labour.

Contractions in this phase are, typically, of 30 to 45 seconds' duration, often mild to moderately strong, and spaced at five to 20 minutes. They will generally progress to longer, stronger and more closely spaced intervals. Towards the end of this phase, you will feel a definite peak, or apex, to each contraction: see 399. For some women, labour does not have a regular pattern during this phase, a strong contraction being followed by a weaker one. You may even be unaware that anything is happening until you are 7 cm dilated.

The contractions in this phase may feel like low back pain, which gradually cramps across the abdomen, or they may feel like a gradual tightening. It is possible to understand how they might be interpreted as something other than pain.

You may well go to hospital only at the end of this phase.

396 What you might feel

You may well have backache with each contraction or, in some instances, constantly; see 359. You may have cramps like those when you are menstruating; diarrhoea, indigestion, a sensation of warmth and a bloody show; your membranes may rupture; see 361. But equally you may experience none of these things.

Dilating cervix

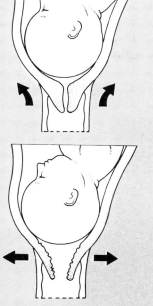

The cervix and its muscular structure can be likened to a bead curtain which hangs down from the uterus. It is pulled in tight at the base to fit snugly on to the top of the vagina. The beads are attached at the top to the fat barrel of the uterus. During labour, the strings are slowly pulled up. As they come up, the gap at the bottom grows wider. You cannot move these muscles as you can the muscles of your arms, but they work in much the same way. At the beginning of labour they are long and thin. During the first phase of stage one, they become shorter and fatter with each contraction, and in doing so gradually draw up and 'thin' or efface the cervix. As the cervix pulls up, it also pulls apart, opening up the birth channel.

You will feel excited, relieved and uncertain; a little anxious and fearful perhaps; or you could feel completely relaxed and chatty.

Towards the end of this phase, the contractions will have become fairlyfrequent and quite strong.

397 What to do

Relax, but don't take to your bed. Make some soup, take a gentle walk, have a warm bath or shower. A light meal is sensible: soup, a baked potato or some toast or sandwiches. Avoid meat, fats, and any food you find hard to digest. Don't overeat, this may give you indigestion or make you sick later.

Try to sleep if it is night time. Not easy, but you may have a long day ahead. Lie on your side, or you if you find it more comfortable, sit upright, well supported.

A glass of wine may help you relax. If you cannot sleep, rest as best you can, or get up and potter, perhaps making a post-birth snack for you both – you may find yourself hungry if you deliver just after the evening meal has been served and you miss it. Check your hospital bag. Go through the relaxation techniques and your breathing with your partner.

If it is daytime, put your partner on alert. He probably does not need to rush home yet, but get him to ring you every half hour or so until you have some idea how quickly things are progressing.

Resist any urge you may get to nest-build. The stove does not need cleaning.

Try to distract yourself from the labour. Watch TV or a video, play games, do crosswords. I found it difficult to read at this stage, even when there were large gaps between contractions.

Urinate frequently to prevent the badder becoming distended. Tell yourself now that you must go on the hour, every hour, throughout the labour. Often the urge to urinate gets lost in the contractions and you could go for 12 hours without noticing.

Time your contractions from start to finish, and from the start of one contraction to the start of the next.

398 What a man can do

Be there. Take the complaints and give in return love and support. Deal with midwives, doctors, machines, forms.

Get involved. Practise timing her contractions. Give soothing and comfort by massaging her back, and stroking her stomach. Run a bath and wash her gently. Hold her against you as the contractions come. Stay calm.

If you are anxious, have a drink. You could transfer your anxiety to her. See 402.

399 Stage one, second phase

This is usually shorter than the first, lasting, on average, two to three and a half

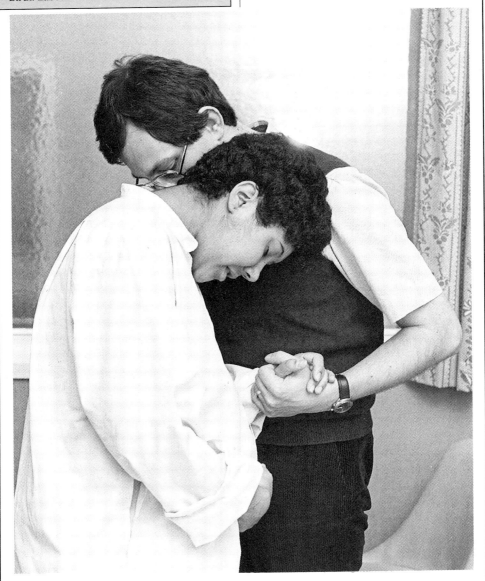

hours. But it is highly variable.

Contractions are much stronger and more frequent; more is accomplished in less time. The muscles of the cervix continue to open the birth channel from 3 cm to 7 cm. Contractions feel much more intense, are about three to four minutes apart and last 40 seconds to a minute. The pattern may still not be regular, but the contractions have a definite peak: a feeling of pull-hold-relax. The peak will feel as if it lasts for about half the length of each contraction. You will begin to understand what is meant by the peak (apex) of the contraction.

You will find that you are no longer able to keep talking through each contraction.

Unless you are giving birth at home, you must move to hospital during this phase.

400 What you will feel

Increasingly uncomfortable. If at first you could understand how contractions could be perceived as something other than pain, now you are probably beginning to change your mind. They stop you in mid-sentence, mid-thought.

You may get increasing backache and discomfort in the top of your legs.

There will be an increase in the level of

vaginal bleeding. Your membranes will probably rupture, or be ruptured for you; see 391.

Your back may still hurt. You will feel restless, and your confidence may begin to waver. Labour may begin to seem endless.

It is difficult to relax or to do anything between contractions. Labour is taking over. Some women find themselves becoming completely absorbed in the work; easily concentrating on the work in hand, relaxing and breathing through each contraction. You may become excited about the job, or you may find concentration impossible.

401 What you should do

Stay as relaxed as possible, especially during contractions. Try to keep moving as long as you can, since labour may slow down once you start to rest.

Sit propped up on the bed or delivery couch and relax with each contraction. You may still be able to walk about. If this is comfortable, do so, falling into your partner's arms for support as each contraction rises. Start the breathing exercises as soon as you are no longer able to talk through the contractions.

If you feel the exercises are not helping, or are making you tense, concentrate on relaxation for a while before starting them again. If these don't seem to help, or you cannot remember what to do, forget them. Worrying about getting it right may do more harm than good.

Don't eat or drink. A damp sponge may be used to moisten your mouth.

Conserve your energy. Think of lying on that beautiful beach with the waves pounding in the distance, the sun beating warmly on your back. Try to relax between contractions; more important, try to relax through them.

Keep on peeing, on the hour.

If you are finding labour is much more difficult than you had imagined, do not be too proud to ask for pain relief.

Most doctors will talk it through with you. You may feel better once you have said "I will if it gets worse"; you may even find you can carry on without drugs.

402 What a man can do

Close the door, turn down the lights; relax and help her to relax.

Continue to massage, hold, stroke and gently talk her through the contractions. If you can, let her sit between your legs,

resting her back against you. Stay calm.

Ask her which forms of massage help most, and try them out.

Take her foot in your hands and press your finger into the ball of her foot. Move it around to find the pressure point which will reduce the pain of the contraction; see 380.

Warm her feet if they are cold.

Time the contractions. If there is a foetal monitor, ask how to read it and warn her of the contractions as they come. If you place a hand an her abdomen, you can act as her monitor by feeling the contractions rise and fall.

Breathe with her through difficult contractions. Tap out the rhymes with her. Sing the distracting songs together.

But don't keep her at it if she doesn't want them any more. Let her say how it should be.

Be her spokesman. Tell the doctors and midwives anything you think might help her. Fight her battles if she wants them fought – but do it out of the room: don't upset her.

If she shows signs of hyperventilating (she will feel dizzy, light-headed and her legs will go numb), cup your hands over her mouth and nose. This way she can re-breath the air she has just breathed out. One air breath, one cupped breath, until she feels better. If you brought your sandwiches in a paper bag, use the bag instead of your hands.

Reassure, praise, remind her she is getting there. Don't pretend there is no pain. Tell her you understand. Know this: she needs your love and empathy.

Ask her if she can really manage without drugs. If you decided together to have a drug-free birth, she may not want to let you down.

Walk around with her and hold her through the contractions.

Help and remind her to relax. Remind her to pee on the hour. Dampen her mouth. Find out if there is any ice for her to suck.

Wash her body with a cool damp cloth; keep rinsing it under a cold running tap.

Try to distract her with games, silly or sensible. "What do you think Queen Victoria said when she was in labour?" Accept her bad temper, irritation and lack of sympathy. It is hard for her to think of anyone else just now. She does need you, even if she does not show it.

Search out the doctor if she asks for medication.

Stimulate her breasts if labour seems to be slowing down. Roll the nipples between your fingers. See 407.

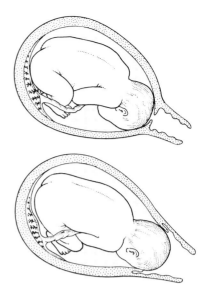

403 What hospital staff will do

Help you to relax. Reassure you that all is going to plan.

Check the baby's condition by looking at the foetal monitor or listening to the heart beat. Check your show for the greenish stain that can indicate foetal distress.

Assess how far the baby has moved down the birth channel.

Check blood pressure, and the strength, timing, and duration of contractions. Assess the progress of labour by internal examination.

If labour slows, it will be stimulated by rupturing the membranes or giving oxytocin. Breast stimulation may be suggested.

Drugs will be administered if necessary.

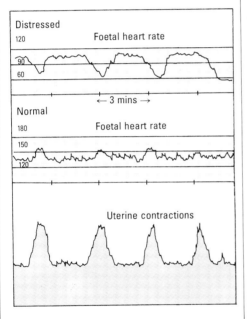

404 Stage one, third phase: transition

This is the most difficult part of labour: exhausting, intense. There is a sudden speeding-up of contractions. They come without mercy. For a description of how they feel, see 399.

Each now lasts about 90 seconds and often the next seems to begin before the first is over. Indeed, you may begin to wonder what they mean by apex. Some contractions have more than one peak. Up it goes again before the first peak has died. There is no time to relax between peaks. That final 3 cm of dilation will take beween 15 minutes and one hour. That is the best thing that can be said about transition.

405 What you feel

You will begin to feel the pressure of the baby in the rectum and the lower back. You may not yet feel the urge to push, but you may feel that the intense pressure may make you soil the sheets. This worries many women. You may well soil them, many do, but no one will mind. It is a trivial detail. Body temperature is erratic: you will feel hot and cold, bathed in sweat, then shivering. Your show will increase as the final part of the cervix is pulled apartand the small blood vessels around the neck burst. You may begin to tremble uncontrollably, especially your legs, which can feel clammy and cold. You may suddenly feel (or be) sick.

The flow of blood and energy to the hard-working muscles of the cervix may leave the brain a little short of oxygen. This is not serious, but it may make you feel sleepy or slightly befuddled between contractions. You will feel exhausted, competely taken over by the labour.

You will probably feel bad-tempered and out of control.

Transition makes you feel vulnerable, overwhelmed and disoriented. Something is almost bound to irritate you. A dirty cup, your partner's touch, the way the curtains are drawn. I remember getting irritated because the picture on the wall was slightly crooked.

Relaxation seems impossible, you may feel the breathing has gone wrong (and that you cannot be bothered with it any more). You may tell everyone you do not want the baby, never did, never will. Ask to be sent home, or demand all the pain relief you can get (which at this stage may be none).

406 What you can do

Hang on. It does not last long. Think how much you have achieved. This is the beginning of the end. It does not go on like this, the next bit is more exciting and easier. Don't worry that you are not coping, few women cope well at this stage.

If you feel like pushing, pant and blow instead. The cervix needs to be completely dilated before you push. If you push too soon, you will bruise the cervix and the swelling will cause a delay in delivering the baby. The midwife will tell you when it is safe to push.

Take what comfort you can, but feel free to say what you want. Many women don't want fussing or touching at this stage. Let your partner know if this is so.

Keep up your distraction techniques. Between contractions, try slow, deep, rhythmic breathing. It may calm you.

407 What a man can do

Stay tuned to her mood. If she wants to be left alone, leave her. Accept her irritation as normal for a woman in transition: there is no need to feel you are failing her, even though you probably feel helpless and left out. (She would almost certainly say you were the lucky one.)

If she wants encouragement, praise, sympathy or someone to cry out to, be that person. If she wants to ignore you, let her.

Give counter-pressure to her back if it aches, but only if she wants you to do so.

Keep warning her about the onset of contractions by watching the monitor or feeling her abdomen.

Tell the doctor if she wants to push. Mop her brow, and wait for the next exciting stage. See 412.

408 What hospital staff will do

Continue as before, supporting, monitoring and checking.

Prepare to deliver the baby. In some hospitals this may mean moving to the delivery room.

Examine you internally to check if you are fully dilated before giving you the go-ahead for stage two.

409 Stage two

Until now you have been simply taking everything your muscles can give.

Now you have a role to play. Although the contractions are still strong. and pushing a 7½-lb (3.4-kg) baby out through your vagina is hard work, many women find the second stage of labour easier than the first.

Pushing, or 'bearing down', is not essential, it only helps the baby out. The uterine contractions are strong enough to expel the baby by themselves. Remember this if you find that you have no urge to push, or feel too tired to co-operate. It will be quicker if you help, but it will happen even if you do not.

The second stage of labour generally lasts about an hour with a first baby, rather less with subsequent births. Two hours is probably the maximum; after this most doctors would use forceps to lift the baby out of the vagina.

Bearing down to push a baby out of the birth channel is an instinctive response. As you feel the urge to push, you will automatically take a deep breath, expanding your chest and pushing the diaphragm downwards, which in turn presses the top of the uterus.

It seems natural to bend your legs, open them slightly and strain. As if, it is often said, you were trying to pass a melon. Except, of course, you are trying to pass it along a slightly different route.

The more upright you are at this time, the easier it will be to push. Lie flat and the baby has to travel uphill; squat and it has gravity to help it.

The contractions are now more regular than in transition, lasting between 60 and 90 seconds, often with longer gaps between them. They are, for many women, less intense than the contractions of transition.

You may feel you have time to catch your breath, even time to think between contractions.

My two sons share a birthday. I clearly remember watching the clock during the second stage of my last labour, having time to wonder how close their birth hours would be. (They were spot-on, to the minute.)

410 What you will feel

An overwhelming desire to push is perhaps the most common sign that this stage has begun, although it is far from universal. You will probably feel you are getting a second wind, perhaps because of the breathing space between contractions. But if the first stage has been drawn out, you may feel extremely tired and unable to summon up much enthusiasm for what follows.

At first you will feel a tremendous rectal pressure as the baby moves down into the vagina. As the uterus begins to expel the baby, you will see the movement clearly if you look at your abdomen.

There will be an increase in the bloody show, as more small blood vessels break and the uterus forces blood into the vagina. Again (see 405), you may unintentionally urinate or defecate. Sometimes you may think you have soiled the sheets when you have not.

As the baby moves into the vagina, you will feel a tingling and burning sensation. Pushing is hard work, but it does not hurt. The powerful pressure of the baby against the pelvic floor has an anaesthetic effect, so this stage is often less painful than we imagine it will be. But for some, the sensation is rather like being split in half from the crutch upwards.

You may feel relief once you can begin to push the baby out, perhaps exhilaration as the baby's head begins to appear. But don't be surprised if you feel disinterested, many do.

411 What you can do

Get into your chosen birth position. See illustrations.

During pushing, the anal area and the pelvic floor should be completely relaxed. Listen carefully to instructions, pushing when told, panting when necessary. It is the smooth co-ordinated pushes that do the job. The midwife may say something like 'Use your contraction'; she means co-ordinate your push with a contraction.

Do what comes naturally, pushing as you feel the urge. Take a few deep breaths as the contraction starts, hold and push down with all your might as the contraction reaches its peak. Push until you need another breath. You may get as many as five pushes from a long contraction. Use them.

If you feel no urge (as, indeed, you may not if you have had an epidural), listen carefully as the midwife guides you through the delivery.

Stop pushing when you are told. Rapid crowning can cause tearing; the midwife will slow things down for a while. You will also need to wait if the cord needs to be freed from the baby's neck. Pant or blow until you are told to push again.

Remember to watch for the head in your

Delivery positions

Squatting or semi-squatting are widely acknowledged to be the best because they use gravity to help the baby on her way.

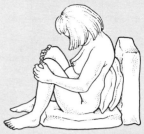

Sitting nearly straight is probably the commonest modern delivery position: you can hold on to your knees during contractions and give some support to your head by dropping your chin to your chest. Relax between contractions by lying back on the pillows. This position enables hospital staff to get a clear view of what is going on.

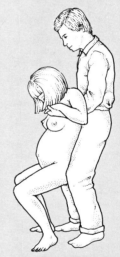

The supported squat: Your partner takes your weight by holding you under your arms and letting you lean back against his thighs.

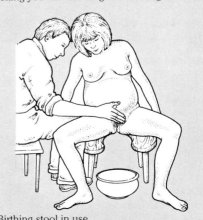

Birthing stool in use

mirror, but don't despair if you see the head disappearing back into the vagina. It is normal to go two steps forward and one back at this stage.

412 What a man can do

You, the father-to-be, have the best view of what is happening.

Enjoy it. Feel the excitement and anticipation. If you find in your excitement that you have almost forgotten your partner, don't worry too much. She is probably too engrossed to remember you, either. Don't be hurt if she does not meet your eye: her energies have another focus.

Guide her if she wants you to: although the midwife or doctor has taken over, you can still reinforce their instructions with a squeeze of the hand or a gentle whisper. Don't feel inhibited by the hospital staff. This is your baby.

If you can support her back, or give counter-pressure, this may be particularly helpful, especially if she has had a 'backache' labour; see 358.

Tell her what you can see and hold the mirror so that she can see too. If you have no mirror, a running commentary is essential. Take her hand and feel the head together.

You might like to ask if you can catch the baby as it comes out, or be the one to place it on her abdomen. You might also ask if you can cut the cord.

It is perhaps symbolically right that you should cut that tie. See 421.

413 What the hospital staff will do

The support, and monitoring of mother and baby, will have continued. Hospital staff have probably visited you intermittently, but now they appear in force and will stay with you until after the baby is born. They will prepare for the birth, if necessary perform an episiotomy (425), and decide whether forceps are needed. If the second stage is long, or the baby is not progressing, they will use forceps to turn the head from a difficult position, or to lift the baby out of the vagina. Once the head emerges, they will free the air passages and make sure she is breathing, taking any measures which are necessary to ensure her general health.

They will assist the birth of the shoulders and the rest of the body, place the baby on your stomach, keep her warm, then clamp, and later, cut the umbilical cord; see 418.

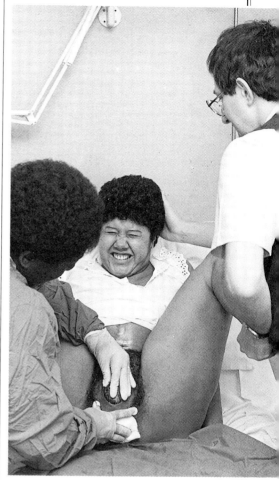

414 Crowning

This is the moment when the baby's head first appears at the perineum. It will slip back slightly before coming forward again with the next contraction. Getting it right out may take a surprisingly large number of contractions. Each time the head reappears, it opens the vulva a little wider. The perineum bulges; and you will look as if you have a ball wedged inside you. It is usual to feel a burning and stinging sensation as the baby is crowned. You can get an idea of how it feels by opening your mouth wide and pulling your lips sideways at the corners.

As soon as you feel it, you should stop pushing and pant, letting the uterus do the work for you. Your additional effort is not needed now; force can cause tissue damage. Make a conscious effort to relax your pelvic floor. As the burning subsides, the baby's head will stretch the vaginal tissue so thin that the nerves are blocked. No pain messages are sent to the brain and you will feel blissfully numb.

Delivery

415 Birth

This is when you may be given an episiotomy. Automatic episiotomies used to be common and still are common in some hospitals, but pressure from women is calling this procedure into question. It is, nevertheless, sometimes necessary. Without an episiotomy, I was badly torn with my first child. A small cut and a few stitches would have been infinitely preferable to the extensive repair job necessary after that birth. See 425.

It is possible to stretch the perineum during pregnancy, and this will reduce the necessity for an episiotomy; see 426.

As the head is born, you will feel as if something is being passed: a feeling, I always found, adequately expressed only by a deep, whole-body grunt. The baby's face will almost certainly be pointing down towards your rectum, but she will quickly turn to one side as the shoulders are born.

It is over. One contraction will deliver the first shoulder, the next the second, and the midwife will lift your child on to your stomach.

416 What the baby does

Some cry as they are delivered; most will be crying within a minute or two.

If she does not breathe straight away, the midwife will clear the air passages and give oxygen. Don't be alarmed by the sudden activity. She will be returned to you as soon as she is breathing normally; see 433. She will soon be looking at you wide-eyed.

417 What you should do

Hold her, and share her. You may want to try to put her to your breast straight away. My first-born and I were both too full of pethidine (and I too inexperienced) to succeed. Don't worry if you cannot manage; see 467-469.

418 Cutting the cord

Some medical staff will clamp and cut as soon as the baby is born, some will wait for the placenta to be delivered. Others wait for the cord to stop pulsating.

Opposite: Contrasting birth positions; see also box on page 148.

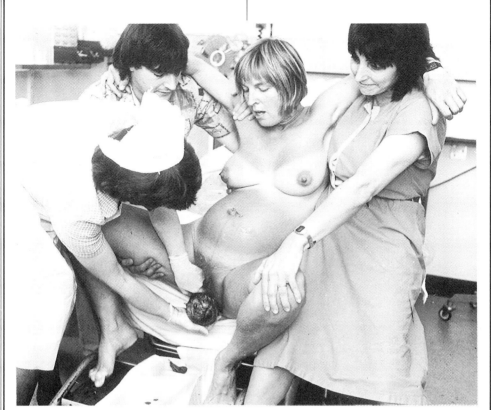

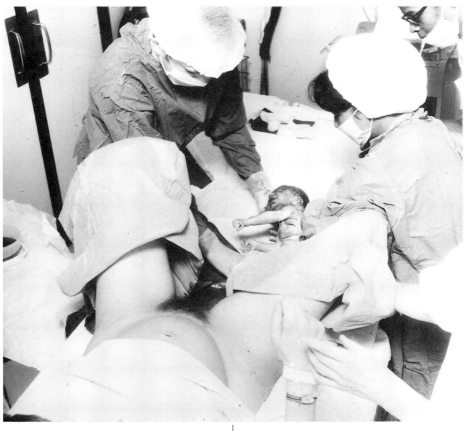

151

419 Greeting the baby

Your hand automatically goes out to touch her gently. You may, or may not, feel a surge of love for this creature; and it does not matter. Many women find the actual presence of their baby something of a let-down; are unsure of how she got there; unsure even, that this one is theirs. Try not to have big expectations of this moment; then, if you feel strangely detached, it will not disturb you.

No one can prove it, but I suspect love for a new child is rarely instant; like all good things, it needs to grow. See 439-449.

420 Stage three

Your attention is elsewhere, but your uterus, working independently of your conscious mind, keeps on pushing and squeezing. The placenta, left behind in the uterus, is wrenched from its wall. The cervix is still dilated, so as the uterus contracts further, the placenta is pushed out into the vagina. With your help it, too, will be forced into the world, its job completed. This whole third stage rarely takes more than half an hour and often considerably less. The midwife may assist the process by pressing on the uterus and pulling gently on the cord. You will usually be given a drug to assist rapid expulsion: either a synthetic form of oxytocin or syntometrine, which combines syntocinon with ergometrine; see 427.

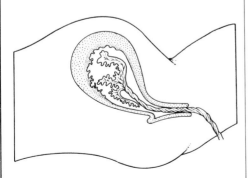

The oxytocin makes the womb contract within two or three minutes of the injection, and the ergometrine causes further sutained contractions for the next seven minutes. The cord will be clamped to stop the drug passing to the baby. You probably will not notice the injection given as the shoulders are delivered.

The placenta will be checked to see if it is complete. If it is not, the doctor will examine the uterus manually for any bits left behind. A retained placenta will usually be removed under general anaesthetic.

421 What you will both feel

Birth takes people in different, often unpredictable, ways. Sometimes you just feel tired; pushing out the placenta is an effort. Sometimes you have a great burst of energy, anything seems possible, and pushing out the placenta is a mere inconvenience. You hardly pause as you chat to those around you and look at your baby.

After a difficult labour, tiredness, relief and flatness are perhaps to be expected, but they can occur after a short labour, too. My daughter was born in 55 minutes, after a wonderful, energetic pregnancy in which everything was possible. I felt so good that I only stopped work six hours before she was born. But immediately after the birth, I felt I could have slept for a year; she was sleepy, too. Two hours later, I was wide awake.

When my youngest son was born, my labour lasted 12 hours. The pregnancy had been exhausting, and yet at the moment he was born, I swear I could have danced all night; so I think could he. He remained awake all the next day, wide-eyed, watching the sunlight through the window. I don't know if this matching of mood was a coincidence. Both labours had been drug-free.

You are, at any rate, likely to feel thirsty, probably hungry too, particularly if the labour has been long. Fruit juice and a light snack are welcome. Some women suddenly get shivery; their legs shake like jelly.

You may feel excited, relieved, unreal. Or you may feel none of these.

How you feel towards your partner could take you by surprise. You may have waited for this moment, seen it as the crowning of the experience you have shared, a time of immense closeness and love. But you may not.

There is nothing wrong: deep emotion is often felt in this strange detached way. We do not all greet birth with ecstasy, just as we do not all greet death with howls of pain. You may both feel an initial emotion almost of disbelief. It will go.

For his part, your partner may also have mixed feelings. He could feel flat; he could feel a surge of love and admiration for the

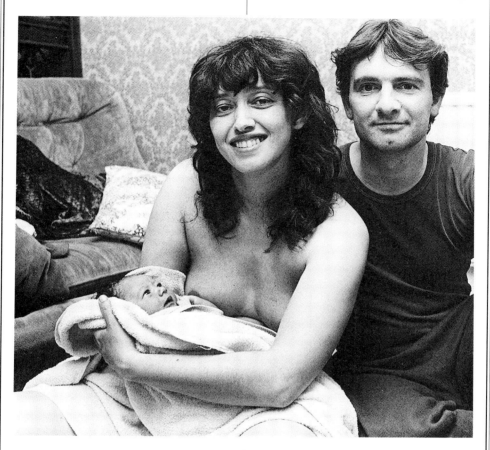

mother of his child. It is not unusual for him to feel a shock of emotion which reduces him to tears. He has witnessed one of life's great moments. Just then, there was pain, blood and mess. Now there is this tiny form; that physical presence and the first cries can carry a huge impact. Before, the baby was an idea; now it is flesh. The translation, before his eyes, is very moving.

If it is your first child, he is seeing, again with a new clarity, that now there are three of you, and life will, indeed, never be the same. See 423.

422 What you can do

Help to expel the placenta; be patient while tears are repaired; nurse the baby; relax and enjoy the moment, don't worry if it all seems such an anti-climax; don't worry if your mood does not match your partner's.

423 What a man can do

See 421. Many men say that the profound experience of witnessing a birth is reason enough on its own to be present. That aside, he can now assume roles that he may find more natural than those of birth attendant. He can find her some fruit juice and a snack; open the champagne; hold the baby; understand; take pictures – if he remembers. See 449.

424 What hospital staff may do

Stitch up any tears; check the level of vaginal bleeding (it should be similar to a heavy period); clean you up; give you a clean night dress; wheel you and your baby to the post-natal ward.

425 Episiotomy

This is a small cut made in the perineum to ease the baby's passage. It is usually given as the head presses down on the pelvic floor, causing numbness, and you will, almost certainly, feel not a thing. If there is time, an anaesthetic may be given a couple of minutes beforehand.

The incision is made either along the

the mid-line, towards the anus, or (most commonly) medio-laterally, slanting to one side. (A mid-line cut can cause rectal damage which is why it is almost universally discontinued.)

Episiotomy should not be performed without reason. If a large tear seems likely, a cut is considered easier to stitch. (Each layer of tissue must be stitched separately, and this can be difficult with a large, jagged tear.) But a tiny tear heals more readily than a large cut, and many people feel that once the cut has been made, there is more, rather than less, likelihood of tearing.

An episiotomy is almost certainly necessary if:

- You have a forceps delivery.
- Labour needs to be brought to a rapid conclusion. If, for example, you, or the baby are in distress, or if she is premature.
- It seems likely that you will tear badly.
- It is a breech delivery; see 428.

You should not have an episiotomy because someone thinks:

- It is routine.
- A stretched perineum might cause later womb prolapse. There is no evidence for this.
- Stitching will tighten the perineum, thereby heightening the pleasure of sexual intercourse. This is a male myth: along with the bigger the better comes the tighter the better.

Better for whom is the appropriate question here. Episiotomy is certainly not better for the one who has to put up with the stiches. It almost certainly makes sex painful for women in the short (and often the longer) term; see 560-562.

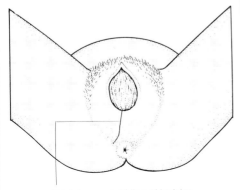

Episiotomy: usual line of incision

426 Avoiding an episiotomy

First check on hospital policy. If they routinely do episiotomies, make it clear that you don't want to be part of the routine.

Take steps to avoid the possibility of tearing by stretching the perineum. This involves perineal massage in the last two months of pregnancy:

Take a large pot of cocoa butter or groundnut oil, and massage the labia, vaginal area and perineum generally until all the oil has been absorbed. This should take four or five minutes. Then, taking more cream, insert several fingers just into the vagina and gently open them, slowly stretching the outer lips. Continue until you feel it beginning to burn, and hold it at this point for several minutes.

Do this every day: you will notice that the burning sensation will happen later and later. The aim is to be able to open the vagina to 2½-3 in (6-7 cm) before the burning begins. It will probably take about one month to work up to this.

427 Syntometrine

The drug was developed to help prevent haemorrage after delivery (postpartum) caused as the placenta comes away from the uterus. The risk increases with each delivery. Syntometrine was originally given to women having a seventh or eighth child or after a twin pregnancy, but now it is quite routine in some hospitals, despite the fact that haemorrage is rare in first and second deliveries. Side effects:

- It can make your blood pressure drop.
- It can cause vomiting.
- It sometimes closes the neck of the womb before the placenta is expelled.
- It may delay milk production.

If you start to bleed, an injection directly into a vein can work within 45 seconds, so unless haemorrage is likely, it would seem best not to give syntomine until bleeding actually happens.

However, if you have had oxytocin to induce birth, or to drive labour, or if you have had an epidural, you are at risk of haemorraging and should not refuse the drug. In any event, having decided not to take the drug, be sure that no one pulls on the cord.

428 Breech delivery

About three per cent of babies are born

bottom first. Properly managed, a breech birth is no more difficult than a normal, head-down birth.

You will almost certainly be offered an epidural anaesthetic if you are to deliver a breech baby vaginally. This is not because it is necessarily more painful; in the early stages, there is no difference between the two presentations. A breech labour does, however, sometimes need emergency Caasarian section, which can be performed quickly if the epidural is already effective.

Breech labours are potentially problematic, especially if the baby's bottom passes into the birth channel before it has opened wide enough to let the head pass through. In a normal delivery, the head lays out the path which the body will follow; where it can go, so can the body. A baby's bottom is smaller than its head, and if the head cannot follow the bottom, the head may come under pressure.

Delivery will almost certainly need the assistance of forceps, which in turn means an episiotomy; see 425.

Most early breech presentations turn automatically to the correct position at about 30 weeks. Failing this, your doctor may attempt to turn the baby manually in the weeks before birth. However, this is not always successful.

A vaginal delivery will not usually be attempted unless the baby is a frank breech – that is, if his legs are tucked up against his face. If the baby is in an open breech position, or is a footling breech, with one leg dangling, a Caesarian is the usual outcome. It will also be considered if the foetus is large, premature, or if there is any doubt that the mother's pelvis is inadequate.

There is an increased likelihood of breech presentation in premature babies. About 40 per cent of breech births are by Caesarian section.

429 Caesarian section

In the past, this procedure was always carried out under general anaesthetic. Today, you can have a Caesarian under epidural; see 377. You will be conscious and can see the baby emerging. In some hospitals, husbands are allowed to watch.

'Caesarian' refers to Julius Caesar, purportedly born in this way: 'section' simply means surgical operation.

Your pubic hair is shaved, and a catheter is inserted into your bladder to keep it empty. A glucose drip will be

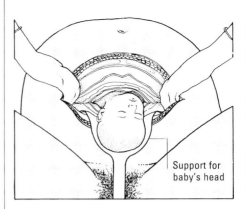

Support for baby's head

inserted in your arm. All this is carried out before you receive any anaesthetic. You need to have the smallest dose possible: no one wants to waste time doing things under anaesthetic which can be done while you are awake, and it is important not to anaesthetize the baby.

If you have an epidural anaesthetic, the needle will now be inserted into your lower back; see 377. A screen will be put up so that you cannot see the operation taking place.

Once the anaesthetic has taken effect, a small cut is made in the lower abdomen, in the vicinity of the bikini line. You may feel this happening, but it will not hurt. A second cut is made in the lower part of the uterus. The amniotic sac is ruptured, and the waters drained. You will hear this happening. It is something like a bath being drained noisily.

The baby is about to be born. If you want to watch, ask if they will lower the screens. The baby is eased out by hand, or using hands and forceps. You may feel pulling and tugging sensations, and pressure, but it will not hurt. You will then be given a dose of oxytocin to help the womb to contract.

It takes little more than five minutes. Next, the placenta is removed, then the doctor will take a quick look at your reproductive organs to check if everything is in order. If all is well, you may be given the baby to hold while you are being stitched up.

Each layer is stitched separately. It will take a little time. Blood and other fluids will be drained by suction before the surgeon finally stiches up the abdominal wall.

Don't worry if you find that the baby has been taken to the intensive care nursery. This is standard procedure in some hospitals, and it does not mean that anything is wrong.

430 No progress

Labour can be slow; it can even stop.

'A prolonged pause' (a latent phase) usually means that the first part of labour has lasted more than 20 hours. It occurs for a number of reasons.

Possibly, labour has not really started. Perhaps you have had too much medication. Panic can also cause delay.

You can help matters along by keeping upright and active. A full bladder will slow things down, so empty it as often as possible.

The doctor may suggest breaking the waters or inducing labour with a drip; or a Caesarian may be considered.

'Dysfunction of the active phase' is said to occur if dilation progresses at less than 1cm per hour with a first baby.

The doctor will consider whether the baby's head is too big to pass through your pelvis. A pelvic examination (possibly using an ultra-sound scan) can assess this. If the pelvis is too small, a Caesarian section will be performed.

When no progress is made over two hours, you are said to have 'arrested dilation'. In about half these cases, the pelvis is too small; in others, the uterus is exhausted. If the baby can be delivered vaginally, you will be given an oxytocin drip, which will, in most cases,re-establish labour.

'Abnormal descent' of the foetus is said to occur when the baby moves down the birth channel at less than 1cm per hour. In most instances, delivery is slow but uneventful. Treatment, both medical, and non-medical, is as before.

A 'prolonged second stage' is one that lasts more than two hours. Many doctors routinely use forceps in such cases. Gravity will help. Occasionally, an emergency Caesarian may be needed.

431 APGAR scores

Your baby's condition will be rated at one minute after birth and again five minutes later.

The doctor will check her appearance (A), pulse or heartbeat (P), grimace or reflex (G), activity or muscle tone (A) and respiration (R). The acronym APGAR is also the name of the paediatrician who developed the scale.

Babies who score between 4 and 6 often need resuscitation. Those who score under 4 need more dramatic life-saving

techniques. A score of 7 or more at 5 minutes means a good prognosis. However, recent research suggests that many babies with low scores at this point do not have any later problems.

432 Forceps

The original instrument was designed in 1598 by the British surgeon Peter Chamberlen, whose family kept it a secret for their own commercial gain until 1800. Nowadays, forceps are used to speed up the second stage of delivery if there is foetal or maternal distress. There are two types: High Keillands or Neville-Barnes to turn a baby's head from a difficult position; and Low Wrigleys to lift a baby out. Vacuum extraction is sometimes used instead if this is the hospital's preference.

433 First breath

We wait for the first cry, because we know that this means life. It may happen even before the whole baby is born. Most babies begin to breath two or three minutes after their mouths leave their mother's vulva.

She may gasp, she may splutter; she does not have to cry. A cry forces open the lungs; that she breathes is important, not that she cries.

Sometimes the airways need clearing before crying begins, and sometimes breathing needs stimulating. She will have been practising breathing movements inside the womb, sucking amniotic fluid in and out. Before the first breath, the lungs are collapsed and sticky; when it is taken, air rushes in, opening up the airways and the tiny air sacs. As the lungs expand, blood rushes to them, and so independent life begins.

434 Stretched

Will your vagina ever be the same again? Strictly speaking, no. Its ribbed structure will not return, and the contraceptive diaphragm you had before you were pregnant will probably be too small. But the vagina can return almost to its former condition. It is a highly elastic organ, capable of gripping a small tampon, and passing a 7½-lb (3.4-kg) baby without tearing.

But will sexual pleasure ever be quite the same? Yes. Perhaps not for a few months, but yes it will. The small

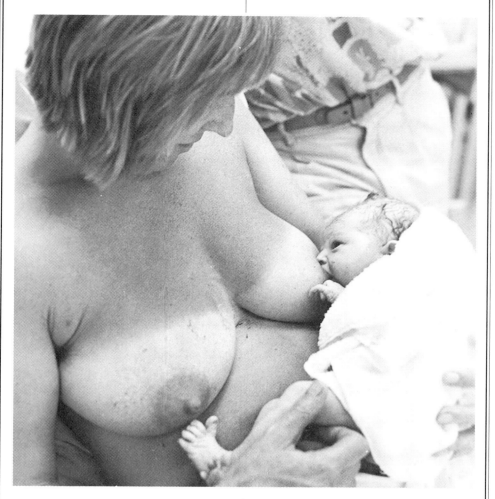

difference in size is more than compensated for by the increased awareness and control of the muscles of your vagina gained by pelvic floor exercises, see page 39.

435 Handicapped

About one in 25 babies has a congenital abnormality. Half of these will be minor, an extra finger, a loose hip, an extra set of nipples. One in 50 will have more serious abnormalities, some inherited, some caused by diseases such as *Rubella*, but most from unknown causes.

If she is handicapped, you will almost certainly feel anger, pity, grief, disappointment and possibly guilt: you will need to talk about your feelings but you will also need practical help in caring for a baby who is different. She may be difficult to handle and to feed, she may cry more. You will also need to know the long-term prognosis.

For now, she will probably be taken to the special baby care unit. Your doctor, midwife and health visitor will all offer what help they can in the first weeks. But it can be difficult to concentrate on a child's positive qualities, difficult to talk about her problems, even with friends. They probably don't know what to say or do.

Often the most realistic help comes from people who have experienced similar problems. Many self-help groups exist. Your doctor may know of one, so may someone at the social service department or the hospital where the baby was born.

436 Still birth

Most mothers reflect on this nightmare from time to time. The loss of a child, even a child you have never known, is the loss of hopes and dreams. It is tragic.

Remember, still birth happens rarely – about 15 in every 1,000 births, most of

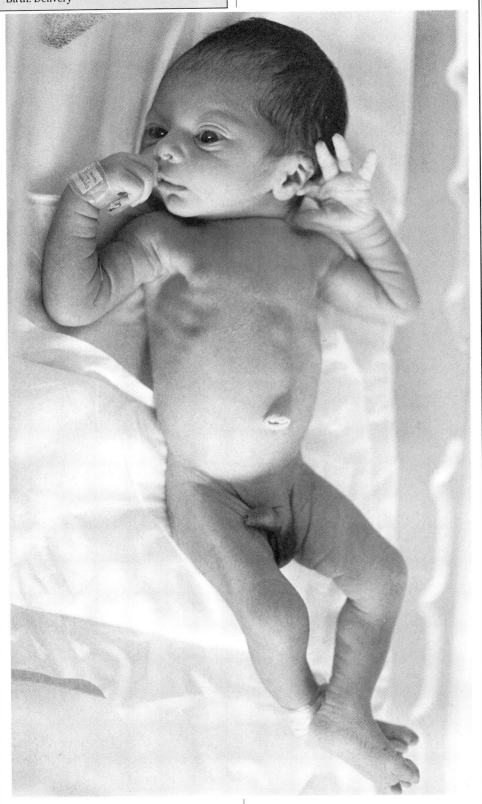

which could not have been prevented. The baby may be severely handicapped, or just too tiny to survive. Perhaps the largest group is those in which the placenta has not been functioning.

Holding and touching the dead baby helps many parents with their grief. When a baby which grows inside you is born, then dies and disappears from your life, it is difficult to have a focus for the grief you feel. There are organizations who can offer counsel and support.

437 Looking at her

New-born babies are always beautiful, however they look, and sometimes they do look a little odd. Most of these oddities are natural.

You might see:

● Swelling of the genitals. Both boys and girls may have surprisingly large genitals at birth. They are normal, and will appear a more normal size in a few weeks time. Girls may have a milky vaginal secretion; again, this will disappear. It happens as a result of the mother's hormones passing to the baby.

● Swollen breasts, and even milk-like liquid (witch's milk) are also due tomaternal hormones crossing the placenta.

● Lanugo: fine downy hair. Earlier in the pregnancy, it covered the whole baby, now it is most likely on the back, shoulders, ear tips and temples. It will disappear.

● Vernix caseosa, usually just called vernix: the waxy substance which covered the baby in the womb: how much depends on how mature she is. It will wash off.

● Hair: newborn hair is often a totally different colour to later hair. It can be short or almost shoulder length. It will fall out gradually over the next months.

● An oddly shaped head: often the head is moulded during birth to fit through the pelvis. Sometimes there is a bump on it, called a caput, caused by pressing against the cervix before it was fully dilated. The bump will disappear in a day or two; the moulded head will become round in a few weeks.

● Eyes of Caucasian babies are almost always blue, but they may go dark later. Dark-skinned races have brown-eyed babies. Watery eyes may mean that a tear-duct is blocked.

● White heads: these will disappear, as will rashes.

● Coffee-coloured spots: usually permanent birth marks.

● Stork marks: reddish blotches at the base of the skull and on the eyelids or forehead. Common in Caucasians, they, too, will disappear.

● Mongolian spots: these bluish-grey marks on the back, buttocks and occasionally the arms and thighs, look like bruises. They are common in Asians, southern Europeans and blacks. They usually disappear before the child reaches school-age.

● Strawberry marks: these raised, bright orange patches usually fade to a mottled grey, then disappear.

● Port wine stains are bigger. Again they often fade. If they persist, ask your doctor about treatment.

● A squint: if is present at birth it will usually disappear. If a squint persists after six months, consult your doctor.

● Jaundice: this is caused by an excess of the pigment bilirubin, produced in some babies by heavy turn-over of red blood cells which causes problems for the liver. Mild jaundice is treated with fluid and sunlight and normally disappears within a few days. If it is serious, your baby will not be allowed home until it is under control.

● Caul: very occasionally, a baby is born with some of the membrane still covering its head and body. Superstition has it that this is a sign of great fortune.

The Newborn

438 The alert baby

In the first hours after birth, most babies are awake and wide-eyed. She will pull faces, even poke out her tongue; she may even meet your eye. Though she can perceive little detail, she will notice the outline of your face, and especially the prominence of your hairline. She may well stare fascinated by the sparkle of a ring as it catches the sun.

Pleased to see you? That is not certain, but interested, certainly. Later she may be sleepy, much more like a doll. Now she is very much alive and loving her and interacting with her are easy. Later it will be much more one-way.

Falling in love is so much easier when you feel you are being loved in return. Wait a few hours and the magic might be over. But if you cannot take this opportunity to give her your undivided attention, don't worry. Time is on your side.

439 What mothers do

If mothers are given their babies immediately after birth, they explore them. If a baby is placed naked on the bed beside her, the mother will start by adjusting her position so that she is looking directly into the baby's eyes. Then she will speak gently and lovingly. Using first finger tips, then her whole hand she will feel the baby's body, smiling, asking questions. Some mothers offer the breast.

No one tells them what to do, they just do it. Middle-class mothers in Britain; poor mothers from deprived areas of the United States: they all behave in the same way.

What does this response amount to? Watch a child with a puppy. Is it much different? Do lovers act like this when they first share a bed? Maybe. Certainly, they do when they come together after separation. The behaviour is a means of rediscovering someone who already has a place in your heart; a greeting.

440 The growth of love

It is essential for mental health that an infant should experience a warm, intimate and continuous relationship with his mother (or permanent mother substitute who steadily mothers him) in which both find satisfaction and enjoyment.

John Bowlby's *Child Care and the Growth of Love,* from which this statement

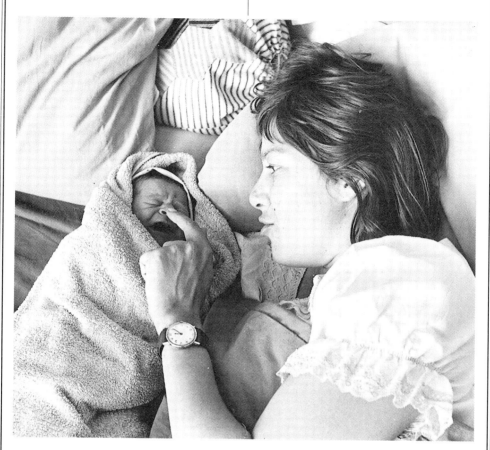

is taken, has probably had more influence on childcare practice than any other book. When your elder child comes to your hospital bed to meet his sister, or if later you stay with her in hospital, you have this book to thank. As you lie with your baby in a crib beside you, you can thank Bowlby too. It was not always so.

441 The bad old days

In the days when ordinary mothers had large families, little household help and few labour-saving appliances, birth was a time for necessary rest – in bed. For most of the population, health care was a luxury, and birth was one of the few occasions when a woman could be ordered to bed on medical authority.

Indeed separation of mother and newborn for long periods of the day and most of the night was, until recently, standard hospital procedure in most countries. It is often described as something done for hospital convenience, but I doubt it was as uncaring as that. Many women did need rest above all else.

And if they did not bond with their newborn in those first weeks, it might have been regarded as a blessing. The infant mortality rate was so high that many parents surely felt it was best not to love too much at first; indeed failure to bond to a very sick infant remains a reality, indeed an understandable defence mechanism.

442 Superglue

It is now almost a universal assumption that cuddling and holding babies in the early hours after birth is essential for the formation of the bond of love between mother and child. Some have even suggested that there is something special, critical, about being together directly after birth: that only then can some superglue bond a mother to her child.

But is the assumption correct? Or, perhaps more to the point, how true is it? It is obviously a key issue; so important, in fact, that in the detailed consideration that follows (443-449) I draw not only on scientific studies, but my personal experience. I honestly feel that in the end this subjective evidence is as valuable as any other.

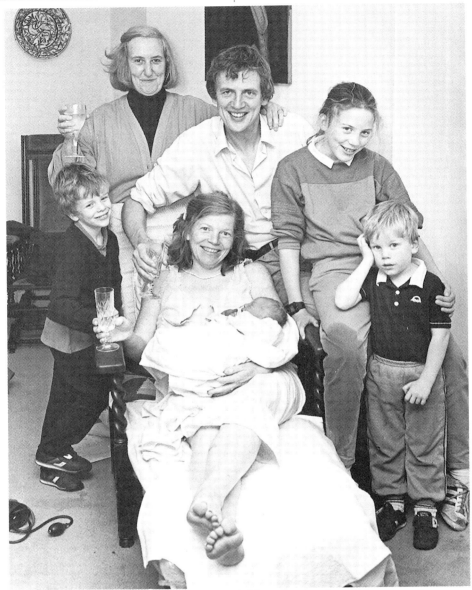

443 Bonding – theoretical evidence

The research that forms the basis of our ideas about bonding comes from many sources: from studies of motherless monkeys, who never form adequate social relationships; from watching geese and chickens imprinting (learning to follow) on their mothers; and from watching what horses and sheep do soon after birth.

In a wide variety of animal species, the mother only accepted an infant it saw in the hours shortly after birth. In others, the young became attached to the 'mother' they saw in the first hours after birth.

These 'mothers' could be research scientists or flashing lights; no matter what they were, they gave comfort to the young.

Researchers began to wonder if bonding was like this for man. They saw that the relationship between mothers and premature babies was often not very close: in those days, mothers might visit the intensive care nursery for only an hour a day, and they were not allowed to hold or feed their babies.

Perhaps more significantly, they noted that almost a quarter of children involved in child abuse cases were born prematurely.

Child abuse is clearly a complex subject, and no one has ever suggested that failure to bond is the only factor involved in it. That a quarter of child abuse victims were premature does not mean that a quarter of premature babies were abused: far from it: 997 in every 1,000 were not. But three were, and that is almost three times as many babies as one would expect by chance.

444 Direct evidence

The next step was to set up an experiment. A hospital was chosen in which mothers and babies were, as a rule, separated for long periods each day. The researchers simply changed the hospital rules for some women, giving them their babies for the first three days after birth.

The effects were startling. Not only were the mothers closer to their infants, and more finely tuned to their needs, but they remained in tune. Even after a year, they were closer than mothers who had been separated.

445 Mothers' evidence

But all this (442-444) is scientific evidence, not mothers' experience of bonding.

When asked how they feel on first holding their babies:

- 70 per cent of mothers say they are not interested.
- 20 per cent say they are are amazed and proud.
- 10 per cent say they are euphoric.

Why are so many disinterested? One factor may be that the drugs commonly used in labour, such as pethidine, make women sleepy and confused. They make babies drowsy, too. Perhaps a sleepy mother and a drowsy baby find it hard to mesh. Perhaps mothers need to be drawn into this first relationship.

But then again, perhaps it is more complex than this.

446 Personal experience

My eldest son was born at 4.15 on a snowy November morning. I was alone: his father had been sent home two hours previously, and I was heavily drugged 'because I was not really in labour'.

We were both very sleepy, and my son was separated from me almost at once while I was extensively stitched. By the time I saw him again, it was light.

What I remember of the time is the brightness: the snow on the roof tops, the white counterpane on the bed; his face, beautiful, and very, very, familiar; his yawn, like his father's; and the feeling of love. It was love without question: the certainty that whatever he did for the rest of his life (and mine) I would always love him, always forgive him. What they call 'blind' love. For 16 years, this child and I have had an often tempestuous relationship: he has driven me wild, brought me joy, sorrow and anger. He could say the same for me.

He is the only one of my three children I have ever smacked, said hurtful things to, or who has made me feel ashamed.

That, as I understand it, is the 'superglue' type of maternal love: emotional, automatic – indeed, pretty hopeless.

When my daughter was born, I expected this love to come again, but it did not. I had waited five long years for her: she was the daughter I had always longed for. Everything was on my side, I had had a wonderful pregnancy, a labour lasting 55 minutes from the first twinge, and no drugs. It was even snowing. I fed her within minutes, and she never left my side. She was tiny, dark and pretty. Her father was present all through her birth.

And I felt no love. Even though she never left my side in the days that followed, I never felt that automatic love I felt for my first son.

For her, love grew slowly over a period of weeks. I can look at her now with love, feel it very strong and sure; it is no less strong than that I feel for her brother, but it is different.

In nine years I don't ever remember feeling angry or resentful towards her. She is pure delight. Sometimes I am cross, but I have never lost my temper with her, and doubt I ever could. She has, in a strange sense, earned my love; that is how it feels.

447 Why so different?

Before Anna was born, I had five years of infertility and had lost one baby. I was, perhaps, too frightened to believe I was really pregnant. I sailed through the pregnancy, almost without admitting it existed. I worked until the day she was born, gave a dinner party for 14 in the final week.

Then, suddenly, she was there, a tiny, dark, stranger. My son looked familiar. She

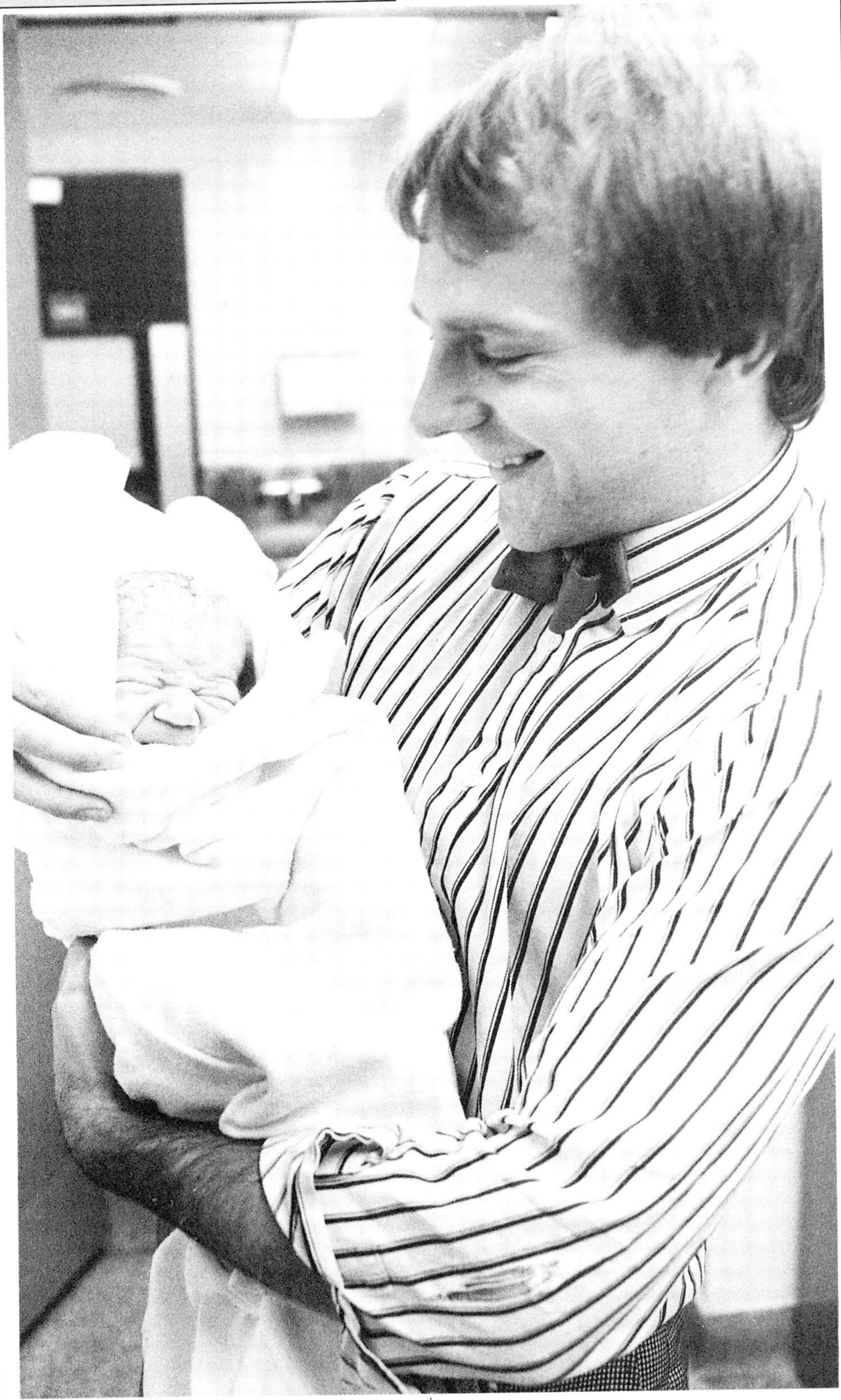

did not (then) look like anyone I knew. Perhaps seeing resemblances between yourself and your children is part of the glue; see in adjustment. Anna's paternal grandmother bonded very strongly to her on first sight.

My son I 'knew' before he was born: not just because he had regular hiccups, but by his large foot poking the right side of my belly. It was as if we had been talking on the telephone each day. We were not strangers when we met: he looked 'right', very fair, like me, like the babies in my family.

448 So what?

Did these two extremes make any difference in the long run? Not, as I have said, in the strength of the love I feel for them; perhaps in the way I love; but I cannot tell. My third child rests somewhere between the two extremes, both in how love came to me and in how I feel about him now. This has always intrigued me; made me wonder if we set the pattern (if not the fact) of love in those early experiences.

My experiences have proved to me that we certainly do not need to bond in the early hours after birth in order to love, and that there is a danger in thinking that we do. Instant bonding is no more essential to a relationship between mother and child than love at first sight is between lovers.

Love can grow, as it does in intensive care units, as it does between sick children and their parents, as it does for adoptive children, and for the large number of perfectly normal mothers and babies. My experience (and much research suggests that I am not alone in feeling this) is that the love that grows is as strong – indeed can be stronger – than the love that glues.

There is, I know, a world of difference between losing one's temper with, and abusing, a child, but it does not seem to me that anger and violence towards children necessarily means a lack of bonding.

449 Fathers bond, too

Research shows that fathers who are present at birth (even if they do not actually see the child being born) are much closer to their offspring, more finely tuned, than absent fathers. But see 341, 451 and 452-453.

450 A modern luxury

Go back three or four generations, and you will find few families strangers to the death of a child.

In 1874, 17 of every 100 infants died in their first year. In 1872, a survey of working mothers showed that of 185 children born to 110 mothers, 127 died within the first five years. Life was a little kinder to the leisured classes among whom 248 of 544 children died. Queen Anne had 14 stillbirths; Louis XVI lost five of his 11 legitimate children.

What could it have been like? *One cannot grieve after her much* said the American Mrs Thale on the death of a baby daughter in 1770. *And just now I have other things to think of.*

Once a child died, she or he was gone. Pictures were destroyed and often the name passed to the next child. Sometimes an infant would be named for an elder sickly child, even before it had died. Four Williams, and one might carry on the father's name.

Did mothers bond soon after birth? Or did they learn to love in later years? One cannot tell. That they loved we do know.

Here is Cotton Mather, the early American colonialist, who lost 13 of his 15 children:

My lovely Jerusha expired. She was two years and about seven months old. . .I begg'd, I begg'd that such a bitter cup as Death of that lovely child might pass from me.

And these words come from what may be some of the earliest literature on childcare, written about 1585:

Of all the misfortunes. . .none is so distressing. . .as the death of children. It preys upon the mind. . .and increases with time. . .nature has not provided a remedy.
– Scevole de Sainte Marthe.

Love of children is not a modern invention.

451 A first parting

The time has come to leave the delivery room. Mother and baby are wheeled to the ward. The father goes too, probably carrying her suitcase. But soon he must go home alone, while mother and baby stay together. Some men say of this moment that it always seems to be three o'clock in the morning: the streets are empty, the house is cold. See 452-453.

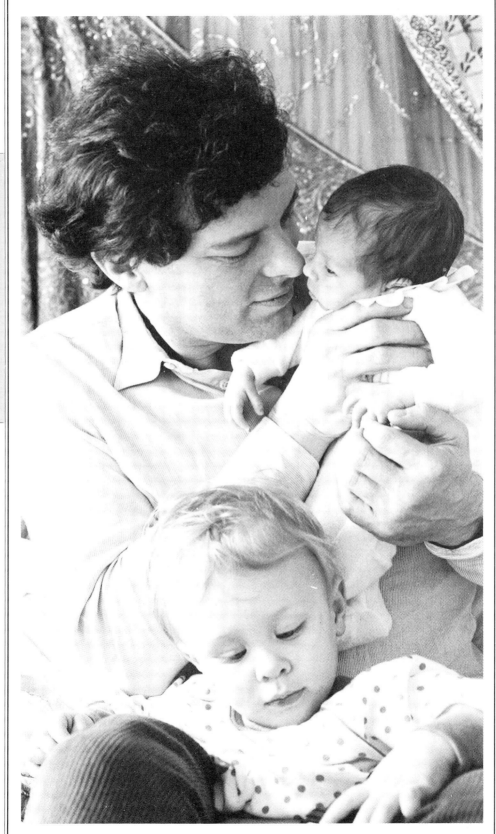

Adjustment

452-485

The First Days

452 First days a father

Walking out of hospital after the excitement of the birth may seem like going into limbo.

Pregnancy and labour may have been 'hers', but at the moment of birth you were two new parents. Now, already, that equality has evaporated. She enters a world of women from which you are excluded; you may visit but never belong. A world in which you feel your inexperience, and your inferiority, as a parent.

'They' all know what to do with babies. Of course they do: they have all day in which to practise. Even first-time mothers learn quickly that babies are tough and will not break. Your first attempt at picking her up is all too public. In fact, probably no one watches, but it does not feel like that.

Men often describe the feeling of being judged when they make public attempts to care for a child. Many women reinforce the insecurity, often without realizing it:

'Be careful you support his head'.

'Now you have woken her. I wish you had left her to sleep'.

'Here, give her to me; she'll stop crying if I feed her'.

The hospital, too, imposes its rules. You can visit, but not stay. Peter Lomas sums it up in his *Childbirth Ritual:*

During this time the husband has little or no influence over the affairs of his wife and baby. He is patronised by the hospital staff who, in the same way as the general public, humorously assume him to be in a state of incompetent dither, best out of the way since liable to be a nuisance, and he accepts this practice.

Most men fill these unreal days by ringing relatives with news of the birth. It is a ritual, and a necessary one, an opportunity to talk. Sharing the great milestones in life is a basic need. For the mother the experience of birth is rapidly replaced by the experience of having a baby; this, not the birth, will almost certainly be the main topic of conversation between her and the father during hospital visits.

However you decide to deal with these first few days (and staying with friends or relatives may be worth considering – at least then you could return home together as a family), it is important to realize that at this stage you are still becoming a father. You will not feel truly a father until you take on the social role of fatherhood,

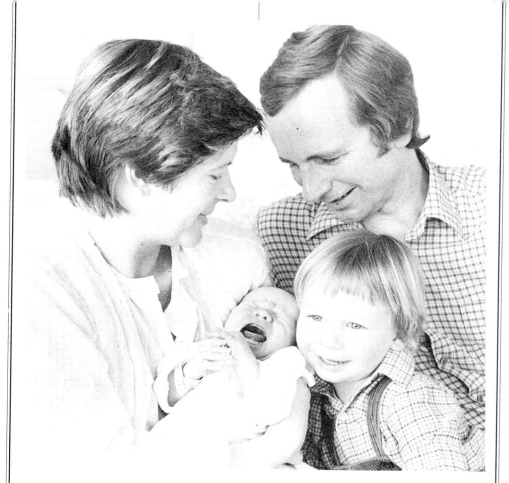

and you cannot do this (indeed, no one will let you) until mother and baby are home with you.

You have a right to feel alienated; a right to feel that it is not as you had planned. Not all men commit themselves to equal parenthood, but today many men want to go some of the way, especially if their partners are intending to return to full-time work. It is unfortunate that the first lesson you learn about parenthood is that motherhood is full time, while fatherhood is, at best, a peripheral activity. The lesson will often be repeated; yet should you heed it, your partner will almost certainly be resentful. You cannot win – at any rate, not without effort, tact and persistence in extraordinary amounts.

It is hard to imagine a more disastrous start to fatherhood. Women, and increasingly society, pressurize men to take on a more equal parenting role. We draw them into the pregnancy, we ask them to coach and comfort us through birth and to share that moment of becoming a parent. Then, one way or another, we shut them out.

453 Postnatal depression – in men

Both men and women can have postnatal 'blues' (see 488-491), although it is perhaps more likely that the male simply feels flat. The more serious and prolonged depression suffered by about one in ten women may also occur occasionally in men, as does the postnatal psychosis that involves partial or complete mental breakdown and normally requires hospitalization. It is not so surprising. Men don't undergo the changes in hormonal balance that affect women, but they do experience the changes in life style and the unfamiliar demands. See 482.

454 First days a mother

The limelight is your baby's. Your physical condition is monitored, your physical ills righted, but your emotional needs are often pushed to one side. When you have been the centre of attention for nine long months, it can be hard to take, especially when you are feeling apprehensive. Your body switches from housing and nurturing the baby to supplying milk, and the attendant hormonal juggling plays havoc with your emotions and moods. Faced with the reality of what you have done, you may feel panic. Your inability to get your baby to latch on to your breast makes you feel deeply inadequate; a problem exacerbated by the difficulties you have in carrying out apparently simple tasks such as putting on nappies. It is like the first days in any job. Everything has to be learned; motherhood is not instinctive. In the past it may have seemed like that, but in the past few women could have reached this stage in their lives without any experience of child rearing. It was learned at their mother's knee, or their elder sister's house. See also 488-491.

455 Lochia

After birth, all women have a bloody discharge, rather like a heavy period, composed of left-over mucus, blood and tissue: a cleaning-out of the uterus after the baby's nine-month stay. Because it is at times inclined to gush, especially when you feed the baby (see page 175), or get up in the morning, it often seems to be heavier than it really is. The discharge rarely amounts to more than one or two cupfuls.

Bleeding that saturates more than one pad per hour for longer than a couple of hours should be reported immediately; see 456. As well as the odd gush of blood, you can expect to see small clots of blood and bits of membrane in the first few days. Large clots should be reported immediately to a nurse, since sometimes bits of the placenta are retained. Knowing what is large and small is difficult: clots two or three times the size of a pea are normal, but check that they consist only of blood and membrane.

In the first days the lochia will be red, but by the third day it should begin to turn a watery pink, and by about day five it should be brown. Over the next week or two, it will gradually change to a yellowish white. Occasional streaking with blood is normal in the later stages, so is a slight back-tracking in this sequence. Bright red bleeding should be reported if it occurs after the fourth day. A heavy discharge of red blood at this stage needs urgent attention.

You should use sanitary towels, not tampons, to absorb the flow.

Lochia may persist, on and off, for up to six weeks.

Breast feeding makes your uterus contract, and you will feel afterpains (457), and often an increase in the flow of lochia.

456 Postpartum haemorrhage

Normally, the uterus contracts after delivery, pinching off exposed blood vessels. Failure to do so produces post-partum haemorrhage. There are many underlying causes: maternal fatigue or illness; a long, exhausting labour; an excessive load on the uterus during pregnancy because of multiple births, a large baby, or an excessive amount of amniotic fluid. It may also occur if parts of the placenta are retained, if you develop an infection, or have lacerations of the vagina or uterus. Report any persistent pain or discomfort in the lower abdomen that occurs after the first few days following the birth.

Occasionally, a woman will develop a uterine infection after birth. It is now rare, but you must report a body temperature of over 100°F (37.7°C) if it lasts more than a day, or lochia (455) which smells foul.

457 Afterpains

These are caused by contractions of the uterus as it shrinks back into the pelvis. You will almost certainly feel the pains quite strongly while you are breast feeding, but they can appear at other times also.

Afterpains are often stronger after a second baby, or if your uterus has been stretched by a large baby or a multiple pregnancy. The pains should subside by the end of the first week. Breathing and relaxation exercises (pages 90-91 and 113) will help to minimize the discomfort, and mild pain killers are often prescribed.

458 Perineal pain

Everyone is bruised and sore after delivery, especially if there has been an episiotomy; it can feel as if you are sitting on a bed of nails. Pain may be eased by:

• Sitting on a pillow or, better still, a rubber ring (the sort used by children learning to swim).
• Cold compresses: fill a rubber glove with crushed ice or use a small packet of frozen peas and hold it in position.

- Warm salty baths.
- Applying comfrey ointment or chilled witch hazel pads.
- Lying on your side, and avoiding long periods of standing or sitting.
- Tightening your buttocks before you sit, and raising yourself into this position. This increases blood flow to the area, thus promoting healing.
- Pelvic floor exercises and bottom exercises (page 39); these also improve blood circulation.
- Keeping the area as dry as possible. Use your hair dryer if you find it difficult to wipe yourself dry.
- Changing your sanitary pad at least every four hours.

Occasionally, infections develop, even in those who have not had stitches. Daily checking of your perineum by the hospital staff means any infection can be dealt with promptly.
- Washing the area frequently with warm water, wiping from front to back. If you can do this each time you urinate or empty your bowels, so much the better.
- Removing your sanitary pad from the front, backwards.

459 Constipation

"Have you had a bowel movement?" is a perennial hospital question; the answer is generally no in the first couple of days after birth. So don't worry. If you had an enema before or during labour, it is likely to take even longer to get the pattern re-established. Activity, fluids and, above all, fibre are the remedy. Ask for bran every morning, or take your own into hospital with you. If you find bran cereals hard going, look out for high-fibre tablets in health food shops and chemists. They look like rat droppings and you may find they taste little better, but they work wonders.

Drink plenty of fluid to make the faeces soft and so prevent fissuring.

460 Bladder

The other perennial hospital question is "Have you passed water?" The answer just now should be yes, plenty. Bladder capacity may increase after birth: there is more room for the bladder in your enlarged abdomen and you may not feel like passing water as often as before. But try to do so. Sometimes urination is difficult even when you do try. There are various reasons: the drugs given in labour sometimes disrupt bladder control; you

expect it to hurt; perineal damage, which can cause spasms in the urethra; bruising, and consequent swelling and temporary blockage of the urethra.

You should mention any difficulties to the hospital staff or midwife, who can empty your bladder with a catheter if necessary. You can help yourself by:

- Drinking plenty of fluids.
- Walking about.
- Passing water standing up: it is often less painful than the usual position.
- Running a tap.
- Asking for privacy if you have to use a bedpan; also a little warmth. A cold pan will not help.
- Sitting on an ice pack, or having a warm bath; both heat and cold are counter-irritants.
- Not panicking; a catheter sounds horrible, but it is nowhere near as bad as it seems.

Not urinating enough is one side of the problem; doing so involuntarily is another. Many women suffer from stress incontinence after childbirth. You will find yourself wetting your pants when you cough, or if you run or jump. Pelvic floor exercises (page 39) will usually cure the problem.

461 Exhaustion

If your labour was long, you will probably feel exhausted: up to 48 hours without sleep is not made any less tiring by the excitement of having a baby. Be sensible. You don't have to have the baby beside you 24 hours a day in order to love it. You are not just a mother, you are a woman who happens to be a mother too.

In an ideal world, you would take your baby in your arms and together you would curl up and sleep, content in each other's warmth. But there will be time enough for this. Now, it makes no difference to her whether you are in the bed beside her or not. She can only see clearly (519 and 521) at a distance of 8-10 in (20-25 cm); she does not yet know your smell or your voice. Comfort for her is being held or wrapped up tightly. Once she is out of your arms she might just as well be out of the room, so take advantage of what respite the hospital arrangement can offer.

Of course, having your baby beside you ('rooming in') is an essential part of bonding; but the crying of other babies will drive you to despair. Many women who later suffer from post-natal depression report difficulties coping with hospital rooming-in policies. I suspect it may arise from a shifting conflict between the desire for sleep and the feeling that you should want the baby beside you. If this is true, it is yet another sound reason for home birth.

But what about the necessity of feeding? Babies are not just beside the bed for bonding; they are there so that demand feeding schedules can be established. It is true that the earlier a woman puts the child to the breast, the easier breast feeding will be; but this, like bonding, does not require 24-hour contact. In the first three or four days of life, a baby lives off fat reserves, she does not need feeding. (Indeed, in the past, babies were often left without food in the early days.) Let your needs be your guide, rather than a feeling of what should be right.

462 Relaxation

Sometimes, insomnia develops because, perversely, you are overtired. Try to relax. Take a warm bath and ask your partner to give you a massage; see page 111. Letting go is especially important if you want to breast feed.

If the sleep problem is really intolerable, the hospital should consider discharging you early.

463 Sweating, hair loss, wind and piles

Most women sweat more than usual in the days after birth, since there is extra fluid to be eliminated. Hair loss and excessive wind are other disconcerting, but temporary, problems.

Piles are also common after birth and may be more painful than the stitches.

464 Left-overs

You may not expect to have your pre-pregnancy figure back for some time; nevertheless you may be horrified by what you see in the mirror. The distension will not disappear overnight, in fact it may only go with effort, especially if you put on excessive weight during pregnancy. But you can have firm stomach muscles, slim legs and hips again. Start your pelvic floor exercises straight away. These, and bottom-squeezing routines, described on page 39, will assist blood flow to the

perineal area, which also helps reduce fat deposits. If your ankles were swollen in the latter stages of pregnancy, they may take a few weeks to subside.

The stretch marks on your breasts will grow pale in the coming months, those on your abdomen and thighs will take much longer; in fact, they may never completely disappear.

465 Routine aftercare

Your general health will be watched closely in the days after birth. Blood pressure and temperature will be checked. Your abdomen will be palpated to check that your bladder is functioning properly and that the uterus is shrinking back. Sometimes the shrinkage is measured with a ruler. Your sanitary pad will be checked, and your perineum. Stitches will be examined. You will probably be given a blood test to check that you are not anaemic.

466 Recovering from a Caesarian

No stitches between your legs or soreness in the vagina, but everything else will be much the same: lochia, afterpains, fatigue, sweating, hair loss. You will, in addition, be recovering from a major abdominal operation and possibly from a general anesthetic as well. If it was an emergency Caesarian, you probably also had a long and difficult labour.

People react differently to anaesthetics. Some feel very sick when they come round, others pleasantly fuzzy, others have frightening dreams. All after-effects are transient. Breathing exercises will help to clear the anaesthetic from your system, but the incision will hurt as you do them or if you cough. It may help if you push a pillow firmly into your stomach before you cough. Analgesics given to ease this pain may make you drowsy, but it is still safe to breast feed.

A catheter and intravenous drip will usually be left in place for 24 hours. After that, you can start eating light meals.

Your shoulders may hurt because of referred pain from your diaphragm, which is often irritated during a Caesarian section.

Surprising as it may seem when you come round from the operation, you will probably be on your feet within eight hours, and breast feeding the baby by the end of the second day.

Prepare for walking by wiggling your

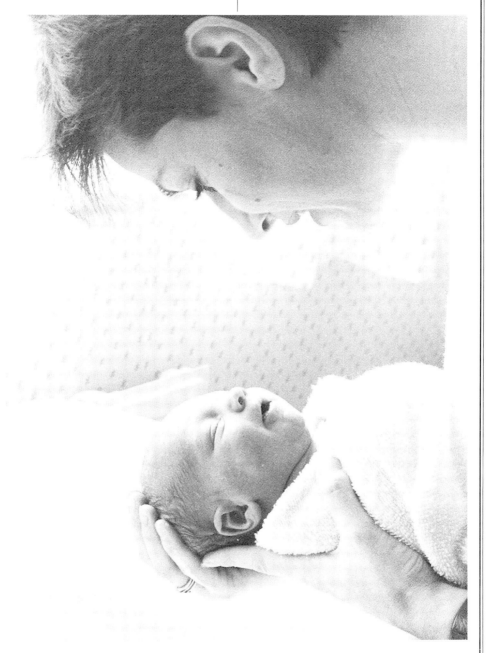

toes and then tightening and releasing each muscle in your body. Starting with the toes, work slowly up the body, then:

• Pull up your knees and lift your head slightly: a half-hearted version of the stomach exercises you did in pregnancy.
• Twist from the waist: staying flat on your back, and holding your abdomen as tight as you can, reach across your body with one arm to touch the other.

Wind is always a problem after abdominal surgery; this and getting your bowels and bladder to work, are generally the most trying post-operative problems. You may find that the milk takes a little longer than normal to come (see 474) and that it is difficult to hold the baby in a comfortable position to feed her. Laying a pillow on your lap, then drawing her into the breast with your arm should help.

Stitches, unless they are the kind which dissolve, will be removed after five or six days. You will probably be allowed to leave hospital after about ten days.

Feeding– Breast and Bottle

467 Breast feeding

'All you have to do is put the baby to the breast and let her suck. Easy.' Well, it is with the second baby, but I found it far from straightforward with my first.

I had breasts full of colostrum (469) – and later overflowing with milk; I had the nipples; he had the mouth and the sucking reflex. It should have been straightforward, but it was not. See the panel on page 176.

468 Milk supply control

The hormone prolactin is the key: the more you release, the more milk you make.

Prolactin is made by the pituitary gland in the brain. The more the baby squeezes the nipple, the more prolactin is released. This is the baby's means of placing her order for meals: the more she sucks today, the more she gets tomorrow; supply and demand, or rather demand and supply, are finely tuned.

Although a ready supply of milk is stored just behind the nipple (see illustration), it is not possible to store all the milk required by the baby at each feed. Most of the milk is stored in the milk glands and is known as hind milk. It is about three times richer than the foremilk. It is squeezed into the ducts by the muscles around the glands, an action known as the let-down reflex. When let-down occurs, you will often find that milk starts to spray from the breasts in spurts, as if being pumped.

Breast feeding often fails because women do not establish this let-down reflex. Indeed, 'establishing' breast feeding means establishing a reliable let-down reflex.

Let-down is under the control of oxytocin – yet another of this hormone's many functions; see 297. It is released in response to nipple stimulation, but this can take time – as long as three minutes. By this time, the baby will have already finished the fore milk and will be left sucking an apparently empty breast. The delay causes frustration; she fusses and stops sucking, the mother gets upset, oxytocin is not released, and the hind milk is not let down. It is a delicate mechanism.

Oxytocin is also involved in the control of contractions during birth, and it is released at orgasm. Both these processes, it is widely acknowledged, can be inhibited by tension, and the same applies to the let-down reflex. Indeed, there are other similarities. Just as sexual feelings can arise without any direct sexual stimulation (just looking at someone, or hearing their voice) so many women find that let-down can occur even before the baby starts to suck. Some may find it happens if they merely think of feeding their baby. I know that I used to let-down to a whole variety of stimuli, including the neighbour's Siamese cat.

469 Colostrum

This is the fluid in the breasts during the first few days of the baby's life. It forms a bridge between the blood that nourished her in the womb and the milk that will nourish her in the next months.

It is yellowish, rather than the bluish colour of mature milk, and it contains nine times as much protein as mature milk, and less sugar and fat. Most important, it contains many antibodies. These give the new-born resistance to infection in the early days; they also coat the lining of the gut, preventing organisms entering the blood stream, and stop the absorption of foreign protein which can produce an allergic response.

470 How often to feed

A schedule for 1906 would recommend ten times a day in the first month. One from 1940 would say at four-hourly intervals.

During the first month (but not necessarily in the first few days) ten feeds a day would be closer to the norm. Most small babies want to feed at two to three hourly intervals by day, and a little less frequently (if you are lucky) by night. Some babies will need feeding more often, some will space their feeds more widely than this.

Your baby is the best judge.

Demand feeding will not continue to be so demanding. All babies settle down to a more or less regular schedule of meals, but there will be days when they are upset and constantly need to suck.

471 Feeding problems

In the early days (especially if you are stitched) finding a comfortable feeding position is difficult. It is no use trying to feed sitting up in bed, or in an easy chair that makes you lean back. The correct

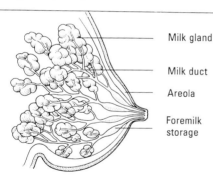

Milk gland

Milk duct

Areola

Foremilk storage

How the baby gets the milk
- **Milking:** Foremilk is extracted by the baby squeezing the areola with her gums.
- **Sucking:** She creates suction on the nipple by producing a vacuum in her mouth.
- **Let-down:** The milk is ejected into the mouth in squirts: all she has to do is swallow. You can see when she is taking this milk: she will take several gulps, then pause with the nipple held loosely in her mouth, waiting for the next squirt.

Milk production
A breast is made up of 15 to 20 segments of glandular tissue, rather like bunches of grapes on stalks. Each 'grape' is a milk gland, each stalk a duct. The duct from each segment passes to the nipple, which means that the nipple is like the head of a watering can fed by several separate streams of milk.

The milk glands are lined with milk-producing cells. Around the grapes there are star-shaped muscles: when they squeeze the milk gland the milk is forced into the ducts.

Each duct has a storage area located just behind the darkened areola which surrounds the nipple. Here the duct widens, and its walls become elastic. An instant supply of milk (the foremilk) is stored here for immediate consumption when the baby is put to the breast. When full, these storage spaces can measure up to about ¼ in (1 cm) in diameter.

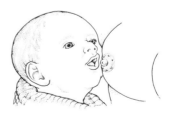

Breast milk's composition
Milk is manufactured from the blood by the milk glands, each gland being supplied by the fine network of blood vessels around it. In the blood are the hormones which tell the milk glands to get to work, plus all the ingredients (water, protein, fat, carbohydrates minerals, sodium, trace elements and vitamins) which it needs to make the milk.

position is leaning slightly forward. Unless you have a straight-backed comfortable chair, you may find lying side by side in bed most comfortable at first. If you lie your baby on a pillow, you can still use your elbow to manipulate her head. If you have had stitches, you will find this is the only position which allows you to relax.

472 Sore nipples
● To minimize the problem, start

gradually: two minutes per breast the first day, adding a minute the second and third day, and two minutes the fourth and fifth day. Add an extra minute on each of the next four days. She should then be getting ten minutes per breast per feed.
● Never let the baby suck on the end of the nipple.
● Never pull the nipple from her mouth while she is still sucking.
● After feeds, dry the nipples carefully.
● Wash the breasts and nipples with water morning and night. You don't need to wash before each feed; soap will dry the nipples so use lanolin as a cleanser

How to breast feed

1 Find a comfortable position. Which breast you offer first is immaterial, although the left one may seem most natural if you are right-handed. Lying side-by-side is worth trying (see 471), but sitting bolt upright also works well. Placing pillows on your lap may make it easier. You cannot feed leaning back on pillows until you are an expert.
2 Undo your bra.
3 Loosen the baby's blanket. This should help to keep her awake. Free her hands; she may like to touch the breast.
4 Support her head and shoulders with one hand and lift her into position.
5 Push the nipple out, using the thumb and index finger of the free hand, and squeeze just behind the nipple. You may find it easier to use your index and second finger, in which case you hold the fingers flat on each side of the nipple and press into the breast until the nipple pops out. Ease the pressure. You can now manoeuvre.
6 Keeping the fingers in position, support the breast from underneath with your cupped hand.
7 Tilt the baby back, resting her head in the bend of your elbow. Practise moving your elbow to change her position.
8 Stroke the side of her mouth with the nipple or a finger to make her root.
9 Manoeuvre the nipple so that it touches her upper lip and then her lower one. You may need to repeat this process a number of times.
10 As her mouth opens, adjust your elbow so that it moves her head slightly towards you.
11 She should then latch on to the breast and suck automatically. It takes a little practice to get the timing right.

● Don't try to force the nipple into her mouth; instead, ease her on to it.
● The nipple needs to go right into her mouth. If you press your upper finger slightly into your breast as she latches on, you will push the nipple towards the roof of her mouth and she may latch on better. She needs to have all the nipple and the areola in her mouth (unless they are very large) in order to compress the milk glands.
● If your breasts are large, she may bury her nose. Give her a breathing hole by pressing the breast gently. It is better not to press the breast too hard as this can compress breast tissue, affecting the milk flow. If slight pressure is not enough, lowering the supporting elbow should free her nose.
● Watch her. Lean forward slightly as she sucks. If she is sucking with a rhythmic motion, she is getting milk. You can see her swallowing (sometimes you will hear her too). After a while, you will be able to feel the milk 'let down'.
● Relax. Don't hunch your shoulders or hold your breath. Think of the milk flowing and try to feel the flow.
● Leave her for two or three minutes. If she is not sucking in a regular pattern, you can leave her longer. Breast feeding is a little like sun bathing: you get sore if you do to much at first.
● When she has finished the first breast, ease the nipple gently to the corner of her mouth. Don't pull, wait for her to pause. It should slip out easily. Never pull out the nipple while she is sucking.
● Dry the nipple.
● Repeat for the second breast.
● It is usual to start with this second breast at the next feed.

instead.

- Don't try to toughen the nipples with spirits.
- Rub in a little lanolin, cod liver oil or mass cream to soothe the nipples and make them supple.
- Never leave the nipples wet: they will crack.
- Don't feed for more than ten minutes at a time, including pauses.

473 To treat sore nipples

- Expose to the air whenever possible.
- Apply massé cream, lanolin or cod liver oil.
- Friar's Balsam may be soothing.
- Use nipple shields for a while. You may find that once the baby has started to suck, the pain will ease. Try starting each feed with the shield, then offering the nipple.

474 Getting milk production under way

- New-born babies do not need any food for three or four days. Relax: you have plenty of time. Your milk will come into production about the third day after birth. Don't worry if she takes only a little at first. Look on early attempts to feed as practice – and as a way of supplying your baby with antibodies. She will take plenty in time – when she starts to get hungry.
- Start as soon as you can. At birth the rooting reflex is at its strongest and the baby is usually alert.
- Take no notice of hospital rules about

Expressing milk

If you can master the technique, hand expressing is the quickest and most comfortable way to collect breast milk for giving later in a bottle.

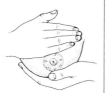

1 Find a comfortable place to sit, and relax. A warm bath is ideal. **2** Holding the breast with one hand, gently stroke with the palm and fingertips towards the nipple. **3** With thumb on top, gently squeeze the areola just behind the nipple. Milk should squirt out. Stop when milk starts to come in drops.

when and where you should feed. You need to feed your baby when she feels like feeding, and where you are comfortable.

- Make sure nobody gives her a feed if she is taken to the nursery. Even a bottle of sugar water can fill her up.
- If she is screaming, wait until she stops. Cuddle her, rock her, talk softly. Wait until you have both calmed down before trying to put her to the breast.
- Stay calm. Send out visitors before you start. Most of us feel a little uneasy feeding in public until we are experienced.

475 Engorgement

As the colostrum (469) of the first few days changes to milk, it is easy for the breasts to become engorged: over-filled with milk. They need to be emptied, but babies do not always oblige.

Engorgement is painful. Your breasts become hot, hard, lumpy, swollen and tense; they feel like lumps of concrete. You wake one morning feeling hot and shivery. Everything about you, apart from your all-too-solid breasts, is fragile. The pain may extend under your arms; you will burst into tears at the slightest provocation.

There are a number of schools of thought on how to deal with the problem. Here (476) is one suggested by a trained counsellor.

476 Treating engorgement

- Find a couple of face cloths, or a nappy, and go to the bathroom.
- Undo your bra and wrap a towel around your waist.
- Run the cold tap until it is really cold and saturate the cloths.
- Place one cloth over a breast and leave it until the breast feels cool and the cloth warm.
- Place the second cloth over the other breast, and repeat. A large packet of frozen peas may work better than the face cloth, since it will not drip. Remember you need to leave the compress in place until it can cool the inner layers of the breast. The treatment is effective for the same reasons that cold compresses work on pulled muscles: besides excess milk, engorged breasts suffer from vastly increased blood supply, and from tissue swelling. The treatment works because cold makes blood vessels, particularly the small capillaries, contract. The body reacts by withdrawing fluid in an attempt

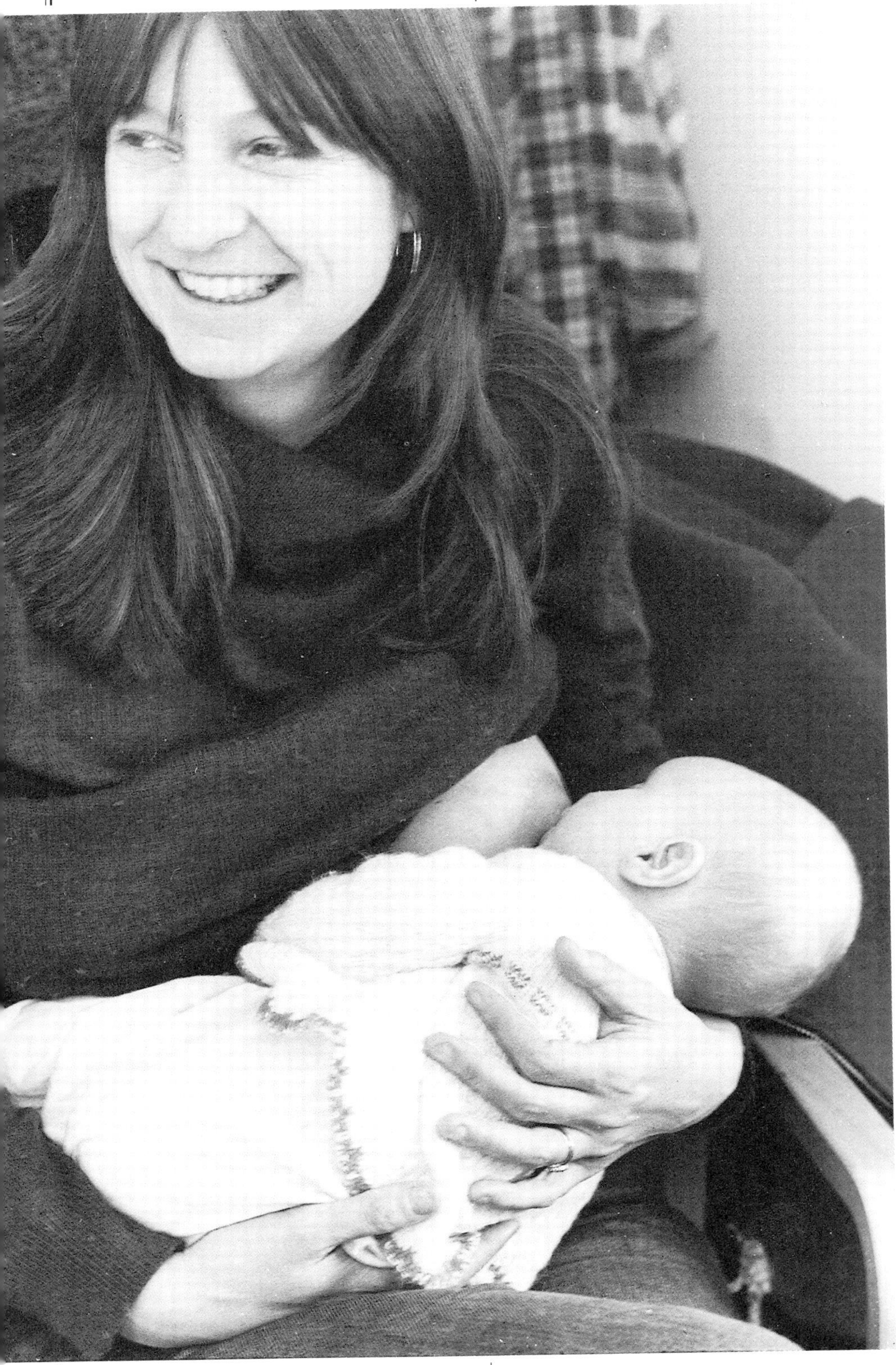

to keep the blood temperature constant. With fluid drawn off, the swelling reduces.

As soon as you feel sufficiently comfortable, let the baby feed from each breast.

Don't express milk. If you already have too much, this will make more, and if the engorgement is due to blood, rather than to milk, it will be painful. Let the baby set the level. You may find feeding little and often is the easiest way.

If the cold compress does not seem to work, and you feel you must let out some milk, try kneeling in the bath with your breasts hanging down into warm water. Massage the breasts downwards towards the nipple, with oil. Some milk ought to flow out without stimulating prolactin release – a better way of getting rid of excess than letting the baby suck, since sucking sets off your prolactin release mechanism, creating yet more milk.

If she cannot latch on to the breast, express a little milk. Try to relax, especially while you feed her. Check your body for tension as you feed. Talk yourself down, it will pass. Listening to music may also help.

Support your breasts at all times until the engorgement has passed. Since your bra will not fit, make a sling for each breast from a crepe bandage or some other soft, light material.

The orthodox treatment for engorgement (which the hospital may suggest) is hot compresses and expressing milk either with a pump, or by hand. I found it much less successful than the cold compress method.

477 Mastitis

This is inflammation of the breasts. It may be caused by an infection or by damage to breast ducts. It usually starts locally, but if untreated can spread to the entire breast, or develop into a breast abscess. You will notice an inflamed red patch on the breast, and you will probably feel feverish.

• Don't stop feeding.
• Lean forwards as you feed to help the breast drain. Drain the breasts by kneeling in a warm bath; see 476.
• Apply cold compresses every hour to reduce the inflammation; see 476.
• Ensure your breast is not constricted by a tight bra. Support it in a sling (476) if necessary.
• See your doctor.

478 Diet when breast feeding

You need simply a normal, balanced diet, but it should have 500 calories over and above the normal intake. If you don't eat enough, or if your diet is unbalanced, you will still make good milk; there won't, however, be enough for the baby. Sometimes babies are upset by certain foods – chocolate and cabbage are often considered culprits – so if she seems upset it is worth keeping a record of what food you eat. If she suffers from colic (543), it is worth dropping all cow's milk protein from your diet. To give this manoeuvre a fair chance of working, persist for seven days. Then re-introduce dairy foods again and observe the result in order to confirm your diagnosis.

479 Advantages of breast feeding

• Breast milk is free, and designed for babies.
• It is always hygenic and warm.
• It can protect against infection, and this protection may last into childhood.
• Breast-fed babies are less likely to get gastro-enteritis, respiratory infections, middle ear disease and a number of other infectious diseases.
• Breast-fed babies smell good. Their nappies are less foul than bottle-fed babies and their posset is almost odourless. They suffer less from nappy rash.
• They are seven times less likely to develop eczema, and may be less susceptible to food allergies.
• They are less susceptible to Crohn's disease, ulcerative colitis; and possibly also heart disease and dental decay in later life.
• Women who have breast fed are less susceptible to breast cancer.

480 Disadvantages of breast feeding

• You have to feed more often.
• The baby is less likely to sleep through the night.
• You cannot share the early childcare with your partner in the way you can when you are bottle feeding.
• Breast feeding binds you to the baby for more or less 24 hours a day.
• Breast feeding reduces sexual interest in most women.
• You know how much food a bottle-fed baby has taken; gauging this can be difficult with a breast-fed baby.

481 Bottle feeding

It is, of course, convenient; not in the sense of feeding the baby on a cold night – putting her to the breast is more convienient then – but in terms of fitting in with life outside baby care.

If you intend to return to work, this is important. Books extolling the virtues of breast feeding often suggest that it is possible to carry on breast feeding after you go back to work by expressing milk for feeds during the day and rushing home to feed the baby in the evening.

I don't know how many of these writers have tried this, but I have, and I found that it simply did not work. Well, in honesty, I did manage exclusively to breast feed my youngest child, but it is the exception that proves the point. I lived three minutes by car from my place of work, my job could be interrupted for half an hour (I just worked a little later); I could go home for lunch and had a nanny who could drive the baby in to me. Also, he rarely wanted feeding at less than four-hourly intervals. On the rare occasions when I knew I would not be able to stop to feed him, I could express milk.

Even with the same job, home and nanny, I could not exclusively breast feed my daughter: she wanted feeding too frequently and liked to take her time. If, like me, you know your career is important to you, or if you want to work when your baby is under nine months old, you must accept that she will need some bottle feeds every day.

You may find, incidentally, that she does not like switching to a bottle when you start working again. Prepare for this by getting your partner to give her a bottle of expressed milk each evening, from the time she is about three weeks old. While he feeds her, you express milk for the next evening's feed, and there is no problem with her looking for the breast. This also enables you to leave her from time to time.

Many of the health advantages of breast feeding remain if the baby is exclusively breast fed in the first six weeks, and partially in the months that follow.

If you did not manage to establish breast feeding, or never wished to do so, it is also important to realize that remaining a happy contented mother probably outweighs all the advantages of breast feeding.

How to bottle feed

● Bottle, teats and all equipment must be well cleaned and then sterilized. This last is very important: you cannot be too careful. Use hot water, detergent and a bottle brush to clean the bottles, and granular salt to clean the teats before you put them into the sterilizer. Also sterilize any jugs and spoons you use in the preparation of feeds. The bottle brush will also need to be sterilized.

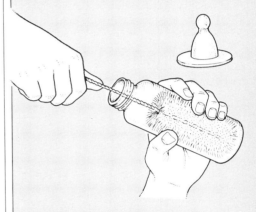

● Wash your hands.
● Bottles come in many varieties. If you are supplementing breast feeds, the baby may find the 'nursers', which use polythene bags, easiest. They can be held at any angle.
● If you are bottle feeding exclusively you will need at least six sets of bottles and teats.
● Sterilizing tablets or liquid are easy to use. Make up as directed and fully immerse the bottles for two hours.

If you boil bottles, say because you have run out of sterilizing agents, you must do so for at least 20 minutes after the water has come to the boil.

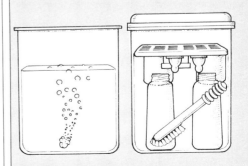

- Equipment does not remain sterile: it should be left in the sterilizer until it is used. Nor will it necessarily remain sterile in water that has boiled.
- Change the sterilizing fluid every 24 hours.
- Formula must be made up accurately. Never add a 'bit for luck' or guess how much powder or liquid is needed.
- Formula must be made up with water which has been boiled. Boil the water and then let it cool to hand heat. Feel the outside of the kettle, not the water.
- If you are using liquid formula, pour boiling water over the can, and punch holes with a sterilized opener.
- Take the jug (or bottles) from the sterilizer and measure the formula into it. Hold the bottle up to check the level if using fluid. If using powder, level it off carefully with a sterile knife.

- Add the correct amount of water. Hold the bottle at eye level as you pour in the water.
- Add sugar if necessary. (Most formula now has sugar already added.)
- Stir the mixture with a sterile spoon, or put the cap on the bottle and shake.
- If you are making up more than one feed, fill each bottle and put them all into the fridge. Never leave the teats uncovered in the fridge. Use the sterile caps provided.

Never leave feeds (or liquid formula) standing at room temperature. Warm milk is a dangerous breeding ground for bacteria.

When travelling (or at night) you can keep water warm in a sterile flask and add this to powdered formula in the bottle. Bottles of liquid formula must be kept cool.

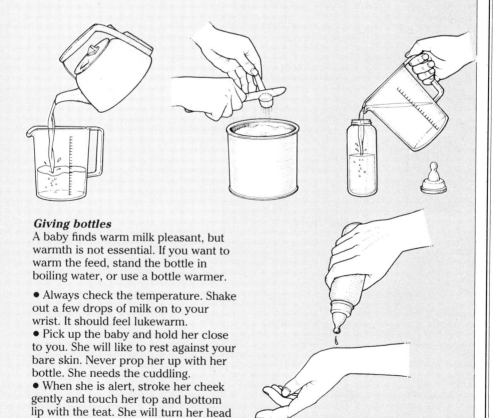

Giving bottles

A baby finds warm milk pleasant, but warmth is not essential. If you want to warm the feed, stand the bottle in boiling water, or use a bottle warmer.

- Always check the temperature. Shake out a few drops of milk on to your wrist. It should feel lukewarm.
- Pick up the baby and hold her close to you. She will like to rest against your bare skin. Never prop her up with her bottle. She needs the cuddling.
- When she is alert, stroke her cheek gently and touch her top and bottom lip with the teat. She will turn her head to you and open her mouth. Slip in the teat. Let her suck. Hold the bottle firmly, and sloping upwards, so that the milk flows down by force of gravity.
- As she sucks, she is likely to produce a vacuum in the bottle, particularly if

she does not pause. This will make the teat go flat. You can prevent this by gently pulling the bottle towards you, so releasing the vacuum.

482 Fathers and breast feeding

Some research suggests that fathers can feel envious of the closeness that grows up between mother and baby as a result of breast feeding. The catch for many fathers is that those who are most committed to sharing childcare are also more likely to be committed to breast feeding.

But there is more to it than that. Most men are clumsy with small babies, and many are uneasy when handling them. Some fathers totally committed to child rearing will neverthelessstill leave bottle feeding primarily to the mother while the baby is tiny.

Some men may not only envy the closeness, but feel sexual jealousy of the breast-feeding baby's access to 'their' breasts. They may also be embarassed by a woman's readiness to expose her breasts in public in order to breast feed. (It is all right on the beach, everyone else is doing exactly the same.)

None of this is surprising, given the role that breasts play in our culture and in the sexual relationship of most couples.

The fact that breast feeding reduces sexual desire in the majority of women, and that sexual activity is in any case unlikely to resume for some weeks after birth, can aggravate the problem. See 560.

483 How often to bottle feed

As with breast feeding, it is best to let the baby set the pattern, feeding her whenever

---

Bottle feeding: adjusting quantity
Bottle-fed babies tend to feed less frequently than breast-fed babies because formula takes longer to digest.

Human milk is designed for babies, who feed at frequent intervals. Formula is based on cow's milk, which is designed for calves who feed only twice a day. Although the formula modifies the milk, basically making it less rich and more dilute than cow's milk, babies still tend to go for much longer periods between bottle feeds.

After the first few days on the bottle, a baby usually settles into a four-hourly feeding schedule.

How much?
She will start by taking about 2 oz (50 ml) at each feed, but this will increase slowly. As the feeds get bigger, she will probably go for longer periods between them, especially at night. It is best, nevertheless, to continue with a demand feeding schedule. Let her tell you when she wants to feed, and how much she wants to drink. Some days she will feel hungrier than others. If she seems well, there is no need to panic if she does not take all of her bottle.

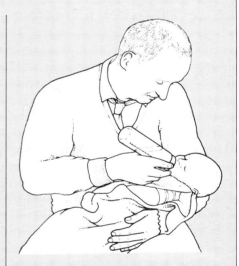

It is always tempting to make her finish the last few ounces, but remember that she had no say in how much you put into the bottle. Overfeeding a bottle-fed baby can easily lead to obesity.

You should, however, also take care not to underfeed. If she always finishes the bottle and asks for more, she probably needs it.

This table gives approximate quantities only:

Age	Weight	Feeds per day	Quantity
0-14 days	7½ lb (3.5 kg)	6	3 oz (90 ml)
2 months	11 lb (5 kg)	5	5 oz (150 ml)
3 months	11 lb (6 kg)	5	6 oz (180 ml)
6 months and over	16½ lb (7.5 kg)	4	7 oz (210 ml)

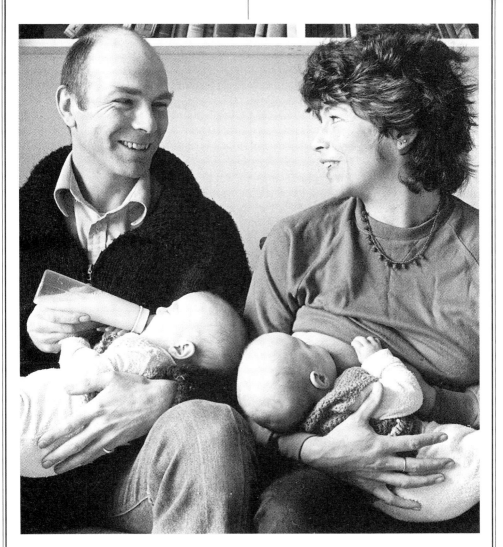

she is hungry. You will find that she soon settles into a routine of roughly four-hourly feeds. Some babies like to feed a little more often by day and wait for longer between feeds at night. There will be nightmare days when you seem to spend all day feeding, but it will settle. By the time the first month draws to a close, most babies have adopted a fairly stable pattern.

There will still be occasional off- days, and days when illness, teething, or holidays disrupt the pattern. If you are combining bottle and breast feeding, remember that breast milk is 'ordered' (468) by the baby. You cannot decide one morning that it would be more convenient to feed only by breast today and expect the system to jump into line. You will not immediately produce enough milk for every feed if you have only been feeding at night.

484 Winding

Simply hold your baby upright after a feed; let her lean on your shoulder: if wind bubbles up, she will belch it out. If not, there is no problem. If you feel happier patting her back or rubbing it, do so, but it is not really necessary. I forgot all about burping with my second two – I don't think it makes any difference at all.

485 Bringing up milk

Almost all babies bring back a little of their feed from time to time; some do it more than others, over-filling themselves and then bringing back the excess.

• The problem is more pronounced if you feed your baby lying down. Sit her in an upright position.

- Don't bounce her after feeds.
- If she cries much before a feed, she will suck in air. When this is released, milk will come up with it.
- Ensure that bottles are held upright to prevent her sucking in air.
- If the hole in the teat is too small, there may also be problems with milk flow. Shake the bottle to test how freely the milk flows. The hole should not, on the other hand be so large that she doe not need to work at sucking. The work is important for the normal development of jaws and teeth; see page 267.

486 Vomiting

This means bringing back digested milk, rather than recently swallowed milk. You can tell the difference: vomit smells unpleasant.

If the baby seems unwell, especially if there is any sign of fever or diarrhoea, consult your doctor without delay. In tiny babies, vomiting with diarrhoea can lead to serious dehydration at alarming speed. But if she seems perfectly well, carry on as usual, keeping your eyes open for illness. All babies occasionally vomit, it is not invariably serious.

487 Projectile vomiting

The baby literally throws back her feed, up to 3 ft (1m) across the room. If it happens regularly, and it is usually a boy who does it, he probably has a pyloric stenosis, a fault in the muscles of the stomach outlet. Tell your doctor at once. It is not dangerous and is easily, and permanently, cured by a minor operation. However, if he is bringing back all of his feed in this way, he will rapidly become dehydrated, and that can cause heart failure. Medication can control the vomiting until the operation is performed.

488 How do you feel?

In the days immediately after the birth, most women float on a blissful cloud of contentment. It was all worth it: everyone smiles, the world seems a wonderful place. Then, something pulls the rug from under your feet.

Round about day four, most mothers suffer from the baby blues. Your breasts may be full and heavy with milk, you are sore, moody and may even be running a slight temperature. Meanwhile, your previously happy baby has used up all her fat stores and is now hungry, tetchy and letting you know she is ready to feed. The contentment of the past few days is lost in a torrent of demands. Moreover, you feel unbelievably tired, dull, fat and flabby.

How could you have been so naïve as to have thought that motherhood was for you? Too late, you long for time, just a little time, of your own. Everyone is expecting you to cope. You may pretend you feel fine, but deep down, you suspect you cannot and will not. Does it help to reflect that almost all women feel this way? Perhaps – only perhaps; when you feel bad, you feel bad. Better, perhaps, to grasp the feeling for what it is: a form of mourning for times past. So try to look forward, and realize that most get over it as quickly as they fall in.

It would be odd if at this stage you did not have doubts about whether motherhood was the right choice, or whether you will be successful in the role. Motherhood is for many women to some extent a bid at living happily ever after: the prince no longer comes, so the baby is elected in his place. The realization that the baby is no prince (nor even a princess), but yet another person making yet more demands, hits hard.

But part of you knows that potentially she is a princess. You have something truly within your grasp. The present feeling of panic is largely fear that you might not grasp it.

It has been suggested that a woman never has so little control over herself and her destiny as in the first days after giving birth.

489 Postpartum syndrome

A small proportion of women find themselves with baby blues which last weeks, months, or even years. You may hear the condition described as post-natal depression, too. Many do not realize what is happening to them: they feel changed, but cannot quite say how. The feelings of despair, when they reach bottom, are unmistakable; the feelings of everyday depression are harder to recognize. Why it happens, no one is sure; the changes in hormone and water balance, in physiology, in social status and in body image all come at once. Because of this, it is difficult to label any of these as the main culprit, and for different women, different factors will be the cause.

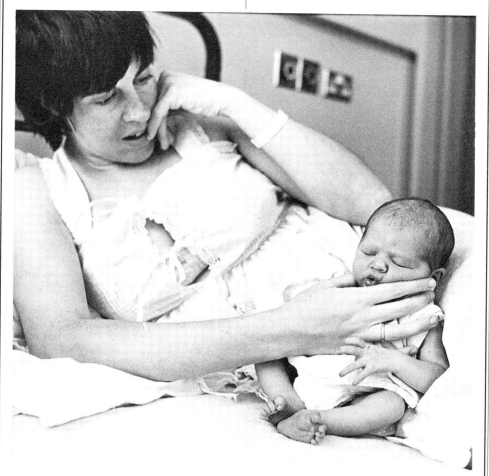

490 Fighting depression

Fighting is perhaps the wrong word. Of its nature, post-natal depression disinclines you to be positive. However, research, for what it is worth, shows that depression is reduced if:

• You are well informed about motherhood.
• You are helped by partner, family and friends.
• You make friends with other couples who have children.
• You consult your partner fully over plans for the baby, and also make a point of discussing plans and worries with family and friends.
• You keep some outside interests.
• You are not too concerned with appearances.
• You can see which tasks are important, and leave the rest.
• Stay put. Moving house is bad news.

Follow the practical steps given in 491 for alleviating depression.

491 If things get really bad. . .

Don't let depression blot out the good things about your baby.

• Try to relax when you are with your baby, especially while you are feeding her. Physical relaxation will help you to relax' mentally.
• Keep a list of the good things that happen in any one day, even if they are fleeting. Tell your partner about them when he comes in *before* listing the bad.
• Talk about your depression to someone. Don't try to hide it or pretend that it does not exist. Sometimes those closest to you are the best confidants, sometimes other mothers will be more understanding. Your clinic, your doctor or the people who ran your birth preparation classes may be able to put you in touch with a support group.
• Try setting yourself a realistic goal: getting a little fitter, perhaps, or starting an evening class; even learning the names of plants in the hedgerows. Every week aim to achieve something concrete, in addition to caring for the baby.

The Early Weeks

492 Your body

When you first catch sight of yourself in a full-length mirror, it may be a shock. Before, your body was firm and round, if large; now the tone has gone, but not the size. What you thought was baby looks much as if it was fat after all. After months in loose clothes, you may be longing for something fitted; but not while you look like this. Something has to be done.

Water loss takes time, but the extra sweating (463) will get rid of much. However, until your hormone balance is settled, you may find water retention remains a problem.

Your stomach muscles have been stretched to fit around the baby: they cannot snap back overnight. It will take time and effort to tone up.

There is nothing special about postnatal exercises, except that you must take them gently. If you have had a Caesarian section, start in the second week and take it even more slowly. Your body must be the judge: anything which hurts is bad for you. But toning up has to be done by exercise: dieting is impossible if you are breast feeding, and is anyway not advisable until your metabolism has settled down after the birth. On the other hand, don't overeat.

493 How many calories?

A useful rough guide to how many calories you need each day is to take your pre-pregnancy weight (real, not ideal) and multiply it by 12 if you are sedentary, 15 if you are active, and 22 if you are especially active. Thus if you were 10 stone (63.5 kg) and spend your days lolling on the sofa, you will need 1,920 calories per day. If you spend your day racing about, you need 3,520. If you are breast feeding, you should add 500 calories.

If you have substantial fat stores, you can drop the requirements a little, but never drastically; if you have no excess fat, you may need to eat a little more. Calories come in all forms, the ones you need come in a well balanced diet (see page 282), not from the sweet shop or the cake counter.

494 Postnatal exercise

The exercises recommended during pregnancy can be used to help you get back into shape; see pages 37-39. If you have continued to exercise throughout

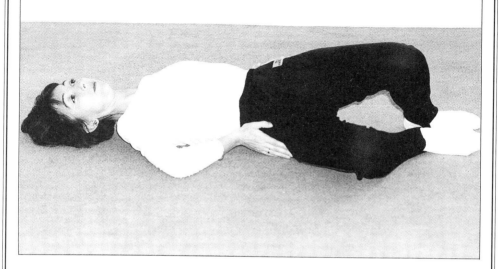

pregnancy, your muscles (apart from those of your abdomen) will still be firm, and you can proceed more rapidly than if you let exercise go in the last months.

Now that you no longer have a bulge, you should find it easier to stretch out the muscles after exercise; this is a key aspect of postnatal exercise. The natural process of recovery after stretching builds muscles, and the body gains in flexibility. Stretched muscles don't ache, either.

Once you are allowed out of bed, begin.

Day one
Sit up in bed and do the first seven exercises from the daily dozen (page 37); get out of bed and take a gentle walk.

If you feel able to complete the dozen, do so, but go easy on the side stretches; and you should just lift your heels off the floor for the running section in the first week.

Days two and three
Build up gradually. Leg exercises will feel much too strenuous at first. Introduce them gradually from the third day. After completing the leg exercises, always stretch out the muscles. Number 11 of the daily dozen is ideal for the purpose. Hold the stretch for as long as you can, then drop into a kneeling position and lean back as far as you can. You should feel this pulling the tops of your thighs. The stretches

suggested as supplements to the daily dozen (see page 189) are also useful.

Abdominal exercises on page 188
These should, like the others, start slowly. Put a pillow under your shoulders for the first couple of days and do no more than five of each at first. Gradually build on this, getting rid of the pillow on the third day, adding one extra lift every other day for the first two weeks, then one a day for the next two weeks, and two a day for the fifth week. By then, you should be feeling rather pleased with your shape.

If this schedule feels too fast, ease up. Postnatal exercises often suggest lifting the head and pushing the arm down by the side of your leg. This is much harder than keeping your arms behind your head. A worthwhile goal is 50 lifts in each position.

Postnatal exercises

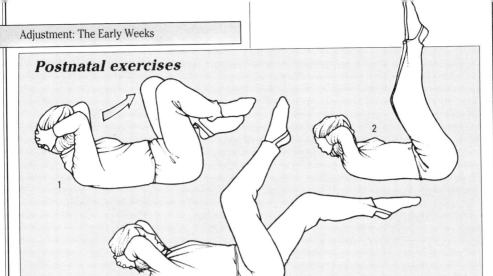

1 Cross both legs and lift them so that your knees are vertically above your hips, rather as if you were sitting cross-legged against a wall. Put your hands behind your head and lift your shoulders.

Aim to do ten lifting straight up and ten moving your right elbow to your left knee (keep your knees still, it is the upper part of your body that moves). Then repeat with the opposite elbow to the opposite knee.
2 Keeping this position, drop your knees towards the floor. Then raise them back into the original position. Repeat. You should feel this in the lower stomach. Take care, never strain.

3 Lastly, lie flat and raise your legs vertically. Now bend the knees slightly so that they are more or less in line with your navel, and point your toes. Put your arms behind your head and lift as usual. As you get fitter, you can move one leg back so that it is almost parallel with the floor. By moving the position of your legs as you lift, you use different abdominal muscles.
4 You should bring your knees into your chest after each exercise. When you have finished, roll over on to your stomach, lift yourself on to your arms, and stretch the abdominal muscles. Hold in position for as long as you feel comfortable.

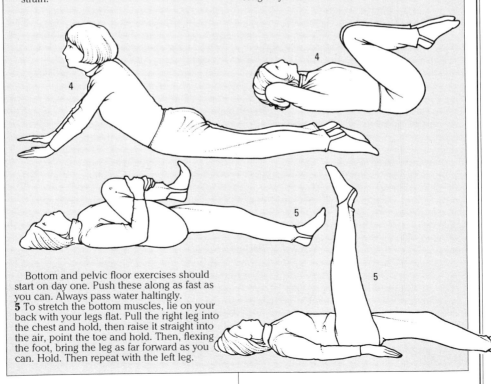

Bottom and pelvic floor exercises should start on day one. Push these along as fast as you can. Always pass water haltingly.
5 To stretch the bottom muscles, lie on your back with your legs flat. Pull the right leg into the chest and hold, then raise it straight into the air, point the toe and hold. Then, flexing the foot, bring the leg as far forward as you can. Hold. Then repeat with the left leg.

1 Standing with your feet hip-width apart, reach up with both arms above the head; reach again, higher, with the left arm, then the right. Now, falling forwards from the waist, bend the knees and push your arms between your legs. Repeat for a count of eight.

2 Now, staying down, straighten the knees and, bending from the waist, touch both hands to your feet. Clap. Repeat for eight. (It may take weeks to get to the foot; meanwhile just go down as far as you can.) Then push your arms through your legs (knees bent) for a further eight.

3 Add these stretches to your daily dozen. The first helps tone up the inner thighs.

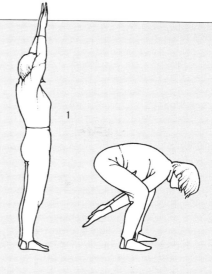

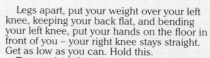

Legs apart, put your weight over your left knee, keeping your back flat, and bending your left knee, put your hands on the floor in front of you – your right knee stays straight. Get as low as you can. Hold this.

Turn to the left and you will find yourself in position to start a race. Hold this. Repeat to the other side.

The best exercise for lower bottom flab is probably 'Rover's return' or 'doggies', so named because it looks like a dog who is undecided whether he wants to pee.

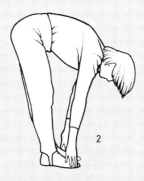

Get down on all fours and drop the right elbow on to the floor. Keeping your leg bent, lift the right leg just like a dog would to pee. You make an undecided move, lifting the leg up as high as you can, then down again. Repeat eight times. On the downward journey, don't let your leg touch the floor. Keep your leg in the up position, then ease it higher and yet higher. Count eight slowly. It hurts, but it works wonders. Aim eventually to complete three sets on each side.

To stretch the muscles you have just worked, sit with your legs crossed. Now take your right leg and lift it to the far side of your left knee. Straighten your back and hold. Repeat on the other side.

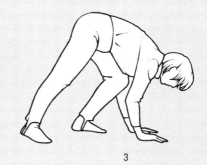

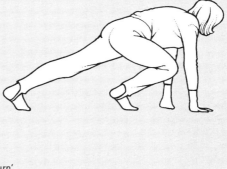

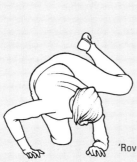

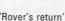
'Rover's return'

495 Lower abdominal muscles

These may have separated during pregnancy. If this has happened to you, it will be obvious if you blow out your abdomen and feel the bulge below the navel. If they have separated, go easy on all exercises that work these muscles. If they have not separated, start working these muscles. The second set of abdominal exercises on page 188 works these lower muscles, but you might like to try the ones in the panel as well.

Exercises that firm up the muscles will make you look (and feel) good, but they will not necessarily make you fitter. This is the role of aerobic exercise, which works both heart and lungs. Running, swimming and skipping are all excellent aerobic exercises. Even someone who is not fit can jog 1m (1.6km) in 15 minutes, which is less than the time it takes to boil the potatoes. As you get fitter, you will find that you can run further and faster. Twenty minutes, three times a week, is usually the recommended minimum for aerobic fitness. It will raise your metabolic requirements and burn off calories. During aerobic exercise, your pulse rate should be between 140 and 180. It is easiest to take your pulse in your neck. See illustration.

> **Other problem points**
> The main problem areas after pregnancy are the waist, thighs and hips. The stretches on page 189 should help the waist and thighs.

496 Cautions

• Never exercise cold muscles.
• Always start with the daily dozen (page 37) – actually now the daily 15.
• Work up slowly to the recommended minimum for aerobic exercise. First time out, jog 100 yards (90 m) then walk 100 yards. Jog again only if it feels easily within your capabilities. From this gentle start, build up over four months to the minimum of 20 minutes three times a week. If you are very unfit to start with, get your doctor's advice.
• Always stretch muscles after you have worked them.
• Cool down slowly, never stop suddenly. If the baby cries, walk around slowly with her against your shoulder for two or three

minutes. If you were in the middle of a session of aerobic exercise, you should make this six minutes. Your muscles will get stiff, and you will feel dizzy if you sit down to feed the baby straight away.
• Don't worry if you cannot find time every day to get through the whole programme. You will get into shape within two or three months even if you only manage two sessions a week.

You may find it easiest to do the daily 15 every morning, followed by a work-out of one body area and a little running on the spot. Wave your arms in the air as you run in order to improve the circulation. Five minutes with a skipping rope is another possibility.

497 Special care babies

Almost one in every seven babies in Britain spends some time in a special care unit. Babies may need special care because they are born too soon, because they are small-for-dates, or because of handicap.

Small-for-dates babies have not flourished in the womb. For some reason (and there are many), the placenta has not worked efficiently. Birth is often difficult because of oxygen shortage, and later breathing difficulties prolong the oxygen deprivation. These babies often suffer from low blood sugar (499) and can also have fits. Because there is little fat on their bodies, they usually look red, and you can often see the blood vessels through the skin. Most newborn babies have difficulty controlling their temperature and for low birth-weight babies this difficulty is increased by the absence of fat stores. They are nursed in temperature-controlled incubators.

There is a great deal of heat loss through the head, so a special-care baby sometimes wears a hat. More often, you will find her with a heat shield over her and a thermostat attached to her stomach. The heat will automatically be switched on if body temperature falls, or vice-versa.

Many low birth-weight babies suffer from jaundice, and all pick up infections easily, a cause of anxiety in parents: she may seem to be doing well, then suddenly become ill.

Breast milk will help protect her from infection, especially the early colostrum and transitional milk which is rich in immunological proteins (469), You should breast feed her, or provide breast milk using a breast pump if you are able to manage it.

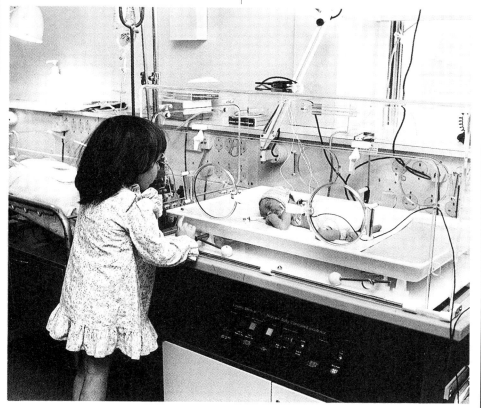

498 Special care equipment

The machinery which surrounds a tiny premature baby in her incubator can seem alarming: the tubes and gauges distance you from her. Remind yourselves that in the womb she would also have tubes attached and that you know her better than you would if she were still inside you. The nursing staff will explain the function of each catheter.

Premature babies are often born before their lungs are sufficiently mature. Surfactant (310), essential for early breathing, only develops in the last few weeks before birth, and babies born before surfactant covers the lung surfaces have to work hard to draw each breath. You can see the chest rising and collapsing each time, and often you can hear her grunting with the effort. She will also look quite blue. The remedy is extra oxygen, but it must be monitored carefully, since too much can damage the eyes.

A catheter inserted into her navel monitors the oxygen in her arterial blood; the oxygen itself is delivered under continuous positive pressure through a small catheter inserted through her nose. Sometimes a face mask or head box is used instead of the nose tube.

Because premature babies often have to work extremely hard for each breath, they can become exhausted and stop breathing.

A small-for-dates baby will also suffer from breathing difficulties (apnoea) in the first days and weeks after birth. She will probably be nursed on a special mat, or have a monitor strapped to her chest to record each breath. If she stops breathing, or has any difficulty, an alarm alerts the nursing staff. Stimulation will usually start her breathing again.

499 Low blood sugar

Limp, apathetic babies have low blood sugar, and so do some jittery, active babies. Extra sugar is usually provided via an intravenous glucose drip, usually inserted into the baby's hand.

500 In touch

How can you hold such a tiny, fragile thing with all those tubes?

You can, and all babies need to be touched and held; all parents need to touch. At first it may not be possible to take her in your arms, but you can stroke her. The seeming brutality of the machinery can be, must be, softened by human contact.

While you are still in hospital you may be able to visit her frequently; later, you may be able to stay in a room next to the unit. Staff are well aware of the value of your care and they understand that under all the tubes and sticking plaster she is still your child.

Sometimes a baby has to be taken to a special care unit in another hospital or for special treatment available only in a certain centre. You should ask to accompany your baby if this is at all possible. Fathers often have to provide the essential link between mother and baby in these cases. Left alone in hospital, a woman may feel inadequate, even jealous, of those (including her partner) who care for and visit the child, especially if she remains in a hospital ward where other mothers and babies are together. Ask for a photograph of your baby: it is better than nothing.

You will need plenty of time alone with your partner; ask the hospital to provide this privacy for you. You need to be able to vent your anger, to feel your misery, without interruption.

501 Being realistic

It is often too easy to hope. Sometimes doctors and nurses have difficulty telling parents how seriously ill their child is, or, in truth, whether she may lead a normal life. It is distressing to have to tell parents who are looking for a glimmer of hope that there is none.

But it is best to face facts now. Hopes are built, dreams are made; few of us can face their continued destruction. Direct questions require direct answers. Ask the paediatrician to give you all the information available, not just about the baby's immediate progress, but about the long-term outlook. You have to know the possibilities of physical and mental handicap in order to plan realistically for the future. In the long run, you will regret being protected from the truth.

502 Losing a baby

For all the care, for all the machinery, sometimes small babies die. If a baby dies,

you should each hold the body before it is taken from you. Grief takes time to work through, but it will, however little you saw her, however little you knew her. Death is easy for a tiny baby, sometimes easier than life. If life was to be lived imprisoned in a severely handicapped body, or a mind too limited to cope with today's world, then death is the way she avoided frustration and pain. Which is not to say it is a happy release for you.

Loss of a baby is the loss of a dream. We all dream of the future, especially while we carry a little of that future inside us. Grieving is coming to terms with lost dreams.

Don't try to forget: it will make you feel guilty, numb, angry, as well as sad. But, in the beginning, you may find yourself totally flat and unfeeling, unable to accept that this has happened. It may take three, even four weeks for you to cry. The hospital will make arrangements for the funeral, or you can ask to do this yourself. The decision is, of course, a very personal one.

503 Going home

Many parents have an idealized picture of what life is like with a small baby; those separated after birth are more likely than most to paint a rosy picture

What is it really like to have a baby home at last? Suddenly, that abstraction, being a family, is a reality.

What you now have in your arms is not just a pretty doll, such as you see in magazines, and indeed some baby books, but a person. She looks at once like any other baby, yet in her familiar, family look, you recognize yourselves. It is not that she has your nose and eyes; rather, there is something you feel you have seen before. As often as not it is an expression – a way of moving her mouth or screwing up her nose. Sometimes it is a fleeting look in her eye.

But it is more than physical features that make her unique. Until now, babies have seemed to you – well, just like babies. Not this one. There is something about her, even with her limited capacities, which you recognize that makes her *somebody*; a member of the family with a will of her own. She is not a blank slate. There is no way you will be able to mould her entirely into the child or adult you want her to be. She is herself: the family relationship will be that of three (or more) individuals all acting upon each other, not simply two parents managing a helpless 'thing'.

504 Individuality

How does this distinctiveness arise? Life, as the Chinese recognized long ago in dating age from conception, has not just begun. In the Middle Ages, it was thought that anything affecting a woman during pregnancy literally rubbed off on the child: her joys, her sorrows, her anger, and also the things she saw, heard and thought.

In modern times we have lost touch more or less entirely with this view of early life. In its place, there is the idea of the fortress womb: one in which the baby is isolated and protected, and which reduces the woman's role from one of central importance to one of being, essentially, an incubator.

The conventional modern medical view can be summed up as: 'Watch your drug intake, eat carefully, and don't worry about what you feel and do during pregnancy, for this cannot affect the unborn child – she is safe inside her bag of water: your only contact with her is through your blood supply. Keep that pure, and all will be well.'

But there is a real possibility (see 285) that the life she shares with you during the nine months, and her experience of birth (see 385), make a small contribution to the child you see before you: small, but nonetheless a contribution.

505 Genetics

Genetic make-up is something else again; see 43. We are all products of our genes and of the environment; a well-known psychologist once said that development is 100 per cent influenced by genetic make-up and 100 per cent influenced by the environment in which we develop. By which he meant that the two factors, heredity and environment, interact.

Take a white Siamese kitten, white at birth because it has inherited the gene for albinism. But the genes' action is directly influenced by the environment, specifically by the kitten's temperature. In the womb, its whole body is warm and the kitten remains a uniform white. Outside, its nose, paws and tail become colder and that makes the underlying coat colour (be it ginger, black, grey or tabby) show through. Raise the kitten in the fridge, and it would be mostly coloured; raise it in an incubator, and it would stay white.

Like the kitten, your baby is as she is because she was made that way, and because of the influences acting upon her even now. She will be the woman she becomes by the way this basic self is allowed to develop in your care; her faults will never be entirely her fault; her virtues will never be entirely to your credit.

506 Elder children

Most of the time, an older child will love having a baby sister or brother. Just as true is the fact that jealousy will also rear its head, and that you will not be able to prevent it; it would be unnatural if you could. Like other emotions, jealousy is something a child must learn to handle; doing so now is hard, but it will make it easier in the future.

Children depend so much on their parents for love, attention, and fulfilment of most of their needs, especially if they are under school age, that it is perhaps not unreasonable for them to feel afraid and jealous of having to share your love for the first time.

A feeling that you prefer the baby is not unrealistic when the elder child (for the sake of argument, a boy) sees you spending so much time tending to her needs, or when he must always wait for attention until you have finished with the baby.

If he is under school age, part of his idea of himself as a person (his categorical self, see 755), is tied up with his belongings. He is the boy with the red hat. He is also the boy with the cot that has rabbits on the side. Remember this when you come to hand it on to the baby. Involve him in preparing the baby's room, but also spend time on his, making it more grown-up. Don't pass the cot straight on to the baby. Make a big fuss of getting him a 'big boy's bed' before the baby arrives. Then let him choose when to move into it.

You cannot avoid changing his routine, but try to keep the changes to a minimum.

With school-age children, jealousy is less likely to be a problem, but don't ignore the possibility. Even teenagers may resent your new unavailability. See 738.

507 Preparation

Be sure that an elder child knows where the new baby will sleep, how she will feed, and how much of your time she will take. It is a shock for the elder child to find that you are always cuddling or carrying the baby.

He may feel left out if he finds that he is the only one not sleeping in your bedroom.

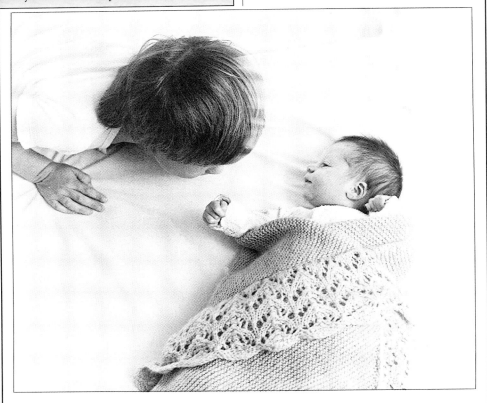

Make sure that visitors don't forget him. Ask grandparents and good friends to bring him a little gift if they are bringing one for the baby, and to greet him first.

● Tell older children you will be tired, that babies cry and make demands. Ask them to let you know if they think they need more attention. Always reserve some time in each day when you can be alone with each child.
● Love uniquely. Make the elder child feel he is special in his own way, just as the baby is special in hers.
● Love fairly. Avoid always putting the baby first. Sometimes it is wise to say "Well, the baby will have to wait until we have done this".
● Don't call the baby by endearing names you no longer use for him.
● Don't belittle him if he regresses: starts acting like a baby. Even 30-year-olds play baby sometimes. If he wets his bed, tell him you did it when you were having the baby. See also 508.
● Don't leave child care to fathers and baby care to mothers. He still needs both parents, and may feel he is getting a bad deal if his father is going back to work after a week.

Timetable
Here is a suggestion – that is all – for how caring for a baby of 12 weeks, and toddler of about two years, can mesh:

7am	Feed baby.
7.30	Get in bed with toddler having a morning drink.
7.45	Get toddler up, washed, dressed and sat down to breakfast.
8.30	Play with toddler
10.30	Put toddler to bed for a nap. Get baby up. Feed and bath her. Sit her in her chair.
11.30	Get toddler up.
12.30	Lunch with toddler.
2.00	Feed baby. Take both children for a walk.
4.30	Tea for toddler.
5.30	Feed baby.
7.00	Put toddler to bed.
8.00	Put baby to bed.
10.00	Feed baby.

Even a two-year-old can help with a baby:
● Carry the bottle.
● Bring a nappy, cream or talcum powder.
● Splash the water when you bath her.

- Rock the crib or pram.
- Hold the baby's hand when she cries.
- Talk to the baby and play with her.

Older children can:
- Hold the baby.
- Help to change a nappy.
- Cool bottles.
- Watch the baby for a moment or so.

508 Symptoms of jealousy
Jealousy takes many forms:

- **Naughtiness:** This is the most common symptom: nine out of ten children show an increase in naughtiness following the birth of a sibling. The easiest way to deal with it is to give the elder child as much attention as you can while he is good. Sitting down to feed the baby, leaving him with nothing to do, is asking for trouble.
- **Aggression:** One minute the child is loving; the next he aims a blow at the baby.

You are angry. But the reason he behaves like this is because he feels uncertain you still love him. Being angry will make it worse. Talk to him; tell him you understand. The baby is rather a nuisance; she does take too much time. But if he makes her cry, there will be less time to play together. Then give him your full attention for a while.

Aggression is the least common of the symptoms of jealousy.
- **Indirect aggression:** He breaks a toy, kicks the furniture, rips his books.

Let him know you understand that life is not so good for him now you have the baby. Make a special fuss. Do something with him while the baby sleeps. Let him have a game with the water at the sink, or making wet footprints all over the kitchen floor.
- **Blaming mother:** The elder child kicks and lashes out at you, and complains about you to others.

You, of course, started it all: you are the one who had the baby. He is hurting, and you should too. In one study there was an eight-fold increase in this type of behaviour in the first three weeks after the baby came home.

It will need much understanding and patience. Try not to worry about this rejection or to take it too literally. It will almost certainly make it worse.
- **Jealousy kept inside:** He looks sad, he is dejected, mopes, looks bored. He has lost his sparkle.

Over half the children in one study became tearful and clinging after the birth. A few are more seriously disturbed. It is commoner in boys than girls.

This needs special care. You will need to talk gently to him, make sure he knows you understand. Encourage him to show his bad feelings, don't condemn them or him for having them. He will keep them bottled up if you do. Make sure he knows that you all love him. If this withdrawal continues, you may need professional help.
- **Reverting to baby-behaviour:** He may wet his bed, (over half the children in one study did), start waking in the night (also common) or say he can only eat mashed-up food. He may try to breast feed.

Reverting to babyhood is, if you think about it, perfectly natural. If the baby is getting all the attention, then the simple answer is to be a baby too. If he wants to breast feed, let him: breast milk comes very slowly, and he will probably go off the idea quite rapidly. Point out how much nicer orange juice tastes. If he wants a bottle, let him have one. If you don't make an issue of it, the phase will pass. Tell him what a lovely baby he was, and how you hope the baby will grow up to be like him.
- **Attention seeking:** He becomes rude and naughty, especially when you are feeding the baby or in the middle of bathing her. In one study, children chose the moment that the mother picked up the baby to do the naughtiest thing they knew. Ensure there are plenty of toys and books about when you are feeding so that he has no excuse. Perhaps put on a story tape or a record.

509 How disturbed?
Most children show one or two symptoms (see 508) of jealousy. No child shows all of them, indeed no child is overwhelmingly jealous. Often the children who seem to be most disturbed by the idea of the birth are the ones who show the most affection and interest when the new baby comes home.

It would be misleading to think the elder child's feelings towards the new arrival are simple. They are a mixture of mature and babyish behaviour, disturbance, anger, affection and interest.

510 How long does jealousy last?
Serious reactions rarely last longer than eight months, but minor disturbances may persist. Fearfulness and anxiety may be

noticeable up to a year, or longer, after the birth. Snakes, spiders or perhaps something as innocuous as the dishwasher could be the source of the phobia. You may have to check the bedroom for creepy-crawlies before he will go to bed.

For many children this is an exaggeration of a common tendency.

Many children also develop elaborate rituals: ways of saying goodbye or goodnight, such as kissing every teddy, only using a certain dish or a special spoon at meal times.

A poor initial relationship does not signal a difficult and quarrelsome relationship as the children grow up, but don't expect jealousy simply to disappear. It will return from time to time, mixed in with all the good feelings, because it is part of growing up. It is inevitable in all relationships, including those of adults.

511 Jealousy and closeness

If you compete for your parents' love with a brother or a sister, you get to know each other very well; your closeness and understanding develops partly because of this jealousy and competition.

You have only to see the precision of siblings' teasing and vindictiveness to understand how well even small children know each other. They know precisely how to make each other cry, how best to undermine security. Know your enemy, perhaps; but that also means knowing your friend.

512 Not all bad

In 506-511 I have concentrated on jealousy, but there is a positive and delightful side to an elder child's attitude to the new arrival.

He will show affection towards the baby; comment on her; share his toys (or give her toys of his own) and help you to care for her.

He will imitate her. Studies of small children with their new siblings show that they copy yawns, grimaces and sounds. They ask endless questions about the baby and often play games in which they pretend to be looking after a baby. They will be distressed when the baby cries.

But it still will not stop an older child doing something mean or deliberately trying to hurt the baby. Ambivalence is part of the sibling relationship: love and

jealousy go hand in hand. See 511.

513 Growth and development

It is often said that you cannot run before you can walk. The reason this is literally true has nothing to do with any physical limitations on running or walking, but because this is how people develop. Within reason, one can generalize about infant and child development, and this book contains many such generalizations. Their usefulness, though, needs to be clearly understood. The point is not in logging a child's progress – metally ticking off the mileposts as they are passed; there is little lasting value in this, and often unnecessary anxiety. The real, underlying purpose of such generalizations is as a guide to meshing your input with her capacity. Knowing *how much* she can see, what she *prefers* to hear, enables you to show her the things which will most stimulate her visually, and to make the noises to which she will best respond.

514 Vision

At birth, or soon after, a baby can:

• Focus her eyes on the same point. Her best vision is 8-10 in (20-25 cm) in front of her eyes. The focus is 'fixed', not rigidly, but the quality of the image falls off nearer or farther away. Eight to 10 in is about the distance of your face from hers when you are breast feeding. Her ability to focus at different distances will improve gradually over the next four months.
• See detail sharply. She could not tell whether the stripes on your shirt were stripes if they were less than 1/32 in (about 1 mm) wide. Acuity improves rapidly over the next six months but does not reach adult levels until after the second birthday.
• Follow a moving object with her eyes – not very well at first, but she improves quickly.
• Tell the difference between some colours by two weeks (and perhaps at birth). She prefers red and blue.
• Show different patterns of interest. Babies will look at some objects for longer than others. They prefer bright objects and contrasts, such as dark hair against a face.
• Perceive depth: babies respond differently to photographs and to real objects at two weeks.
• Respond to parts of objects rather than whole objects. When she looks at a picture of a face, she does not mind if the eyes are

jumbled up with the mouth and nose. By about five months, however, she much prefers to see a whole face.

• Reach out in a primitive way, but not monitor what her hands are doing. In fact, for some time yet she will be distracted if she sees her hand as she reaches out. She does, however, expect to find something when she reaches out, and is upset if she reaches for a shadow.

The accuracy of reaching improves in the first weeks and months; she can monitor her hand by about five months.

515 Hearing

At birth, or soon after, a baby:

• Responds to various sounds, particularly those in the pitch and volume range of the human voice; high-pitched voices are clear favourites.
• Starts at loud sounds.
• Turns away from unpleasant sounds.
• Can locate a sound in front of her, and roughly tell if it comes from left or right.
• Is soothed by rhythmic sounds.
• Can discriminate sounds with different initial letters such as bah and pah.
• Can recognize her mother's voice by two to three weeks.
• Can reach for a noisy object in the dark.
• Can move in time with speech.

516 Smell and taste

At birth, or soon after a baby:

• Reacts to strong smells such as ammonia.
• Can tell the smell of her mother by the first week.
• Can tell bitter from sour.
• Can tell salt from sweet, and prefers sweet.

517 Touch

A newborn baby will respond to touch all over her body, but particularly to touching of the hands and around the mouth.

518 'I like people'

Most interesting of all is that babies seem especially atttuned to people. They are attracted to the human face and to the human voice, especially women's voices. They can even imitate some facial expressions: try putting your tongue out to a baby, she may put hers out in reply. She might raise her eyebrows or purse her lips, too.

When two people talk they move very slightly, keeping time with each other as they talk. They begin and finish each movement in time with the major breaks in speech. Babies do this within hours of birth.

519 Motor ability

She needs to take in and absorb the world around her, especially the world of people on whom she is totally dependent. Because we must love her (for how else would she survive) she needs to show particular interest in us. If she looks alert when we talk to her, if she looks into our faces when we are near, we are more likely to respond.

But she does not need to be capable of much. We feed her, we carry her, we keep her warm. Her motor abilities reflect this: they are pretty poor. She cannot hold her head up, roll over or sit. She cannot co-ordinate looking and reaching or use her hands to explore. But she will improve.

By one month, she can lift her chin off the floor; by two months she will take a swipe at a toy tied to her cot; by six months she will roll over, sit with support and may even begin to crawl.

520 Learning

Babies can learn almost as soon as they are born. She can, for instance, learn that a bell is always followed by a little food, or that when you pick her up she will be fed. She may also learn that you are a good thing.

She learns how you smell, and soon she knows that she feels secure in your arms. By the end of the second week she has probably learned that when she can smell you nearby she will be comforted. Soon she feels comforted whenever she smells you near. Later, she will feel insecure without that comfort.

She may learn to associate other people with anger, anxiety, fear or frustration. This is what psychologists call a 'conditioned emotional response', and it is probably the basis of a 'parent's touch': the special ability parents have to sooth and comfort their own children. Our emotional responses are often automatic, even as adults. We don't always know why it is that we suddenly feel anxious, or why something (or somebody) makes us feel secure. Perhaps they smell like a long-lost comfort.

If your smell can make your baby feel secure, she can also smell your anxiety. A baby with an anxious, nervous mother will probably associate that smell with her behaviour.

521 Other ways to learn

We all reinforce or encourage certain behaviour in our children: you smile when she does what you want; look away when she does something of which you disapprove. She learns to please you, but that is not the full story. Experiments have proved that this learning starts, in a humble way, during the earliest months. Connect your baby's wrist to a mobile with a piece of wool in such a way that the mobile moves when she waves her arm, and soon her arm waves more. She is beginning to make things happen, and it is but a short step to making *you* please *her.*

She stirs; you say "Hello".

She looks wide-eyed; you say "Hello darling, have you woken up?"

She looks right into your eyes and smiles; you pick her up.

She has learned that if she interacts with you, you pick her up.

Actually, the process is two-way: by picking her up you reinforce wide-eyed looking and smiling.

Another example:
She wakes.
You ignore her.
She stirs.
You carry on dusting.
She cries.
You go over and rock the pram.
She quietens.
You go away.
She howls.
You pick her up.

You may not think you are encouraging her to cry, but it might seem different to the baby.

522 A social being

What do you conclude from 521? Essentially, I think, that she is not a doll, but a tiny, if unsophisticated, human being, with the emphasis heavily on one word: human. She is already acutely attuned to people. Whenever she learns something new in the next year or two, she will learn it first in a *social* – a 'people' – context. She is, above all, a social being.

523 Baby reality

Many parents start out firmly convinced that once the baby is home, life will return to normal, but somehow also be richer.

There is a story told of an American professor who wanted to try and convey to students the ties and demands of parenthood. He asked each of his students to be parent to an egg for a week.

The egg had to go with them wherever they went, carried carefully in case it broke, and kept cool (but not frozen) at all times.

It did not need feeding, but in order to keep it cool in the hot American summer, it had to be kept in a box with some ice. Since the box needed to be small enough to take anywhere, the ice needed replenishing at regular intervals, including during the night. After a week of caring for these fragile eggs, most of the students had a much increased respect for parents.

In reality, being a parent is even more demanding – and far more rewarding.

524 Day four – what went wrong?

Around the fourth day after birth, a baby often goes through a period of restlessness. The fat stores on which she has lived for the last days have gone, and she feels hungry for the first time. She will probably fret and cry a good deal.

Mothers are, in principle, ready to breast feed. The milk has 'come in' and you are beginning to get the hang of feeding.

But in practice you are not used to feeding a hungry, fretful baby, and if you have just arrived home, you are none too sure of your ability. Add to this the difficulty of feeding from a rock-hard breast (475) and a touch of the baby blues (488) for both parents, and no wonder many despair of ever getting it right.

Tense and nervous mothers may find that they do not let down the hind milk (468); as a result, the baby stays hungry. Unused to feeling hungry, this previously contented baby cries and cries. A vicious circle develops in which feeding (or its failure) is followed by tears and by total disbelief (on the part of both parents) that two intelligent adults cannot care for one small baby for 24 hours.

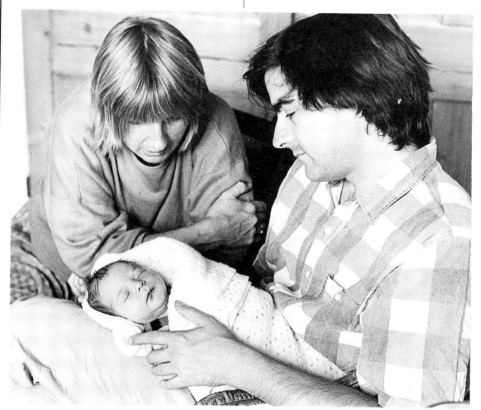

525 Adjustment

Waiting to give birth in the long months of pregnancy, it is easy to lose sight of the goal. The goal is parenthood; most of us arrive unprepared. We went to classes, we read books, but it was birth we prepared for, not childcare. We planned a 'good birth' and we ended up with a child. Perhaps that is why women often see a bad birth as the focus for all the ills that follow.

Suddenly finding yourself in charge of a small baby is alarming. It is hard to imagine how something so small who, after all, does nothing except feed and sleep could take all your time. But she does; if she is your first, she certainly does.

526 Where the time goes

It is not that actually caring for the baby takes much time. Count up the contact hours feeding, burping and changing and it probably is nowhere near eight in 24. But it feels far more exhausting than an eight-hour day of work. Why?

Sleep is, of course, disrupted, but many women have had their sleep disrupted in the last months of pregnancy. The fundamental problem, I suspect, lies in the radically different way you have to organize life with a small child.

Childcare is not something we can cordon off into short, well-defined periods of effort. Babies cannot be organized to fit into a schedule. They are the schedule, the rest of life has to be fitted around them, from sleeping and love-making to eating and (if you should be so lucky), reading the newspaper. Everything is negotiated with a baby. Few of us have ever had to deal with this level of demand.

Caring for children is the most tiring job in the world because you never get a run at anything else to relieve the effort.

527 Making time

Accepting that your time will be monopolized is the first and most difficult step you have to take in adjusting to a baby in the house. Until you have learned not to fight this basic reality, you will find childcare a bind. Once you have accepted the status quo, you can loosen the knot by learning tricks to maximize your time. I never fully made the adjustment with my first child, but the next two, who came in quick succession seven years later, were no trouble; I sailed through their babyhood, enjoying them immensely. Looking back, I know that they were no less demanding than the first. All that had changed was me. Here are some examples:

I used a papoose while I did housework, tried to write, or entertained. But the way I used the sling differed with each child, and my attitude with it. With Daniel, my first, I would start the housework (something I hate doing), while he was asleep in the Moses basket. He would wake; I would pick him up, put him into the sling and carry on cleaning in a bad temper.

My attitude was 'Can't you even let me clean in peace? Do you think I enjoy it?'

With my younger children, I accepted that they would wake and put them into the papoose before I started cleaning. My attitude was 'I hate housework, come and give me a cuddle while I clean'.

If I wanted to think something through when Daniel was small, I would lock myself in the study and concentrate while he was asleep. He always woke. By the time my third arrived, we had no room for a study, so I would sit him in his bouncing cradle chair and work beside him at the kitchen table, or put both children in the pushchair and go for a walk. If I wanted to read the paper, I would lie with the baby on the sofa. Often his elder sister would get her doll and a book and lie on the other sofa 'being like Mummy'. Of course, I didn't read much, but I never expected to; I had learned not to fight, and as a result, I was able to win some time for myself. I would not say that the whole problem is one of attitude, but it does account for a good deal. If she wakes and you think 'Not again, please let me sleep', you both have to calm down before you can sleep again. If your attitude is 'What's the matter? Come and have a cuddle', you are probably both asleep again within a few minutes.

528 Give and take

You could say it all boils down to accepting that people who love each other have the right to make demands on each other.

It really must go for you both. Don't fit your life entirely around your baby; let her fit her life around you as well. There has to be give and take in any relationship.

Don't feel guilty if you make demands on her.

Don't feel resentful when she makes demands on you. See also 558.

529 Bill of rights

There is a section from Kahil Gibran's *The Phrophet,* often read at wedding ceremonies, which talks of the need for separate growth and development, and makes the point that trees do not grow strong in the shade of other trees. It might just as well be read at birth.

A family is one, but it is made up of separate individuals, each with their own rights to growth and development.

- Men have the right, should they wish, to grow as parents, to take an equal (or negotiated role) in the parenting of children.
- Women have the right to grow as individuals, a right not to be entirely subservient to the demands of family life. They have the right, should they wish, to share the parenting of children with fathers.

But these rights, in as far as they go against the traditional expectations of society, require negotiating and need to be consistent. It is no use saying 'This is my baby, hands off', but then expecting a man to take equal responsibilty when the baby grows into a toddler; at any rate, not without further negotiation. Nor has a woman the right, if the relationship breaks down, to say 'It was our baby, but my child.'

Within a family, it is not only children who develop.

The problem, of course, is that at the time we forge this bill of rights, two of the parties are suffering from depression and exhaustion, and the third is incapable of rational thought. No wonder most of us get it wrong. It is tempting to go along with whatever seems easy at the time; but in the long term, failing to think the matter through will lead to unhappiness and resentment. See 666.

530 The Capability view

New parents have, I suspect, something to learn from the achievement of Capability Brown.

The great English landscape gardener created majestic parks in which each separate feature contributes to a landscaped whole, but each also retains its own individual splendour. For all the artificially contrived effects – he moved hills, dug valleys, dammed streams and created lakes – his landscapes seem natural.

And he did it knowing that he would never see the full fruits of his creative skills.

531 Work and play

Before industrialization, most people worked at home or in the immediate vicinity. Eating, sleeping, childcare, play, socializing and all other aspects of living shared the workplace.

Today, most people separate work, which one goes out to, from 'living', which goes on at home. This makes it especially difficult not to see children as confining. They become associated with all the other essential chores, such as washing-up and laundry, that go on at home.

Of course children interfere with leisure, and with work; but if you have set ideas about when and where work and play should happen, children will seem all the more limiting.

532 Your perineum: continuing care

Don't give up looking after yourself when you get home. If soreness persists between your legs, repeat the measures suggested in 458. If you are short of time, try sponging the area with warm water to increase blood flow and promote healing. Either do this over a bidet or the lavatory bowl, or, if you have time, get right into the bath and soak. One and a half cups of dried comfrey root, or one cup of fresh ginger root (peeled and chopped) added to the bath water will relieve itching and irritation.

• It is safe to take the baby into the bath with you, as long as the bathroom is warm. Just lie her between your breasts.
• If you have had an episiotomy, fresh air and sunlight promote healing. But how? Exposing the perineum in the garden may well be impractical; but a sun-ray or heat lamp directed at the perineum for 20 minutes twice a day is a fair substitute. Or put a 60-watt light bulb into a small table lamp and sit with it between your legs, just near enough to feel the warmth. If you feel a bit silly, simply laugh at yourself.
• Apply wheat germ or vitamin E oil to the perineum.
• Put your feet up every hour or so, even if only for a couple of minutes.
• Breast feed the baby lying down: 471.

533 More massage

Massage and relaxation exercises have just as much use now as during pregnancy. Try for at least 20 minutes of total relaxation every day to help dissipate tension. It is probably impossible to use sex as a form of release just now, but massage is a good second best.

534 Acupressure to assist feeding

See the diagram. Does it work? Sometimes I found it did. Is it psychosomatic or does the stimulation really release the body's natural painkillers, the endorphins? I think the explanation is less important than simply having something to do and being able to do it for yourself, or for your partner. There are no drugs you can safely take to treat a tender breast, or to increase your flow of milk. Pressing a few points in the body will do no harm, whereas powerful drugs can, and do. If acupressure does not work, you have lost nothing except a little time spent on yourself or your partner. Hardly a waste.

Milk production: natural remedies
• Peppermint tea to soothe your digestion.
• Carrot juice.
• Fresh lemon juice.
• One teaspoon of dill, one of sweet marjoram and one of aniseed. Steep in water for five minutes, and sip slowly.

---

535 The bundle

Now she is a little bundle who stays where you put her, but you will soon start noticing her develop physically; see 588. Resolve from the start not to worry whether next door's baby does it sooner; much more important is whether you encourage her. You will notice quite soon that progress is never steady. She comes along in leaps and bounds, then seems to have weeks when nothing much changes. She is learning; it takes great concentration; after each effort she switches to automatic pilot.

One of her first milestones is learning to support her own head. If you lie her on her tummy, she may try to lift her head and move it from side to side. Look closely. Recognize it? It is, of course, the rooting reflex, stimulated by her cheek touching the sheet.

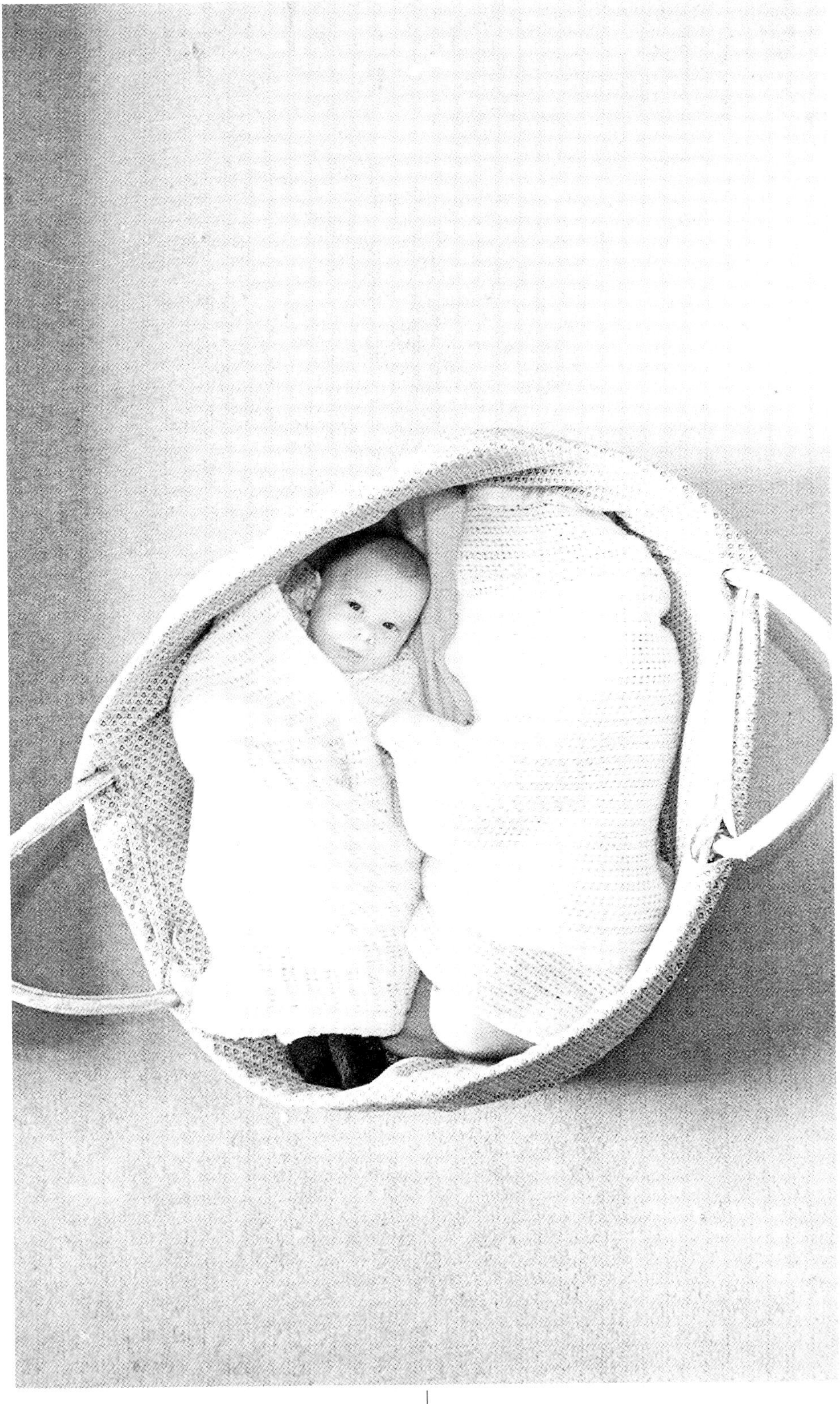

536 Keeping her warm

Tiny babies cannot control their body temperature. They do not shiver or move about to keep warm. The smaller you are, the less internal core you have to keep yourself warm. As fast as new babies heat up, they lose heat again.

The danger is hypothermia. She will become sluggish, her hands and feet will look red and swollen, and she will feel cold to the touch. If you find her like this, call the doctor at once.

A new-born baby must be kept in a warm room, ideally where the temperature is 85°F (29.5°C) or above. Remember, the temperature in the womb was 97°F (36°C). The ideal range in the first weeks is between 80 and 92°F (26.5 and 33.5°C).

Few of us keep our houses as warm as this, especially at night, indeed many of us would find this temperature unbearably hot. Keep the figures in mind. Combining clothing and background heat will provide enough warmth.

Warmth: basic steps

● Asleep in your bedroom, where you feel comfortable under a duvet during the winter, she will need a vest, nightdress and cardigan as well as a shawl to cover her head.
● Bedding can slip off, or be kicked off; fix it or put her in a sleeping bag.
● Remember that she can get too hot as well as too cold. Check simply by feeling her forehead: if she is too hot, she will feel it.

---

537 Elimination

A baby develops selectively; so sophisticated in some respects, yet unsophisticated in others. Even after she has learned to walk and to talk, she may still be in nappies.

What goes in has to come out, and what comes out can become quite an obsession. Perhaps it is because we tend to think of urination and defecation as such private functions. Pushed into the public domain, as they must be with babies and small children, we often go overboard.

Before birth, the slimy lining of the gut is digested, together with any other material the foetus swallows, in the amniotic fluid, which she drank throughout the later stages of pregnancy. Together this forms a sticky tar-like substance called meconium. It is greenish-black in colour and will fill her nappies three, even four times daily in the early days after birth. Then there will be a gradual change to more normal stools. At first these may be passed equally frequently, but by the end of the first few weeks, most babies have settled into a predictable individual pattern.

538 Typical patterns

What these are, and how the stools look, depends on what she eats. With a breast-fed baby, the colour and texture of the motions change from black and sticky to soft and curdy, a little like scrambled eggs. They are never hard and smell not unpleasant. Once she has settled into a rhythm of feeding and digesting, she may go two, three, even four days before letting it all out in one nappy-blowing motion. She may go again that day, then wait for a few more days.

Other babies perform little and often, some once every day. The frequency and pattern is irrelevant, even if it changes. If you are breast feeding her, she will not become constipated. Bottle-fed babies (or those on the breast supplemented by bottle) have harder, smellier, more child-like stools, firmer and browner than those of breast-fed babies. They are produced more regularly, often once or twice a day; but equally a baby may go for a day or two without a stool. If a motion every 36 hours is normal for your bottle fed-baby, so be it. Constipation is a question of how difficult it is to pass stools, not frequency: if she finds it easy, she is not constipated.

539 What are stools?

The waste products of what we eat, which is why they differ in bottle-fed and breast-fed babies. More of the breast milk is digested by the baby and little is wasted. Cows' milk was designed for calves, and even when modified by man still contains some things that babies cannot digest. There is more waste, which makes the stools more 'adult'.

Food is broken down in the stomach, but digestion takes place in the upper part of the intestine. You can think of this as a sieve: as food passes along it, all the goodness flows out, a process aided by bile (which breaks down fat) and other digestive juices. What is left over passes into the lower intestine, where most of the water is absorbed. The remnant becomes mixed with mucus, and the colour changes from green to yellow and, if there is much waste, to brown.

540 Hygiene

Digestion relies not only on digestive juices (539) but on harmless bacteria which live in the gut. Antibiotics can kill them, which is why antibiotics can cause stomach upsets.

In the early days of life, the baby's lower bowel becomes infected with these bacteria. This is as it should be, but if they get into the upper bowel they can cause problems. You should always wash your hands (and the baby's) if they get anywhere near her nappy.

Green stools, hard stools, and other problems:

● **Hard and green, first week:**
In the early days, normal motions can be greenish. This is probably caused by over-production of bile. If they are otherwise normal do not worry, they will settle down.

● **Hard and green, after first week:**
This is a feature of bottle-fed babies and could mean she is not getting quite enough food. Try giving a little more.

● **Loose, green and smelly:**
If the stools are loose, green and smelly, she probably has a bowel infection. The food is rushing through the system without remaining long enough for the water to be extracted or the mucus mixed in. This is potentially dangerous because of dehydration. Call a doctor without delay.

● **Hard and brown:**
This could mean she is not getting enough sugar. Don't add extra sugar to the formula at each feed, but give sweetened fruit juice in a bottle once a day.

● **Soft and brown:**
This may signify too much sugar. If she is listless, or you are at all worried about the condition, get medical advice.

● **Soft, brown and smelly:**
This probably means that the fat in her formula does not suit her digestive system. You may need a formula with less fat or one which is made of skimmed milk, or soya, plus added vegetable fats. Your doctor may suggest diluting the formula, in which case she will need feeding more often. Don't do this without checking with your doctor.

● **Blood in stools:**
If this occurs in the first few days, it comes from the mother, having been swallowed by the baby during delivery. Keep the nappy to show to the doctor or midwife. If there is blood at a later date, tell your doctor.

● **Changes of colour:**
Anything which goes in can come out. If your baby drinks blackcurrant juice, it may make her stools reddish; rosehip syrup may make them purplish; iron, blackish.

● **Constipation:**
If a bottle-fed baby needs to strain, she may need extra fluid or sugar.

● **Diarrhoea:**
If a bottle-fed baby starts to have diarrhoea, goes off her food and/or vomits (see 486), call the doctor at once. She may have gastro-enteritis; most loose stools are, however, due to diet, not infection. See 'Soft and brown' above.

Laxatives

The only people who need laxatives are those ill-advised enough to have used them all their lives. Laxatives upset the normal rhythm of the bowel. Never give laxatives to babies or children.

For the older baby on solid food, the best treatment of constipation is to increase the natural fibre content of the diet. Prime sources of fibre are:
● Whole grains and wholemeal bread.
● Baked beans and other pulses.
● Dried fruit such as raisins, figs or prunes.
● Apples and oranges.
● Bran. Mix it into her cereal each morning: with luck she will not notice the taste, which some find disagreeable.

Urine:
● **Too wet:**
Babies may pass water as many as 30 times in 24 hours. It does not matter how many wet nappies she has but it may matter how few. The way we regulate the intake of fluids is to absorb as much as we need (or can) and to eliminate the rest.

● **Too dry:**
A new baby who is still dry after a couple of hours needs watching. She may be starting a fever, she may be sweating because it is a hot day or

because you have over-dressed her. Feel her body. Is she hot and clammy? If so, loosen her clothes and sponge her. Then give her extra drinks of water or juice. If she is still dry after two hours, call the doctor. She probably has a blockage.

● **Very concentrated:**
Too little fluid, especially in summer when it is hot, can make a baby's urine concentrated. She needs water in order to sweat, in order to cool down. If she is short of fluid to sweat out, she has to save it from her urine.

● **Fishy smell, and concentrated:**
Almost certainly she has a urinary infection. Give her plenty of extra water – boil it first – and take her to the doctor. Untreated infections can affect the kidneys.

● **Urine smells of ammonia:**
This is caused by bacterial action in the nappy, not inside her gut. It causes nappy rash (see 'Sore bottom') but is otherwise harmless.

● **Red urine:**
Urine of newborn babies often contains urates, by-products of urine, which look red on the nappy; show this to the midwife if you are unsure. Urates are nothing to worry about, the system will soon adjust.

● **Blood in the urine:**
First check where it is coming from. In girls, vaginal bleeding is normal in the first few days; it is caused by hormones passed from the mother in the last days before birth.

If bleeding is not from the vagina, the next question is whether it is blood. Have you just started giving blackcurrant juice? It can look a little like blood.

If it is blood, or you are uncertain, call your doctor at once. Blood in the urine may mean a kidney infection.

Sore bottom
What makes bottoms sore?

● **Thrush:**
A common infection of the mouth, which can pass through the digestive system and cause a very red bottom. The redness spreads out from the anus. Consult your doctor. You can usually see thrush, which is a whitish fungus, in the baby's mouth.

● **Washing bottoms with soap:**
Use plain water, oil or baby lotion. Wipe a baby girl from vagina to anus.

● **Ammonia:**
If babies remain in wet and dirth nappies for too long, especially if well sealed in plastic pants, the bacteria in the stools react with the urine in the absence of air to produce ammonia. This irritates the damp skin. You can often smell the ammonia when you take off the nappy. It happens most often in bottle-fed babies because breast milk makes the motions more acid, which slows the action of the bacteria. Try adding vinegar to the last nappy rinse, leaving the nappy slightly acid. This will slow the bacterial action in the same way; but, of course, it can only work with towelling or muslin nappies.

● **Detergents:**
These are difficult to rinse out of nappies completely. Soap powder may irritate less.

● Biological washing powders cause very severe rashes in some babies.

Avoiding nappy rash
If you use towelling nappies:
● Use barrier cream at every change.
● Sterilize them.
● Put a little vinegar into the last rinse.
● Use a liner.
● Keep plastic pants loose.

If you use disposable nappies:
● Do not fasten them so tightly that air cannot get to the baby's bottom. In any event, all babies should spend time with their bottoms open to the air.
● Protect her bottom with a barrier cream such as zinc and castor oil. Silicone-based creams work better on highly sensitive skins.
● Avoid washing the baby too often with soap. If the rash develops into sores, consult your doctor. Let her lie on, rather than in, a nappy and don't use plastic pants or protective creams until the rash is better.

Nappies

Paper or towelling?

Paper and towelling nappies both have their problems.

A paper nappy is always sterile, always free from detergent and soap. But it is always neutral, never a little acid (which slows the action of bacteria), and has to be fitted to the bottom in such a way that air is largely excluded. Loose paper nappies do not work well, although some modern paper nappies are designed with folds which reduce this problem. Towelling nappies are a good deal of work, difficult to rinse, and need sterilizing, but they can be made acid, and above all can be put on loosely. If your baby frequently has nappy rash, they are worth seriously considering for night-time use. Line with a one-way liner and enclose in a pair of baggy plastic pants.

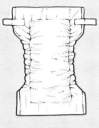

Disposable, elasticated legs

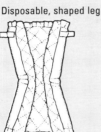

Disposable, shaped leg

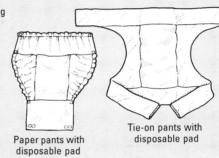

Paper pants with disposable pad

Tie-on pants with disposable pad

Advantages of disposable nappies:
• No soaking, washing or drying.
• A neat looking baby: the nappy is not so bulky as a towelling one.
• Less restricting than towelling when a toddler starts walking.
• Convenient when travelling or visiting.

Disadvantages of disposables:
• They cannot be worn loosely.
• They cannot be made acid; see 'What makes bottoms sore'.
• Expense: new-born babies may soil their nappies up to ten or 12 times a day.
• They sometimes leak, especially if you use the cheaper pad type with new-born girls.
• Less absorbent for night use.

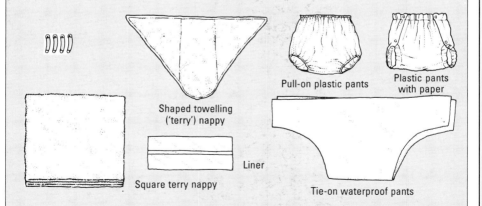

Shaped towelling ('terry') nappy

Square terry nappy

Liner

Pull-on plastic pants

Plastic pants with paper

Tie-on waterproof pants

Advantages of towelling nappies:
• Cheaper than disposable.
• May be worn loosely, or simply placed under the baby if she has a sore bottom.
• May be made slightly acid.

Disadvantages of towelling nappies:
• Work: ideally, you will need a washing machine and a dryer.
• They need soaking in order to be sterilized.
• Bulky.
• Inconvenient when travelling.

It is not surprising that more and more people use a mixture of disposables by day and towelling by night, or if the baby develops nappy rash; or disposables just for outings and travel.

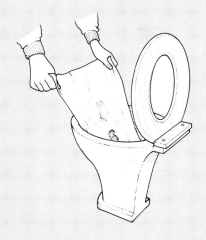

Washing nappies
1 Before attempting to wash dirty nappies, sluice off the mess. The easiest way is to hold the nappy in the W.C. pan and flush.
2 Towelling nappies always need sterilising. Sterilising solution is convenient, but you need to make up a new solution each day. Soiled nappies will need washing; wet ones may simply be rinsed – but thoroughly.
3 Nappies remain softest if you dry them outside on a line, or in a tumble dryer. They get stiff if dried on a radiator. Be careful which powders you use for washing – see 'What makes bottoms sore'.

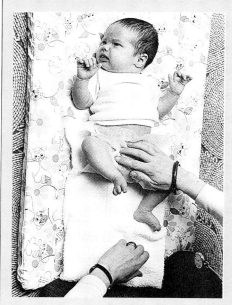

How often do you change her?
There is no evidence to suggest that babies mind wearing filthy nappies. You change her to prevent a sore bottom, and because the smell is disagreeable to those around her. So, how often depends on circumstances.

The nappies of bottle-fed babies and of those on solid food can smell pretty foul. You will probably change her as soon as you can smell the stench. From the point of view of hygiene, you should change her a little more often. A quick sniff around the nappy area is usually infallible.

But what about a nappy which is just wet? I feel it makes sense to change her when you want her to be awake and lively: before each feed if she is not howling, or after if she likes to play then, or at any other time you would like her to be awake. It makes no sense at all to change her at night, unless she is dirty, or her clothes are wet.

If she has nappy rash, one-way liners, not wearing plastic pants and going nappy-free whenever possible are as important as changing her often. A small baby is usually wet within half an hour of a nappy-change. There is no point in getting up at night to give her a dry bottom for half an hour when she is perfectly content with a wet one. Your sleep is more important than this.

Nappy-free playtime
Once she begins to enjoy nappy changing, prolong one of her changes every day by lying her on the changing mat without a nappy. Spread a clean nappy out under her bottom first. She will be safer on the floor, and she can get a clear view of her surroundings.

Nappy changing is a time for play and conversation: actually, it is hard to change a nappy without talking, smiling and telling her what you are doing. (Perhaps we feel we ought to chat in such intimate moments, rather as doctors do when conducting internal examinations.) Whatever the reason, these early conversations are essential to you and the baby, a line of communication which should not be hurried.

Changing a nappy

1 Have everything to hand including somewhere to put the dirty nappy.
2 Plastic changing mats are cold: rest her head on a muslin nappy.

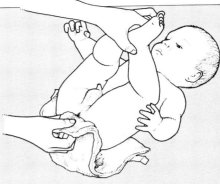

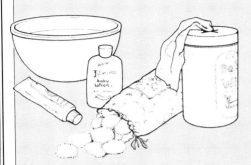

Bottom cleaning kit: water and cotton wool (for especially messy nappies) oil or lotion and cotton wool or tissue; alternatively baby wipes.

Nappy and nappy liners: you have a choice of one-way liners which let moisture out not back through, and can be sterilized for re-use; or disposable paper liners, which can be flushed away. Many prefer to use one-way liners the whole time because they help prevent nappy rash.

Plastic pants (essential with towelling nappies).
Nappy rash ointment, zinc and castor oil barrier cream, or bottom cream.

A change of clothes in case of accidents.

3 Operate on a firm surface.

4 Pick her up gently and place her on the changing mat.

5 Undo the old nappy. If she is soiled, use the nappy to scrape away the worst of the mess. Put it straight into the bucket to soak.

6 Clean her bottom using either cotton wool and lotion or oil, or a baby wipe. Make sure you clean all the creases, and the whole area covered by the nappy. If it was a towelling nappy, this includes most of the upper legs.

Start at the front and work down and under. It is easiest to lift the baby by her ankles. Use a new piece of cotton wool or baby wipe for each area. If you use water, she must be dried, especially in the creases. Some bacteria flourish in damp conditions.

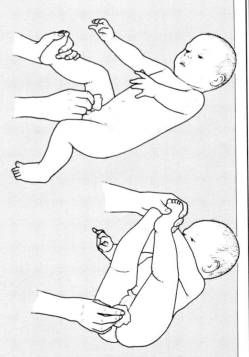

7 Put on barrier cream or nappy rash ointment as appropriate. Spread it all around the baby's anus and genitals.

8 Put on the clean nappy.

There are many ways to fold a towelling nappy: see the diagrams.

Some makes of disposable nappy still suffer from sticky tape failure: any grease on the plastic nappy surface prevents them adhering properly. It is essential to thoroughly wipe your hands on absorbent cloth after applying barrier cream and before securing the nappy by its adhesive tapes.

9 Having dressed her, put her somewhere safe and wash your hands thoroughly.

Triple fold

The most absorbent; fits a newborn baby neatly.

Fold in four, with open edges to top and right.

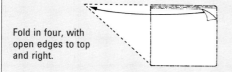

Draw right hand corner of top layer to left, forming triangle.

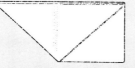

Turn whole nappy over, so point is on right.

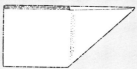

Fold two top layers inwards: use a third of the material.

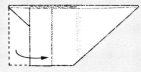

Fold the third inwards again forming thick central panel. Fix with pin.

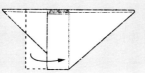

Kite fold

Use when the baby outgrows the triple fold. Adapts well to growing baby.

Lay out nappy as shown. Fold sides in, forming kite.

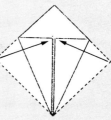

Fold top down.

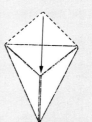

Fold bottom end up. Fix with pin.

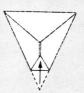

Parallel fold

Alternative to kite fold.

Lay out nappy as shown.
Fold top and bottom points in to centre.

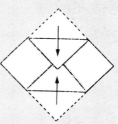

Align left point with top edge.

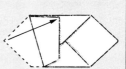

Align right point with top edge. Fix with pin.

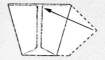

541 Crying

To say that it may affect your nerves is an understatment. It can cut through you; make you feel angry, reduce you to tears. So why do they do it?

In one study, researchers found that one-month-old babies cry for about three hours in every 24 – a good deal of crying.

Babies cry when they want something. It is their best way, often their only way, of telling parents that all is not well. It works because it is difficult for parents to ignore. A baby who is not crying is a happy and contented baby whom it is safe to ignore. Only a baby who is seriously ill, severely chilled or smothering, would fail to cry – unless, of course, she had learned that crying did not produce results, and that takes time.

It is not good for babies to cry for long periods. It does not exercise their lungs.

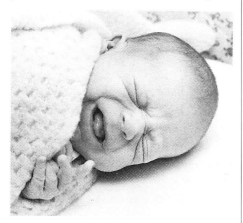

542 In need of what?

Does she know? – Probably not. She responds to inner sensations which she does not understand. She knows she needs, but not always what she needs. She will, however, know what she needs when she gets it; and she will stop crying.

A tiny baby shakes and sobs, her inner feelings are certainly strong, even if she does not understand them. As she gets older, she will know what she needs, and develop a language of cries which can give you quite a precise message. A warning cry, or fretful sound, may just mean 'come'; a loud bellow may mean 'please come quickly'; a cry with a hand wave may mean something different; a whimper something else again.

These signals, which parents pick up, are part of the baby's learning to communicate; see 567.

● Hunger:
A baby signals hunger with a warning cry which soon stops if you feed her. If you try to impose a feeding schedule, you may find that by the time feeding can go ahead on schedule she is too upset to feed. If she is hungry, only milk will do: a dummy or water will stop her only for a moment.

● Pain:
Sometimes it is easy to recognize a cry of pain: she will sound as if her heart is breaking. At other times, pain may go unnoticed. The odd bump, even a pin prick, will produce no response. Sometimes, you assume pain is the cause of the crying when it probably is not. If you pick her up and she burps, you say "That was the problem"; but a baby often brings up wind when you pick her up – tears or not.

● Comfort:
There must be few babies who don't cry because they want to be held. Babies who cry more than average are often those who get less than average human contact time, while those that cry less than average get more cuddles. In the first three months, babies cry most often when they are out of sight, sound, smell and touch of their mothers. Only some of these cries have to do with hunger or pain. See under 'Picking up'.

● Cold:
Babies who are too cold do cry – if they are awake. If you take them out in a push-chair in winter, they will cry because of the cold air on their faces. They will also cry, in an irritable, tetchy way, if they are too hot.

● Fear:
Babies cry when they are frightened by loud noises or shouting, by being suddenly dropped. Some small babies cry when they are washed or bathed; some when they have no clothes on. Most of these fears pass as babies begin to enjoy the social interaction that goes with these activities.

● Being misunderstood:
If you don't get the message, she will cry harder. She is hungry, for example, and you change her. She will also cry if you misread her mood, for instance by trying to play when she is tired.

Wet nappy:
If she cries when her nappy is wet and stops when it is dry, you might reasonably conclude she dislikes being wet. But in a recent experiment, nappies were taken off, then put back on without being exchanged for clean ones. The babies were perfectly happy. Presumably what they like about being changed is the social interaction and the physical attention.

Colic:
If your baby cannot settle in the evening and screams frantically, with her knees drawn up to her stomach, she probably has colic. If nothing you do seems to comfort her for more than a minute or two, and if this crying happens at much the same time every day, suspect colic and see 543.

Loneliness and boredom:
Even tiny babies get bored. There is not much to see when you are lying on your back looking up at the ceiling. Babies like something to look at and listen to: she may be asking for stimulation.

Picking up:
Most babies cry most often because they want to be picked up. Not that your baby has worked this out, but like most small animals, she craves body contact.

There are two time-honoured strategies for comforting babies. Carrying, as African, Japanese and Eskimo babies are comforted; and swaddling (wrapping up tightly), as some American Indian and most European babies are, or rather were, comforted. In modern times, Europeans have tended not to swaddle young babies, putting them to lie in cots as if they were older children. See under 'How to comfort'.

How to comfort
Keep in contact:
Hold and carry your baby as much as you can. A papoose is the easiest way. It leaves your hands free for gardening, cooking, housework and shopping. Buy one that you can wear on either the front or the back.

Read with her lying beside you, or across your knees. Relax or sleep with her in your arms. Bath together, walk together; even eating together is possible. Sometimes she will want to lie playing by herself, or sit in her chair. Use these times to do the things you like to do alone.

Stay close:
Most babies under three months cry less if their mother is close, even if she is not holding them.

Respond quickly:
Persistent crying in babies has been linked with parents who ignore their cries.

Wrap her:
Wrap her up in a warm, soft shawl; it should stretch. She needs to feel as if she is being held firmly. Don't straighten her out; wrap her in a curled position; leave her hands so she can get them to her mouth if she likes to suck them.

Rhythmical sounds:
You can buy a cassette of a mother's heart beat, which is said to be effective. A fan, the vacuum cleaner, a car engine, soft pop music, air conditioning and musical boxes can soothe her, too.

Rhythmical movement:
Rocking through 3 in (7.5 cm) at 60 rocks per minute is supposed to be the optimum. Walking up and down a room with her has roughly the same effect.

Prevent boredom:
If you are leaving her to her own devices, give her some devices: see the illustration. Stimulate her sense of hearing, too: a radio tuned to a chat show can work wonders.

Warmth:
Cold babies are fretful. If she does not sleep well in an unheated bedroom, or in her pram when out of doors, she is probably cold.

Gripe water:
This, and colic mixes, work for some babies, especially if (and maybe because) they contain alcohol. A finger dipped in sherry works in the same way. Obviously, any more than a drop or so of alcohol is undesirable.

Lamb's wool:
Lie the baby on the (washable) fleece to sleep or play.

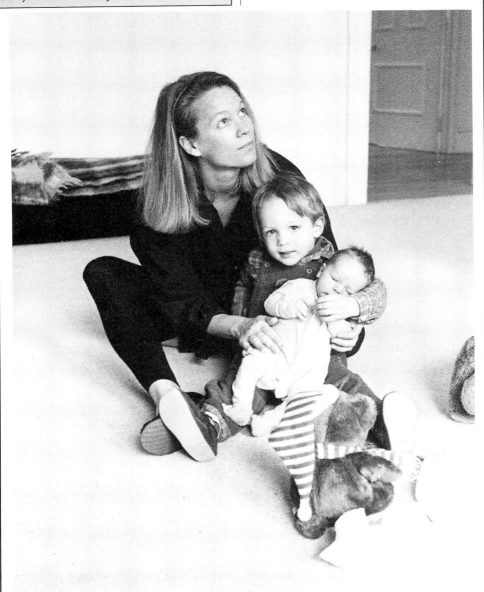

543 Colic

Just because your baby cries in the evening does not mean that she has colic; see 541. But if she has, she will cry as if in pain for long periods, and nothing you do will comfort her for long.

Colic bouts occur most often in the early evening, but also at other hours. The problem tends to start suddenly in the second or third week and, once established, usually recurs at about the same time every day. It often stops as suddenly as it started in the second or third month, but it can go on for much longer.

There is little that can be done for a baby with colic. Walking up and down helps for a while, so sometimes does a noisy fan or a little gripe water. But at best these provide a pause, time to catch your breath. Merbentyl, and other muscle relaxant drugs, used to be prescribed for colic; however there is now a question mark over their safety for babies under six months.

Many parents believe that the root cause lies in an allergy to cow's milk protein. Some babies do improve if switched to a soya milk formula, or if the breast-feeding mother stops eating any cow's milk protein: in other words, anything containing milk, cheese, yoghurt, cream or butter.

Don't feel guilty if you get angry or upset about colic and don't worry that your baby is ill. She will need plenty of comfort, and so will you. Share the care with your partner; if you can each have a day off, you will probably retain your sanity for longer. If your anger frightens you, ask your doctor if he or she can help.

544 Aftercare for babies with colic

Babies who suffer from colic in the first few weeks of life often become restless and poor sleepers in later months. This is probably habit. Try to find something to comfort your baby in the evenings: a fan perhaps, or a lambskin, after the colic has subsided. Try to vary the routine. She no longer has the pain, but something in the environment may make her feel uneasy – just because it was there when she felt so desperate.

545 Spoiling

You cannot spoil a baby, but you can spoil your relationship with her. One experiment showed that the fussy, demanding one-year-old is not the 'spoiled baby' but the one whose parents ignore all demands or delay answering her call. It makes sense: if you are in tune, you don't have to make unreasonable demands, you anticipate each other's needs.

Perhaps in not responding you teach her that all demands are unreasonable, and so they have to be made in an unreasonable manner. Or that she has to make demands persistently in order to get them answered.

Maybe you teach her that demands don't have to be answered, and that also goes for demands made upon her.

Whatever, or however, the lessons were given, the 'spoiled' babies in the experiment (the ones parents picked up or fed on demand), were more independent, had more ways of asking for attention, and were more content with less contact from their parents.

It is true that if you totally ignore a baby's crying all the time you can make her completely apathetic; but I doubt that is what parents want to do.

546 Coping

Not until you have had a crying baby do you begin to understand those who have actually 'battered' a baby. If she is crying so incessantly that you feel you cannot endure another moment of it, call a friend who can watch her while you walk around the block to calm down.

And if there is no one to turn to, don't be ashamed of closing the door on her screams; or turning on the radio loud enough to drown the sound and dancing or exercising it out of your system. Even scrubbing the kitchen floor may help. There is probably little point in trying to relax, to read or to engage in any intellectual pursuit; your inability to concentrate will only make you feel worse.

Remember, too, that no one is a perfect parent. You cannot always get to your baby at once, sometimes you should finish what you are doing. At times, babies have to go to the back of the queue like anyone else. If you are normally responsive to her needs, quick to comfort and cuddle, you are justified in making your own demands. If it is important to have your evenings free, be firm about bed time, even if it means leaving her to cry once in a while. It is much easier to give attention willingly and lovingly if you have set a limit that leaves you some time of your own. If she is not ill, you can say, as all loving parents do: "It is grown-up time now".

547 Communicating

It is not always possible to feel loving towards a crying baby; it is not even possible always to feel loving towards a baby who is not crying.

Tiny as she is, she may well sense how you feel. You hold her differently, less close, or perhaps you pick her up roughly. Maybe you speak differently, or smell differently. Whatever it is, and however you signal it, she will know. The arms that so often comfort offer less, and she may cry with unease. Sometimes this understanding of your mood can be disarmingly perceptive; you feel that she is aware of your withdrawal; and she probably is.

Bathing

It is not necessary to bath a baby every day. In fact, most small babies find it a fairly traumatic experience. They hate to be undressed and are not always comforted by water. Wet babies can also get very cold. Unless you have a really warm room, it is best to keep bathing to a minimum in the winter. Two baths a week are quite enough for hygiene.

A special baby bath is not essential. If the kitchen is warm, the sink is probably adequate, especially if you have work surfaces around it on which to set out all the bits and pieces of equipment you will need.

A proper baby bath has the advantage of being shaped to fit a baby and of being non-slip, but don't overfill it. You can use your own bath, but you will find it difficult to hold her in place until you are skilled at handling.

You will need:
- Apron and a large, soft towel.
- Soap or a liquid cleaner. The latter may be easier to use than soap, since you don't soap the baby, making her slippery, but just squirt it into the water. In the first six weeks it is best to use only water.
- Face cloth or small, soft sponge.
- Cotton wool, tissues.
- Clean nappy and changing kit.
- Talcum powder, baby oil, cream (optional).

A couple of inches (5 cm) of water in the bath is plenty for a small baby. Put the cold water in first, especially if you are filling the bath by kettle, to prevent the sides and base of the bath itself heating up too much.
- Test the water temperature with your elbow. You hand is accustomed to water much hotter than blood heat, your elbow (or wrist) is not and will respond with greater sensitivity. The water should feel warm.

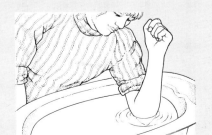

- Clean the baby's bottom, undress her and wrap her tightly in a towel.
- Clean her face.

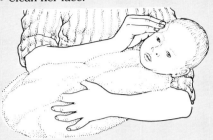

- Wash her hair. Hold her as shown. Splash her head with water. If she has cradle cap, put oil on her hair before washing it. You don't need shampoo or soap for a tiny baby.

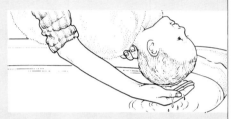

- Now remove the towel. Supporting her head with your arm, grip her upper arm and shoulder with your hand. Using your free hand to support her bottom, lower her into the water, and rest her bottom on the base of the bath. Only the lower half of her body should be submerged.

Talk to her reassuringly all the time.
- Wash her.

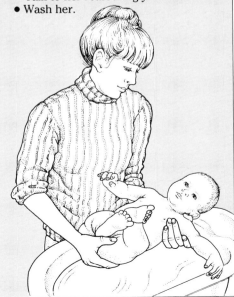

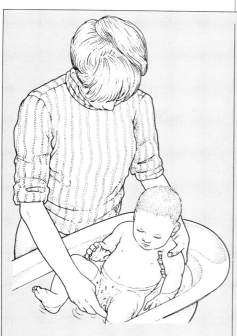

Howling at bath time
Don't be surprised if she is frightened by being bathed. Many babies become extremely distressed when you take off their clothes, partly because they chill so quickly, but the main reason is probably that they feel exposed. If swaddling (579) comforts, it is not surprising that lying without clothes makes your baby insecure. You cannot avoid changing her clothes, but you can keep bathing to a minimum. A sponge bath will suffice if she is really unhappy.

'Topping and tailing'
A useful alternative to a bath.
● **How to top and tail:**
– Put her on the changing mat in her vest and nappy. Wrap her in a towel.
– Wash her eyes, using a fresh damp pad of cotton wool for each eye, working from the nose outwards.
– Wash each ear, gently, and the area behind each ear.
– Wash the forehead, cheeks and neck.
– Wash around the mouth.
– Now carefully dry her face.
– Unwrap the towel and wash each of her hands.
– Clean the nappy area; see 210.
– Dress her as usual.

Sponge bath
Use water alone at first; later you will find it easiest, and quickest, to use a liquid cleaner in the water.
● Prepare everything as if you were going to bath her. See opposite.
● Fill a bowl with water; test it as recommended. See opposite.
● Undress her top half and wrap her in the towel.
● Wash her hair. See opposite.
● Wash her face and neck. See opposite.
● Still keeping her bottom half well covered, unwrap the towel enough to wash her front gently. Wipe her dry, turn her over; wash and dry her back in the same way.
   You can do this with her on a changing mat, or across your lap.
   Talk to her all the time.
● Now dress her top half.
● Undress her bottom half. Wash her legs and feet.
● Remove the nappy and clean as usual.
● Dress.

● Rinse her by splashing water over her gently. Keep smiling, and reassuring her.
● Lift her out carefully: the easiest way is to place your arm under her bottom and grip the top of her thigh. This means you can hold her shoulder and her thigh, so you will not drop her, even if she slips.
● Place her on the towel and quickly wrap her. Cover her head, especially if her hair is wet.
● Give her a cuddle.
● Put her down, still snug in the towel, and carefully dry her, keeping her well covered by the towel as you do so. Dress her as usual.

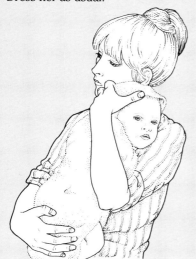

Dressing and undressing

In the first weeks you will find it easiest to dress your baby in a vest and nightdress. It makes nappy changing easier while you are still inexperienced at handling her, and she will need her nappy changed often in the first week or so. Later on, you will find stretch towelling suits with leg poppers the most convenient form of clothing.

Undressing a new-born baby:

• Warm the room.
• Put the changing mat on a firm surface and lay a towel or terry nappy on top of it.
• Gather together everything you need to clean her and to dress her again.
• Lie her down; smile and talk to her.
• Change her nappy; see ???.
• If she is wearing a stretch suit, unbutton it and gently pull out her legs. Then push the suit up to her shoulders and ease out the arms, one at a time.
• For a nightdress which fastens at the back, lie her on her tummy and undo all the fastenings. Roll her over, gently ease out her arms, and pull the nightdress down over her bottom.
• Gently ease her arms out of the sleeves of her vest, open the neck, and pull it over her head. Keep the material of the vest in a tight bunch. She may hate having her face covered.
• Cover her immediately.

Dressing a new-born baby:

• Gather everything you need before starting.
• Lie her down.
• Cover her while you change the nappy.
• Bunch her vest up, pull the neck wide and quickly slip it over her head, lifting her slightly. Ease each earm through its armhole. Again, bunching up the fabric will speed the operation.
• A stretch suit goes on most easily sleeves first. Lie it flat on the changing mat and lift her on to it. Ease her arms into the sleeves, holding them open with your hand as you do so. Then slip in her legs; lastly, do up the poppers.
• Cardigans can be put on similarly.

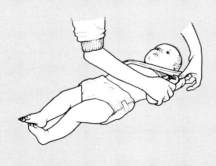

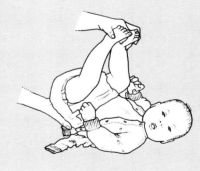

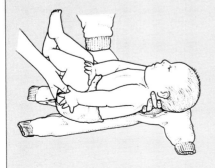

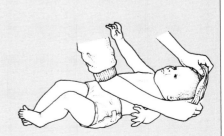

Ears, nose, nails, navel

The ears make wax to keep themselves clean and to protect the ear drum from dust and dirt. Some babies make plenty; even so, it does not need removing. If you push a cotton wool bud into her ear, you are likely to push dirt in with it; if you remove the wax, the ear will make more. If you are worried about the amount being made, consult your doctor.

The same goes for the nose. It will run and clean itself. There is no need to poke anything in to keep it clean, and you could hurt her.

Some babies have nails so long that they scratch themselves. Nails are easily cut, but the operation is worrying when they are so tiny, and you may find it easiest to do it when your baby is asleep. Use a small pair of blunt-ended scissors. Actually, biting them off is simplest.

In the first weeks, you may need to clean the area of her navel with a little surgical spirit on some sterile cotton wool.

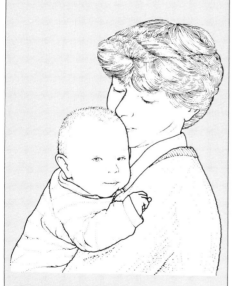

Caring and loving

There is nothing more delightful than cuddling a sweet-smelling baby – and little that delights her more.

I feel that there is only one place to put a baby in the morning after you have changed her: in bed with you. She will like to feel your skin next to hers. Sitting in bed together as a family, baby feeding, the rest of us drinking tea, was always the first social occasion of our day: mundane, but precious.

548 What sort of person?

– "A cry baby. . .Very bad tempered."
– "She's stubborn. She has a temper. When she is content she's a perfectly wonderful person to have around; when she is out of sorts, she's a monster."
– "An angel."
– "When she makes up her mind she wants to do something, she sort of keeps on."
– "The first week I thought she was me; it was really strange: such a strong feeling."

Mothers' comments on their babies at five weeks, from Ann Oakley's *From Here to Maternity*.

549 Little people

It is not so very long ago that babies were thought of as no more than little bags of reflexes not yet ready to be called people. You may have thought so too, until you began to know your own child.

One of the great joys of these early weeks is the realization that she is an individual. 'I never expected her to be so interesting' is the typical comment. She is interesting because, although immature, she is whole: every element of her identity as a person is there in seedling form.

550 What every baby needs

The onslaught of stimulus hitting a baby as she enters the world defies the imagination; but luckily, nature 'filters' the input. She sees and hears best what she needs to know. In the first weeks, it is her family. Her vision is restricted (514); her reactions to touch or pain are slow compared with yours, indeed, she may not react at all unless stimulation is prolonged.

But her selectivity has an even more interesting side.

If you study a video of people talking to each other, you will find that they sway slightly in time with their speech. Within hours of birth, a baby will move in the same way; within weeks, she will wave her arms as you talk together and move her lips as if mimicking patterns of speech.

This choice she makes, from all the stimuli on offer, is so significant not just because it shows she is an active, rather than a passive, being.

It means that she learns by watching and imitating others – which principally means you.

551 Self regulation

This early selectivity (550) has other, even more fundamental aspects. From her first moments, she has to face the challenge of not being overwhelmed by her new environment; but it is no use her simply switching it off. To survive, she must take a vital interest in the world around her. That she can balance these conflicting forces is remarkable, considering how immature are most of her other skills. But, of course, she has to be capable of this because otherwise she would be but a poor learner.

552 Grand circle

The senses that help us to become interested in the world also help us to stay calm. The unknown makes us fearful; familiarity reduces that fear. So exploring the unknown amounts to conquering fear, increasing one's ability to stay calm.

You might indeed say that a baby who uses her senses well will stay calm and attentive; and that a baby who is calm and attentive will use her senses well: the development is self-reinforcing.

In this lies the fundamental importance of parents. You are a large part of that calmness; you are also one of her major interests. From the rock of your security, she can feel her way out into the world. From the knowledge of that world her confidence and security will grow.

For a parent to live with this knowledge requires a degree of self-confidence. But this does not mean confidence in one's ability as a parent; you can never suddenly become good parents – you learn as you go along. But you do need to understand yourselves, your motivations and limitations.

553 Dance

Each step your baby takes is the preparation for the next. Her progress, and yours, in the coming months and years will be like a dance: the whole show can be undermined if one of you gets the steps wrong. Easy babies do tend to have easy parents; but it is not always possible to say who calls the tune. Babies are not blank slates, and difficult babies are not always produced by difficult parents.

A child's own inborn anxiety and fear can influence her parents, just as a

Picking up

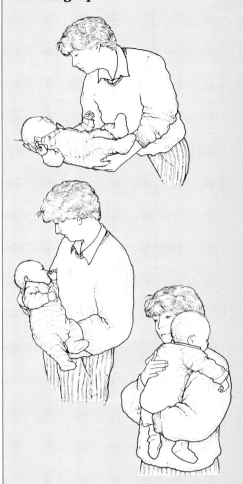

Babies are not cream cakes and hate being held as if they were; they find it reassuring to be held tightly. At birth, your baby cannot support her own head. And although it will do her no harm if you fail to support her head, she will be frightened if it flops backward, since she will feel as if she is about to be dropped.

Even so, picking her up is easy:
● Slip one hand under her head and neck, using the palm of your hand to support her neck and the fingers to hold the base of her head. The wrist should support the top of the back. Her bottom sits in the palm of the other hand, and her lower back is supported by your fingers. Lift her up and in towards your body.

Men, who usually have larger hands than women, should find this simple.

Holding
There are two positions.
1 On the shoulder:
As you lift her towards you, slip the hand supporting the head towards her shoulder. Your arm should now encircle her back, and your fingers still support the head, which rests on your shoulder. Your other hand can support her bottom.

You will find this the best position to use when comforting a crying baby, or moving around with a sleeping baby. It is also a stable position in which to hold a baby when you are climbing stairs. With a little practice, you will be able to free one hand to pick things up, support yourself, or even eat your lunch.

2 Cradled:
How to cradle a baby in the crook of the arm hardly needs describing. The baby's head lies on your upper arm just above the elbow, and the rest of the arm lies along the baby's side, with the hand holding her upper leg. The second arm comes up under the baby's bottom so that she sits on your wrist, She should not lie flat, but with her head slightly higher than her bottom.

This is the best position for rocking a baby and for talking to and interacting with her.

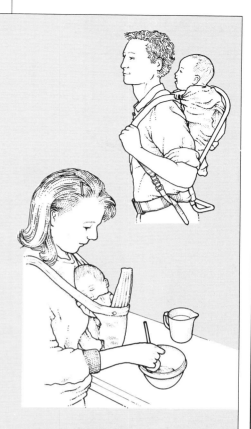

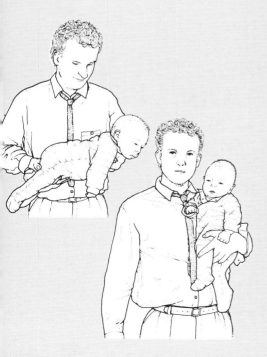

Slings and shawls
You can use these even with a new-born baby. The major problem is getting her into the sling single-handed. You can try tying the papoose loosely in place, easing her gently down into it and adjusting her position after she is inside. Or you can 'dress' the baby in the papoose while she lies on a bed. Then, kneeling by the bed, lift her on to your shoulder, supporting her with one hand and moving the straps into place with the other. It is not strictly necessary to use a bed, but it is reassuring at first to know it would not be a disaster if you were to drop her.

Lying her down to sleep
It is safest to put a baby down to sleep on her stomach or her side: this will prevent her choking if she vomits. A swaddled baby (see 579) may, however, rest more easily on her side. You lie her down holding her just as you would to pick her up. Always give her something to look at when she wakes. When she is awake she will probably be happiest lying on her back, which is safe if you watch her.

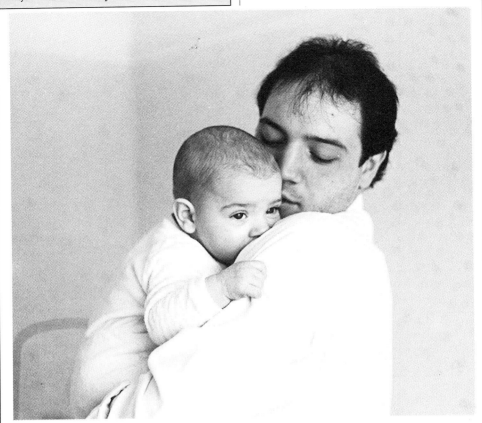

parent's anxiety can influence the child. Life will always be difficult for some children, however perfect, however understanding the parents. Life will always be easy for some children, however impossible the parents.

There are also influences outside the control of parents which shape these initial relationships. It is hard to be easygoing and loving to a baby who screams and howls for hours at a stretch, as a sick baby can, as a baby with colic will. It is hard to be confident and loving when deeply depressed, as some women are after childbirth.

554 Easy? Difficult?

Children are often described as being easy or difficult. What does this mean?

An easy child approaches new events positively, takes new food, likes new toys, sleeps well. eats well and is generally happy.

A difficult child cries, sleeps poorly and reacts to new food and new experiences irritably. Once she adapts, a difficult child can become easier. Often the difficulty seems to lie in the length of time it takes for her to feel secure. A fairer description of this type of baby might be over-excitable.

There are, indeed, under-excitable babies who are slow to warm up. They respond to anything new not by crying or exploring, but by looking the other way. These differences can persist throughout childhood. Again, they can either come with the baby, be in-built, or be made by the parents.

555 Helping over- and under-excitable babies

Gently introduce the new *in combination with* other pleasurable and comforting experiences. Always stay calm, and accept that your baby may need holding when anything new enters her life.

You can help her overcome under-arousal by making new experiences interesting, and plentiful, by finding games that delight and surprise. Observe her carefully: what excites her? What calms her? Use this as a basis for teaching her self-regulation.

556 The wakeful baby

Some babies need little sleep. Do you sleep little? Perhaps she takes after you. You cannot force sleep on an unwilling baby. Once she is able to amuse herself, life will be easier; until then you may find that carrying her with you, as African and Japanese mothers do, is the answer.

Providing stimulus as she lies in her basket or cot may also help, as may warmth, subdued lighting and gentle background sounds before sleep.

557 The sleepy baby

The baby who sleeps for 22 hours in 24 may not seem to be a problem, but it is sometimes difficult to relate to her. You need to accept that she wants to come gently into the world. Give her plenty of attention when she wakes, but don't cram too much stimulation into those two hours; see 555.

558 Self assessment

Sometimes it is worth standing back and looking at what sort of parent you are, or think you ought to be.

● **Withdrawn:**
Anxiety and worry can often make you withdrawn. The excitment of having the baby is rapidly replaced by feelings of inadequacy, and anxiety about facing up to her dependence on you. Once you enter a cycle of depression it is difficult to escape. You begin to treat the baby in a mechanical way. You feel guilty. She senses your withdrawal. You get off to a poor start.

● **Over-stimulating:**
Is she ever left to sit peacefully? Do you let her take turns in 'conversations'? See 567. Do you, perhaps, want success at all costs? It is easy to wish away her babyhood in a mad rush to get to the next stage of her development.

● **Subdued:**
Emotional flatness inhibits enjoyment of the baby; you may well be depressed. We all display elements of each style in combination, and at different times. Some days too bossy, some days too dull. . .

559 Worried

Worrying about children is an integral part of parenthood. If the seed of worry, common to all, grows out of hand, consider these points:

● **Hurting babies:**
To feel that you could throw her at the wall does not mean that you will, or are ever likely to do so. It is a rare parent .pawho has not felt this emotion. But if you find yourself keeping away from the baby for fear you will harm her, seek help from your doctor. Likewise if you find yourself handling her roughly, or if feelings of violence are irrepressible.

● **Sexual feelings:**
Incest is such a strong taboo, sexual abuse so abhorrent, that sexual feelings towards our children naturally alarm us. But are they always so very strange?

Few of us are unaware of childhood sexuality, and most of us accept that we probably had sexual feelings towards our parents as children, even.if we cannot remember them as such. If we accept that there were sexual feelings on our side as we climbed into our parents' bed, perhaps we should stop and ask ourselves an important question. Have you ever shared your bed with anyone for whom you have not had sexual feelings? If warm soft skin against yours as you lie half awake in the morning has produced sexual arousal in the past, why be surprised that the conditioning is so strong? This is probably the first time in your life that you have shared a bed with someone who is not in any sense a sex object.

The same reasoning can be applied to breast feeding. If sucking and stimulating the breasts have formed an intrinsic part of your sexual behaviour, it would be surprising if the baby's sucking never produced sexual arousal.

Sexual arousal does not necessarily mean that sexual feelings are *directed*. Most of us are quite capable of feeling aroused, even when we have no one to feel aroused about. Bringing the feeling into the open is the safest way to deal with it if it worries you.

● **Not enough to give:**
Who does not feel inadequate at times? Often these feelings are intensified by a helpless baby who is totally dependent. Asserting your own needs is probably the best way to deal with this fear. Sometimes a fear that we do not have enough to give masks a fear of rejection.

• **'I am being selfish':**
You are not only a parent; you are a person, too.

• **'I am a bad parent':**
Your baby's behaviour is never all your fault. If she cries, she is probably asking for something, not judging you. Feeling that you are a bad parent can become a self-fulfilling prophecy.

• **'I am losing myself':**
It is easy to lose your independence when you fall in love, whatever the age of the person you love. If you give up your whole life for that person, as many mothers do after the baby is born, it is realistic to feel like this. In time you will probably see it as a new beginning. But don't expect miracles overnight.

Sometimes the fear of losing oneself makes us fear closeness. Recognizing the cause is often the cure.

• **'I am being controlled':**
To a large extent, you are, especially in the early weeks. It will be easier to give willingly if you plan your life so that you have some time to yourself, however short, each day.

• **'I'm jealous':**
Fathers can feel jealous of the relationship between mother and baby; a mother can feel jealous of the things he does with 'her baby'. The first, and most difficult, part is recognizing those feelings. Make it a priority to do things as a couple; on this rebuild your life as a pair.

• **Resentment:**
The man resents his partner's closeness to their child. The woman resents the man's ability to escape the feelings of being taken over and controlled. And sometimes it feels as if the baby resents everything you do that is not central to her life.

560 "Tonight"

Six weeks after birth is not a magic date, but at the medical check-up around this time you will probably be given the go-ahead to start making love again. The vagina may, however, still be sore and intercourse painful. If so, it is unwise to attempt it. There are other ways of giving and taking sexual pleasure.

For some couples these weeks are, in fact, a time of closeness and intense sexual pleasure. For others, sex becomes messy once the milk begins to let down. And for some, sex becomes an issue.

Many women find that their libido has never been so low.

561 "Not tonight. . ."

Love-making expresses and celebrates closeness, mental dependence. It is more than simply a sexual release. Disrupting the normal pattern of love-making can have far-reaching effects, especially if viewed in the context of the growing love between woman and child. For a man to feel rejected when his partner has no desire to make love is natural. Whatever the cause, withdrawing from sex amounts to rejecting him.

On one level, as a woman cuddles and feeds her baby, the reason for the rejection could not be clearer.

But, of course, it is more complex than that.

562 The problem

Quite simply, many women feel reluctant to resume sex after childbirth. A long labour, a difficult birth and the physical exhaustion of being in charge of a baby makes sleep a major preoccupation. If you are in bed, and the baby is asleep, why waste precious sleeping time?

The soreness of the perineal area makes fear of being hurt a real anxiety. Also, many women find that the hormonal balance after birth is not conducive to sex; just as pregnancy can make sex enormously enjoyable, so breast feeding can make orgasm more difficult. It can also reduce sexual libido almost to zero. But there is more to the problem than even these obvious causes.

A woman's sex organs are private, even, in a sense, from their owner. In giving birth, you not only make public the perineum but you have suddenly to accept as commonplace procedures such as a daily rating of blood on your sanitary pad. Some of the essential privacy of your body is lost and with it some of your mystery and sexuality.

There is, too, the growing physical relationship with the baby which gives a sensual pleasure all its own. A baby's skin is soft and silky; holding and touching her surely fulfills some of the sensual needs we subsume under sex. And for many a woman, sexual desire requires a degree of contentment with her body; few are happy with (or in) their bodies in the weeks after birth.

For all or some of these reasons, a woman may feel happy to delay the resumption of sex until after the six-week check. The idea of six sex-free weeks may have seemed unbelievable even a month ago, now it seems perfectly natural.

563 Long-term sexual problems

Few couples expect these problems (560-562) to last, but for many they do, sometimes for six months or more after the baby's birth.

Women are not always willing to admit they do not need or want sex during this period. They may also not want to understand their partner's need. A woman feels herself at the centre of a demand system: the baby wants the breast; the man her body; so why should not she want something for herself? It can easily get out of hand.

If the father shared her lack of libido it would, of course, not be a problem; but male libido rolls ever onward. Having been pushed out into the cold after the birth, it is natural for him to want to re-establish closeness with the mother.

There are no easy answers. As the tension rises, desire grows; as desire grows, the woman feels more and more that she is being put under an obligation; that she is being forced to reject.

564 Palliatives

- **Air the problem.** Pretending everything will be all right next time helps nobody.
- **Don't rush:** It does not have to be in the second week, or the sixth. Start by courting each other again, stroking and petting. If you want to give, you can give, but it does not have to be your bruised vagina.
- **Negotiate:** Instead of "Not tonight", it is sometimes easier to say "May we cuddle this week and talk about it again on Saturday?" or "Give me until next month".
- **Communicate:** A relationship is built on communication: on being able to say why.
- **Don't worry:** It may take time; you may not reach orgasm until you stop feeding, but it does return.
- **Find alternatives:** If intercourse does nothing for you, see if something else does. You may find that you can build a pattern of pleasure based on orgasm for one and loving physical contract for the other.

- **Lubricate:** Until the baby is weaned, the juices probably will not flow.
- **Have a drink:** It will relax you both.
- **Vary position:** Those which allow the woman to control penetration (304 and page 112) are essential in the early post partum period.
- **Contraception:** Yes. If you are breast feeding, you will probably not ovulate until you start to introduce mixed feeding, but there is absolutely no guarantee of this; see 565.

See 666.

565 Contraception

- **Coitus interruptus** is unreliable. Hoping your partner will withdraw is unlikely to make sexual adjustment in the post partum period any easier.
- **Rhythm method:** Until you start ovulating again there is no rhythm; by then it may be too late.

- **Diaphragm:** Your old one will not fit. The cervix rarely goes back to exactly the same size. You can have a new one fitted at your six-week post partum check.
- **An IUD** is easily fitted after birth and this can be done after your six-week check. But it does carry an increased risk of pelvic inflammation and of tubal pregnancy.
- **Spermicides:** Alone, these are unreliable, and there are some doubts about their safety should you conceive when using them; see 218. The foams are more reliable than creams or pessaries. If you find they irritate, switch brands. The main problem with spermicides in the early weeks is that they tend to run out unless you lie flat on your back. And this precludes positions which allow the woman to control penetration.

- **Sponge:** One of the few reliable methods: it is inserted in the same way as a diaphragm and left in place for 24 hours. It is, however, less reliable than a condom.
- **Condoms:** Probably the best method in the early postpartum period. There is no danger of infection, they are reliable and can be used in positions in which the woman can control penetration. You will probably need to use a lubricant.

- **Oral contraceptives** are the most reliable, but they may disrupt breast feeding in the early weeks. If you developed diabetes, high blood pressure or varicose veins during pregnancy, your doctor may advise another method.

566 Postnatal check

All women who have given birth should have a check-up at six weeks. The doctor will check blood pressure and urine; he will palpate the abdomen and make an internal examination to check that the uterus is involuting: going back to a normal size and shape. He will also check the condition of the uterus, which may still be engorged. He will check the condition of the vagina and that stitches are healing. A look at your breasts will reveal any problems if you are still feeding, and that lactation has ceased if you are not. You will be weighed: you should have lost about 17-20 lb (7.7-9 kg). A blood test may be taken to check for anaemia, and a pap smear for cancer of the cervix if this is due.

Finally, the doctor should advise you on birth control and any other problems.

567 Taking turns

Conversations consist of more than words: they depend upon lip movements, expressions and body language. Into all these signals which say 'I'm listening', 'I'm interested', adults can slot language or smiles. Before a baby learns to talk, she relies solely on lip movements and body language.

"Do you want feeding?" you say, pausing, and looking at her as you wait for her reply. "You do? Come on then."

When you talk to a baby, you automatically offer her a turn, and she nearly always takes it. One-way conversations never last long, indeed if you talk at her without pausing, she will fret; this may be why some over-stimulated babies are so fretful and nervous.

Each baby has her own rhythm for taking turns; tuning into your baby's rhythm, or she tuning into yours, is the beginning of the long road towards speech. You should not underestimate its importance.

568 Play

If a baby's first games are social, her best toys are her parents. The ideal form of play at this stage is simply to keep her close to you, and when you cannot do that, to provide plenty for her to see and hear.

569 Smiles

What makes a young baby smile? Wind is the usual answer, but it is wrong. Smiling is smiling. Those little flicks of the mouth, often one-sided, are immature smiles. She will make them in her sleep, as she comes out of a deep sleep into a lighter level of sleep, or vice-versa. All babies smile this way in the first week or so, then they start to smile when things happen in their sleep, say when their faces are touched.

A little later, between three and six weeks, your baby will begin to smile when she is awake. A high-pitched voice, a tinkling bell, a nodding head or a touch of her cheek will all bring a little smile to her mouth. Her face does not yet light up, but later she will brighten to your voice and to your face moving, later still to your face even when it does not move. But as yet there may be nothing special about your face or voice: a doll may make her smile, so might a musical box, so may change.

You may find she smiles more if you put on a hat or take off your glasses. At three months, though, she is smiling at you and soon after that she can manage big, 'whole face' smiles.

All this has been established through research with blind babies. They smile just as much as sighted babies up to three months, after which they almost stop smiling.

570 Back to work: but when?

Not before eight to nine months is a baby firmly attached to her mother. If you want to return to work, should you wait until after this? If you do, you would, in theory, be serving her well by ensuring that the essential bond is allowed to develop. But on the other hand, you will almost certainly feel guilty.

Is it better to return to work earlier, leaving your baby to become attached to a substitute? If you leave her to a surrogate in working hours, will there be any bonding potential left over for you?

571 Clinging baby

The fact that babies form multiple attachments and thrive on them, is borne out by some interesting studies.

In an attempt to capture the nature of the relationship between child and mother, Mary Ainsworth, the American developmental psychologist, set up a 'strange situation test'.

Early stimulation and first toys

In the early weeks you need simply to show her a wide variety of objects, particularly things that move. Encourage her to reach out and swipe at objects by tying toys to the side of her cot, or string them across her pram. You can hang a toy on a long piece of elastic so that it dangles down just above her face. If it is within arm's reach, she will soon take a swipe at it. Wrist rattles and bell mittens draw attention to her hands. Once she is reaching out, provide some firmer toys to touch: things that will not always escape her grip when she tries to hold them.

She needs to experience the weight of a toy in her hand: you can easily help her in this. When she starts to take objects to her mouth, watch that she is not doing so with something that could poke into an eye.

Once she begins to reach, hold toys out for her to take. Give her time. Don't take pity and put the rattle into her hand. It looks painful as she adjusts her hand to reach; but it is not. Rattles with a well-defined 'waist' are easiest to hold: dumb bells, rings, and shapes with substantial handles.

As her skills develop, give her an increasing variety of things to hold and to look at, both when lying and sitting.

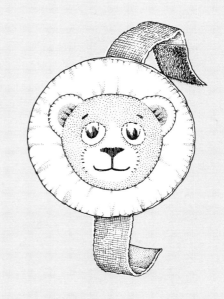

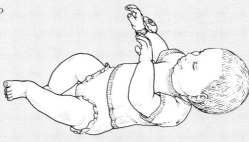

Wrist rattle, fastened with 'Velcro'

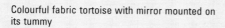

Colourful fabric tortoise with mirror mounted on its tummy

- A coloured cot bumper, a face stuck to the roof of her pram hood, a new toy close by when she opens her eyes.
- Pram beads or simply a string of miscellaneous objects, changed frequently, gives her new objects to see, and later something to reach out to touch.
- A mirror reflects movement and light and can show her a face when she looks into it.
- The most interesting mobiles have the figures at an angle so that she can see them as they turn. Mobiles are expensive to buy, but you can make her one by sticking shapes to the bottom of match boxes. A noisy mobile is a bonus. Hang it where it has a chance of moving in a draught, for example above a heater.
- Fix a soft toy to the side of her cot so that she can take a swipe at it.
- Let her be near you when you prepare meals. She will hear you chopping and mixing, stirring and scraping. She will hear the water in the sink and perhaps the bubbling of the pots. She will smell what is cooking, and she will see you as you go by.
- Let her hear the vacuum cleaner and the radio; she may even like the high-pitched hum from the TV, and its flickering screen.
- Let her feel textures: a dress, a blanket, the softness of a lambskin.
- What happens if you don't give her any of these things? Nothing much. She will probably not be so content to lie in her cot, she may get bored. She may lie and watch her hands, but she will not lose I.Q. points on the way. There is no need to play her Bach or to show her beautiful pictures; she will get all the stimulation she needs, and all the right stimulation, from simply being included in household activities.

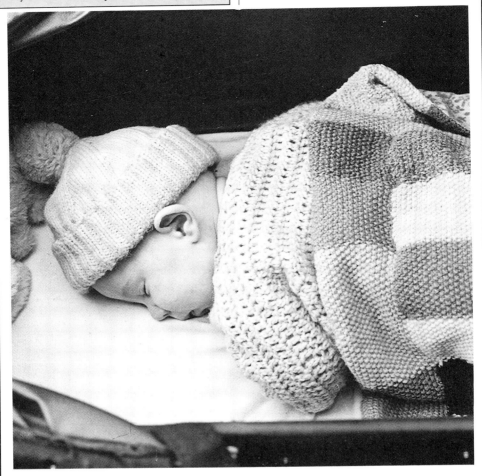

The mother takes her baby into a strange room where all sorts of things happen: a stranger comes in; the mother leaves the child alone with the stranger; the mother comes back to her baby, and so on.

By observing the babies, Ainsworth's team arrived at a definition of what a well-attached baby should be like.

She should, according to these tests, nicely balance independence and dependence. She should not scream as soon as she goes into a new place; but it is natural for her to protest when her mother suddenly leaves her with a stranger.

In fact, this is how 65 per cent of middle-class American infants behave. You might reasonably regard this as the scientifically established norm.

But is it? When the tests were carried out in Japan, it became quite clear that what was normal for a middle class American baby was horrifying for a Japanese baby. There, a traditionally reared child never leaves its mother's side. She sleeps with her mother, she is carried everywhere by her mother; she is never left with a baby sitter. Naturally, the baby screams as soon as her mother walks to the door.

But do we conclude from this that all mothers should be like Japanese mothers? Of course not.

572 Safety in numbers

The research evidence (principally by Rudolf Schaffer of Strathclyde University) shows that children with many attachments are happier than single-attachment children when they visit friends, start school or have a younger sibling. They feel secure with people generally, not only with their mother.

Given the choice (570) of whether to return to work before or after eight months, I would always go back before, encouraging multiple attachments in the process. *Of course* the substitute care has to be good (647-653); *of course* the substitute carers should not come and go too frequently; but provided your baby can fall back on you, and on other people with whom she has formed attachments, this last is not a major issue.

This debate is continued at 645-663.

573 Sleep

You wish your baby would sleep through the night and probably have an exaggerated view of how much other people's babies sleep. If yours does not measure up, you think something is wrong.

My first child slept no more than two or three hours at a stretch, day or night, until he was 18 months old. I was constantly tired and irritable, ill prepared to meet his demands. I had seen a baby as enriching my life, but basically fitting into it.

Our culture presents an idealized view of parenthood, a cosy glow of happy parents and pretty children that does not prepare us for the realities. Becoming a family is difficult enough; trying to do so through a haze of tiredness and resentment is almost impossible.

There must be times when all of us doubt that it is worthwhile. A cynical friend once remarked that it is a baby's business to ensure a comfortable future for himself, and that means making sure parents are too tired even to think of making love, thereby eliminating competition.

574 A norm for sleep?

Most new babies sleep for 12 to 14 hours out of 24. Inexperienced parents often imagine, however, that in the first weeks their baby will wake only for feeds: be awake only one hour in four.

By the time she reaches her first birthday, that 12 to 14 hours will have dropped to ten or 12. Compare this with your own daily sleep requirement – eight or nine hours. Now rethink all the plans you had for the times she was asleep. The most you can reasonably expect is that a newborn will be asleep for five hours longer than you.

575 Patterns

Moreover, this (574) will not be five hours at a stretch. Babies, like adults, have a rhythm of sleep and activity. Within a week of birth, most babies are beginning to develop their pattern; by eight weeks, some babies are sleeping for up to nine hours overnight, but most will have only one long sleep of between five and six hours. The length of this long sleep will gradually increase over the first year so that most babies will sleep through the night by their first birthday; most, but not all: one in five does not.

576 Types of sleep

There are two. One is peaceful sleep, when she really does look as if she is 'sleeping like a baby', body still, breathing regular, peaceful and relaxed. The other is dreaming sleep, in which breathing is irregular, (and may even stop for a few seconds, which is alarming but normal); her eyes move rapidly and her body twitches. She will move, suck, smile and show all manner of facial expressions. Adults dream during this type of sleep, but no one knows if babies do. However, it is clear that up to 70 per cent of their sleep is of this kind, much more than in adults.

The phases alternate. When a baby drops off to sleep, often at the breast (her principal way of controlling how much she takes is to fall asleep while feeding) she will go into a light, peaceful sleep. This will gradually become deeper until she looks completely peaceful.

Then, a period of 'dreaming' sleep will begin – eye movement is the best indicator of this. It may last for up to half an hour, after which she will revert to a quieter phase.

577 Where to sleep

As long as a baby is warm, she will sleep almost anywhere:

● **Pram:** The rocking motion will often send her to sleep. Babies don't have to be put outside in the fresh air; sometimes it may be too cold. However, in the warmer months, she may like to watch trees moving when she wakes and to hear different sounds out of doors.

Remember, she loses heat from her head, and will need a hat on if it is cool. Put up the pram hood if there is a breeze, and turn the pram so the hood shields her from the wind. Shield her from direct sunlight, too: it could cause overheating. Protect her from cats with a cat net: there

is a remote chance that a cat sleeping close to her face could smother her.
- **Carry cot:** Use it day or night; move it from car to bedroom; it is convenient. You can also put it inside a cot, and it is more draughtproof than the traditional drop-sided cot.
- **Baby nest:** Useful in the early weeks: put it inside a cot, the pram or carry cot.
- **Adult's bed:** Until she can roll, this is safe.
- **Warm room:** See 536.

578 Night clothes

Nightdresses make nappy changing easier at night, but see 584. Once she starts to kick and move about, ensure that her bedclothes stay in place, especially if you have no overnight heating. A sleeping bag is the best way to ensure that she stays snug and warm.

Lie her down so that her head touches the top of her crib: it is comforting. Some babies like to have their feet touching, too. In winter, a cloth bumper is warmer than a plastic one. She should be able to sleep anywhere, and through the general hubbub of the household. Encouraging her to sleep in a quiet room is asking for trouble. You may spend the rest of her childhood creeping about in the evenings.

579 Getting her to sleep

Things that soothe:

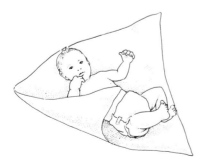

- **Swaddling:** Fold a shawl or cellular blanket into a triangle and lie her in the middle so that her head is just below the longest edge. Roll each of the pointed sections around her fairly tightly. She should make a stiff little parcel.

- **Dummy:** Banning dummies is often the one irrational stricture parents make. Why? Perhaps because you find the obvious sensual pleasure of sucking makes you uneasy? Also, of course, for snobbish reasons: there is almost certainly a link between parents' social class and possessing a dummy. But there are some practical objections, too: so strong can be the attachment to a dummy that weaning a baby off it can be difficult. You may not relish the idea of her going about with it as a toddler. The other practical objection is hygiene: it will need periodic sterilization.

The value of a dummy lies chiefly in the fact that it works.

Don't forget that baby or toddler may find similar comfort in sucking on a bottle of fruit juice or milk. But letting her take one to bed, or letting her suck a sweetened dummy, is to ask for early tooth decay.
- **Changing position:** A baby is more likely to sleep when she is lying down, so putting her down – and leaving her down – can work. Rocking and comfort objects also play their part; see pages 219 and 288.

580 Naps

In the first three months, your baby will usually have a short nap between each feed, longer ones at night. Gradually, over the first year, the naps, and the number of feeds, will be reduced so that at the end of the first year most babies will be taking at most a morning and afternoon nap.

581 Early wakers

Many babies greet the day before you are ready for it. You may be able to squeeze an extra half hour by taking her into your bed for a cuddle, but if this does not work it is probably best to leave her where she is and encourage her to amuse herself.

Don't lie there waiting for her to wake: put your head under the covers when she starts to shuffle and murmur. It is bad for you to feel tense in this way and may affect your subsequent treatment of her.

Wait to see if she really is awake for the day before you get her up. In a close and loving relationship, a baby can do without you for short periods.

582 Night wakers

Night wakers don't have problems, but their parents do. It is essential you get enough rest. You can do little, or nothing, about her sleeping pattern, so concentrate on yours.

When she wakes, try not to wake up more than necessary. Once you are wide awake, it will probably take you much longer to get back to sleep than it will her.

So, respond quickly to her needs before you are fully awake, giving her something to do while you go back to sleep. If the going gets rough, take it in turns with your partner to sleep out of earshot.

Always go to the baby if she cries. By the time she has cried herself into a rage, you will be wide awake and bad tempered. It will take two or three times as long to pacify her, and three or four times as long to go back to sleep.

Take it in turns with your partner to have an early night or a late morning. It may mean expressing milk to bottle feed, but this is worth the effort. A baby will happily take a bottle in her first few weeks, but you may have problems introducing it after, say, the first six weeks.

If you breast feed, cut down on caffeine and nicotine intake: stimulants pass directly to your baby in your milk.

Try to relax after you have fed her, but if you cannot get to sleep, accept being awake. Catch up with some reading, working or thinking; anger will make you even more tired. Take catnaps during the day, linked with the relaxation sequence described in 302.

See also 583.

583 The family bed

My favourite solution to the problem of the wakeful baby is the family bed: it needs to be big – say 6 ft (1.8 m) wide. The crib is kept beside it. When she wakes, you pick her up, put her to your breast, and then do your best to go back to sleep. More often than not, one of you will wake with the baby in your arms: a pleasant way to greet the morning.

Sharing the family bed is safe: remember how easy it is to wake to her cry; it is impossible that you will roll over on top of her without noticing. In the past there appear to have been instances where babies have been rolled on in bed; investigation suggests they were, in fact, either cot deaths that occurred in the parental bed or cases of deliberate injury to the child – disguised as accidents.

Of course, grandparents may view infants in the marital bed with horror. For them there was the unstated problem of what the child might witness there.

The other worry is that once you let your baby into your bed, she will never go to sleep anywhere else. If this concerns you, make an informal survey of friends and colleagues: the evidence will never prove this to be the case.

Some children still want to share the parental bed at the age of three, despite being kept in their own as babies; others, regularly allowed into the parents' bed as babies, stay in their own most of the time after six months.

Failing the family bed solution, it may be worth trying these:

● Taking it in turns to sleep in her room.
● Reaching out and stroking her, or putting her comforter into her hands as she stirs.

Sleepless babies run in some families. Accepting the inevitability of sleepless nights may in the long term cause less strain than fighting the problem.

584 Changing nappies at night

Don't do it. It will only wake her. A towelling nappy with a one-way liner (page 206) and loose plastic pants will keep her freer of nappy rash than frequently changed disposable nappies.

585 Routine

While it is basically impossible to make a baby fit a pattern not her own, there are compromises.

Many will adapt to being left up longer than usual in the afternoon or evening, provided they can enjoy the quid pro quo of being close to you, with plenty of stimulus. Keep your baby in a bouncing chair in sight of you while you cook the evening meal; or have her strapped to your back or front in a sling while you work or relax in the evening. (Or take a relaxing bath together.)

Also try:

● Giving a comforter to suck before you put her to sleep.

● Setting up a routine of a happy playful time – perhaps a bath or a change of clothes – then to bed; but before sleep let her sit with a board book while you tidy her clothes. After, say, ten minutes, turn on the fan, the mobile or the radio and leave her. It is worth giving such routines a fair trial, since it may take time for her to accept them.

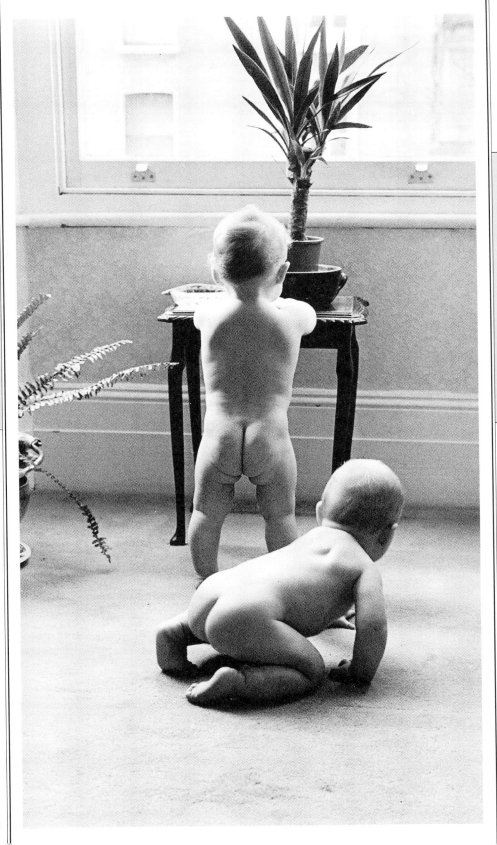

Baby- and Childcare

486-820

The Settled Baby – Three to Six Months

586 Three months old

In the early weeks it seemed at times as if you and your baby might never adjust to each other. Now, suddenly, you do.

It is not that she sleeps through the night; rather, it does not matter as much that she does not. You may still be tired, lacking drive, but you are no longer desperate. She feeds easily, and it is hard to imagine why you found it so difficult to bath and change her. As you dress her, she smiles at you, moves her lips, looks into your eyes and coos. She is a pleasure to have around. Even when her demands seem outrageous, you remember her as a person. She has a great deal of confidence in you (which is reassuring) and you now feel confident in her. You usually know what she wants.

As you both settle with the baby, you also begin to settle down again as a couple: sharing her helps you grow closer again.

Well, that is how it could be if you were that non-existent phenomenon, 'an average family'. Any comment in this book about development is bound to be a generalization: a guideline to provide food for thought, not a standard against which to measure performance.

587 Soap

She is lying in her bouncing cradle chair which has been placed safely on the kitchen floor. Her father is washing the vegetables at the sink. He turns, and moves towards the cradle, catching her eye. She rewards him with a beaming smile, so he moves in close and says "Boo". She turns slightly and the cradle begins to rock. He looks at her again, and rocks the cradle a little more. She looks right into his eyes and moves her mouth. "So you like that?" he says, pausing for a reply. She reaches an arm towards his face, squirms and coos.

Somehow she has you hooked.

588 Growth

Babies don't grow evenly. If they did, we would all look like over-grown babies. Your head is about 1/8th to 1/10th of your height, your legs about half. A toddler's head is about a quarter of her height, a new-born baby's even more.

If her head is comparatively large, her legs are minute: not much longer than her head. You may not find this particularly

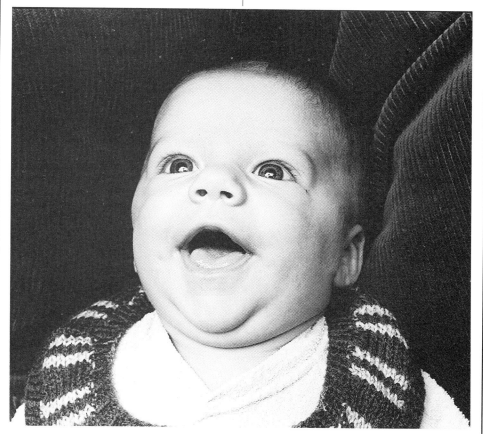

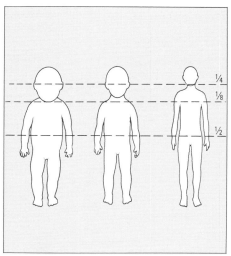

589 Bones

During childhood, bones change in three ways. They develop: there are only three bones in the wrist at birth, 28 by adulthood. They harden: the flexibility and toughness of babies and children is due to the pliability of many of the bones. And they grow: muscles will develop with the bones, too.

590 Taking control

There are natural developmental steps that determine how a baby comes to control her body. She starts at the top and works down (cephalocaudal development) and she starts in the middle and works out (proximodistal development). She controls her neck before her back, and can raise her chest before she can aim her hand.

By the end of the first three months, she will be holding her head up quite steadily and beginning to support her back and shoulders on her own. She will feel altogether less floppy.

If you watch your baby as she lies on her tummy, you can see the gradual development of the muscles. Try it once a

remarkable, except that she seems to fill out the legs of her stretch suits at amazing speed. When she reaches puberty, her legs and arms will grow much faster than anything else, which is what gives teenagers that awkward look. Like foals, their legs look too long for their bodies, and indeed they are.

week. In the first weeks she will begin to lift and move her head, using the muscles of her neck. Later, she will use the muscles of her trunk to squirm forward and turn from side to side. By four to five months she may well be able to roll over. If you lie her on her back and pull her up by her arms into a sitting position, you can watch the gradual development of the trunk muscles: when you first pull her up, she will flop forwards like a rag doll. Later, as she gains control of her head and body, she will hold her head steady as she comes up and will use her arms to balance and support herself so that her body leans forwards on to her knees.

591 Keeping her awake

When babies lie flat on their backs, they tend to go to sleep, perhaps because there is nothing much to see compared to the view from a chair. In a sitting position, she will be more alert and stay awake longer. Try to prop her up – see the illustration – if you want her to save her sleeping for night time.

It is often easiest to swipe at things in a sitting position. Remember she reaches best at objects directly in front of her. If her back is supported, she will be free to use both her arms for reaching.

592 Not sitting?

Babies sit when they are ready, give or take a little. It is not important when she learns, only that she does. There is almost certainly a significant inborn factor affecting how fast babies develop physically. Early sitting and walking seems to run in families and races: black children, for instance, are often physically more advanced than white at a given age. But speed of physical development seems to be independent of physical excellence. Children who walk earliest don't necessarily make athletes.

593 Does she need practice?

A baby will walk, even without practice; she will sit too. But it will take a little longer. Babies who lie on their tummies often crawl sooner than babies who don't; those who lie on their backs are often ahead when it comes to reaching out for objects.

594 Do parents need practice?

Two studies carried out in the U.S.A. examined all aspects of child care in three large cities. One of the most interesting findings was that care givers who interacted more, who played constructively and could comfort and respond to children best, had had some kind of education, formal or informal, in child development. It did not matter how long they had been in school, or how much time they had spent with children: only how much they knew about the way children developed. Children in their care scored better in language and intelligence tests, and were better adjusted socially. The moral must be that although first-time parents clearly cannot 'practise' childcare, by seeking to understand how children develop, they can usefully train for it.

595 Teething?

Is she chewing and sucking objects because she is teething? It is true that many babies teeth at this stage, but this is purely coincidental. She sucks in order to explore. Her mouth is much more sensitive than her hands in these early months. Until she can oppose her thumb with her fingers and poke with one finger (see holding sequence, page 238) she cannot use her hands as effectively as her lips and tongue.

Safety
How safe it is for her to put objects into her mouth depends on the objects:
● Too small and it could be swallowed.
● Mouth-width objects may get stuck.
● Loose and furry, and she may choke on little bits.
● Long and thin, such as a wooden spoon, and it may get stuck down her throat.
● *Anything* sharp can cut.
● Match boxes and cigarettes are not good for babies to chew. The compound on the sides of match boxes is poisonous; and a single swallowed cigarette delivers, for a baby, a dangerously large dose of nicotine.
● If you are worried about germs, sterilize her toys.
● Remember her neck is near her mouth: string, nylon, wool and ribbon could all get twisted accidentally around her neck. It is safest to use wool and elastic to tie toys to her cot: wool breaks and elastic gives if it ends up around her neck.

596 Chewing newspaper

Babies of this age often love to chew paper: it is a wonderful toy because it is noisy and easy to handle. It changes shape, it rips, it changes texture inside her mouth.

Is it dangerous? Newsprint in large quantities is poisonous, but an occasional chew does little harm. Swallowing any paper is best avoided; since it has a texture similar to food she will probably keep it in her mouth, rolling it around until it is small enough to swallow: it makes sense, therefore, never to leave her alone with paper, indeed to watch her extra carefully as she plays.

597 The nature of babies

The brain is structured something like a toy mouse: there is a 'head', a 'body' and a long, fat 'tail'. In man, the head grows so big that it flops back over and almost completely covers the body and tail. There is no other way to store all the grey matter. At birth, the fat tail is well developed; so is the middle, body section. But the head has a long way to go. Although most of the brain will be in place by the time a child is six, it will not be fully developed until puberty. The tail manages all the body's automatic functions, such as controlling breathing, digestion and sleeping. The body deals with reflexes and many additional automatic responses: when you turn towards sudden flashes of light or movement, it is this area of the brain that perceives and organizes your response, which is why babies soon react to rattles and movement. This part of the brain can learn simple causes and effects, such as associating smells or lights with food, or your picking her up with the smell of your body.

By contrast, the head (the neocortex) is the area of the brain that controls thinking, speech, pattern vision, motor control and most decision-making. It follows that your baby will not think as you do, reason, remember, or understand like an adult; indeed, for the first two months of her life, she functions with very little neocortical brain. She sucks, but does not think 'If I want food I just have to suck'. She sucks because the nipple is in her mouth; put her to your cheek and she will try to suck just as if it was a breast.

She can adapt her sucking to suit a bottle teat (as most mammals can), and can learn that milk is coming when she hears you approach (as a cat does when you open the door of the fridge), but such learning remains simple.

She does have a healthy instinct for self-preservation. She will hold her breath under water, lift her hands to protect her face, turn her head if you cover her mouth and close her eyes if you move too quickly towards her face.

The brain is made up of neurones, special cells which communicate with each other. Some of the cells constitue what we call nerves, and some form 'brain cells'. In a baby, neurones looke a little like tiny seedlings: a little seed, (the cell body); a little shoot (which takes messages) and a large number of roots which gather information from other cells. As they develop, neurones become even more plant-like, the roots and shoots dividing again and again so that they make a whole network of connections.

At birth, the seeds are just beginning to sprout; in the weeks that follow, they send out shoots and roots, they form connections with other areas of the brain and begin to communicate.

The shoots can become quite long. The longer shoots from many cells collect together in bundles, which we call nerves (in the body) or pathways (in the brain). They can send information to every part of the brain, making millions upon millions of connections. Many of the cells have roots more complex than a mature oak tree's; indeed, if you traced an oak branch right down to the veins of a single leaf, you would still not begin to perceive the complexity of some of the cells of the human brain. The millions of cells in the neocortex grow and connect throughout childhood, changing your baby slowly into a mature, thinking, socializing, rational (and irrational), logical (and illogical) adult.

It is a long and fascinating journey to watch. When you have a baby, you buy yourself a front seat on the observation deck.

Even at three months, she really does not know who it is out there, or even that the rest of the world exists. She takes it for granted that someone is caring for her; she is delighted that you do, but she will not panic when you leave because she is incapable of considering that you could disappear. She does not even think you exist: you simply turn up every so often.

When she does realize that you are a person who comes and goes, someone with an independent existence, she will start to panic when you leave her. She may yell as soon as you move out of your seat.

Sitting

At birth she will have limited control of her head. It will flop when you try to sit her.

At one month her back will be rounded but her head will be held for a short period.

At four months she will sit while you hold her hands.

At six months she will sit without support, but not steadily.

At seven months she will sit firmly. but with her back still quite rounded. she will brace herself with her hands.

At eight months she will sit up straight.

At nine months she will be able to reach for toys as she sits.

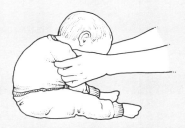

One month

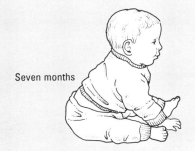

Seven months

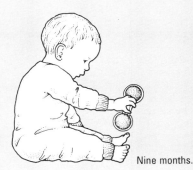

Nine months.

Rolling

At birth she will lie on her stomach with her head to one side. She will still be quite curled up, as she was in the womb. Her bottom will stick up.

At two months she will lie flat and lift her head from the mat.

At three months she will begin to lift her shoulders.

At four months she will push up with her arms, and lift both legs off the mattress.

At five months she will push up, taking the weight of most of her body on her arms: she will soon roll over.

By about five months she will be able to lift up her head while lying on her back and peep at her toes. She can also roll to both sides in order to reach out. She usually learns at about the same time to roll from stomach to back and vice versa.

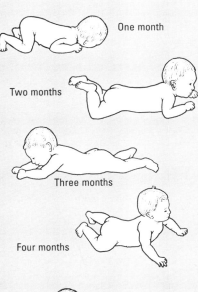

One month

Two months

Three months

Four months

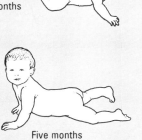

Five months

Safety

She will often roll over without warning though you may learn to recognize when this is imminent: often, it is when she reaches out for something. The soft surface of a sofa, chair or bed can assist the rolling action: many a parent has found the baby screaming on the floor when just before she had been left safely in the centre of the bed.

Propping

Long before she can sit alone she will enjoy being propped in a sitting position. Or you can use the bouncing cradle chair, one of the most popular pieces of baby equipment – and rightly so. Later, a lie-back plastic chair makes an alternative: as she gets stronger it can gradually be adjusted into a more upright position than the bouncing cradle chair.

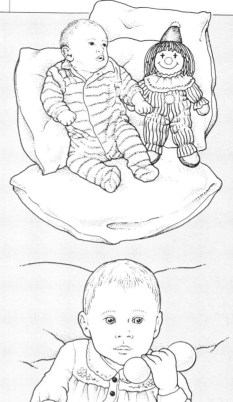

Grasping

At birth she can:

Make rudimentary swipes at objects; hit an object if it is right in front of her, but swiping is her best if it is off the body's mid-line.

She cannot: monitor her hand once it begins to move; grasp objects in a sophisticated manner: she clings to them much as a baby monkey does to its mother's fur: she holds or clasps rather than grasps. She does not adjust her hand in response to the object she is holding.

She cannot pick up an object. She will close her hand around anything which falls into it: with luck, interesting objects such as blankets and rattles will do just that.

She cannot let go. She drops things purely by chance, often because she now wants to clutch something else.

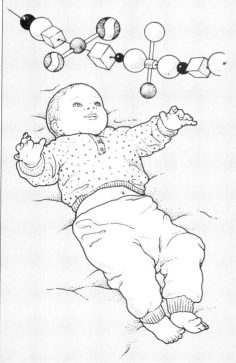

Reaching

She gets to know her world by reaching out to it: the eyes and ears are involved, as well as the hands. Adults reach out automatically, but it is really quite a complex skill. When you give her a toy from the toy box, you look at the position of the toy and program your reach unaware that you are doing so.

You reach out with your hand to grasp it, adjusting the angle and size of your grip as you reach.

You take it in your hand, clasping it with your fingers.

You move your hand towards her, adjusting your movements as she waves her arms in excitement.

You place the toy in her hand.

You let go, helping her to close her hand around the toy.

It is simple for you, but to do the same she has to learn to reach, to judge distance and program precise movement, to adjust grip, to move her arm from one position to the next, to alter the path of movement in response to visual information and to let go.

Hands into view

At first, she does not see her hands; she gets to know them by touch. She moves, and by chance, touches one hand with the other. This usually happens at about six weeks: she still does not seem to know the hands both belong to her: she has found something convenient to play with, and that is that.

Replace one hand with a rattle, and she may like it even more: she naturally turns towards sound, it is one of her reflex actions.

By 12 weeks, the movement of her hands is enough to interest her for its own sake. She will watch them waving in front of her eyes. Her eyes, meanwhile, have been developing; she is becoming increasingly aware of her surroundings. She will perhaps already have learned to swipe at an object; she can certainly reach towards a noisy one.

At first, when she begins to reach for objects, she will be totally distracted by her hand coming into view; but slowly, she learns to ignore this. You will see her reach out and look between the object and her hand, perhaps making adjustments for a second go. At about five months she is ready to reach out in one movement, and at about the same time, she begins to take things to her mouth.

She will start by taking her hands or her fingers into her mouth and using her lips and tongue to explore them. While she still clutches at objects she cannot move them about, poke them or pass them from hand to hand. Thus she must use her mouth instead.

Only when all the stages are complete will she reach out, grasp, take to her mouth and explore.

Eye-hand sequence

At birth she will reach out and touch an object or sound source directly in front of her. She can reach to the left or right, but inaccurately.

● She can focus on objects about 10 inches (25 cm) away.

● At ten to 12 weeks, she will start to swipe at objects.

● At three to four months she will lift her hands and bring them together around an object.

● By four months she will reach towards an object, though inaccurately, and adjust her hand under visual guidance until she makes contact with it.

● By six months she can move one hand directly to an object. She does not watch her hand; she knows where it is.

Hand-eye co-ordination

Does it seem a long-winded phrase to describe something as simple as looking and doing? If so, you have a poor misunderstanding of a baby's mental status: in the beginning, she does not know that her hands are part of her; she does not even know where she ends and the rest of the world begins. 'Hand-eye co-ordination' is actually an apt description of a complex achievement.

Holding sequence

At one month, a baby haphazardly grasps anything that enters her hand by folding her fingers over it.

By two months, she can deliberately hold her hand open, though otherwise it is usually kept 'closed', but still grasps haphazardly.

By three months, her hands are usually open; she still grasps haphazardly and drops objects after a while. The dropping is not deliberate.

By four months she can bring her hands together deliberately.

By five months she can grasp with both hands.

By six months she begins to use her thumb to grip.

By seven months she uses her thumb in opposition to all fingers: a power grip. She can pass objects from hand to hand.

By eight months she can use her thumb in opposition to one finger: a pincer grip.

By eight to nine months she can deliberately drop.

By nine months she can poke her finger into holes.

By 11 months she can hold a crayon, and feed herself.

By her first birthday she is moving her hands in readiness to grasp an object. (Try reaching for an imaginary broom: look at your hand. Now reach for a football: look again.) We prepare our hands in readiness for the objects as we reach out.

By 14 months she can put one brick on top of another.

By 18 months she can build a tower three or four bricks high.

By her second birthday she can turn the door knob to open the door.

Toys for sitting and standing babies

Once she can sit, she can hit with a hammer and push along a toy with wheels: chunky cars, drums, hammers, pots and pans all delight at this age.

At about eight months, she enters a new phase, in which she begins to find out what objects can do for her. She will look at a new toy as if it presents her with a problem; She may try it out in her mouth, then she might bang it or squeeze it in her hand, touch the edges with her hand and then put it back into her mouth. She will turn it over, look at it this way and that.

Why? Psychologists believe that it is because she is beginning to realize that the object exists in its own right. It is the first stage in realizing that it exists even when she is not looking.

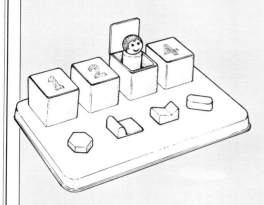

A pop-up toy with built in long-term interest. The challenge is to discover the different method of releasing each pop-up animal by means of a colour-coded button. The button on the left is simply pushed; the next must be slid to left or right; the next works like a light switch, rocking left or right; the last is turned. At one year, or even just under, a baby will release the pop-up mechanism by accident – entertainment in itself. Later the toy will enable her to explore cause-and-effect at several levels.

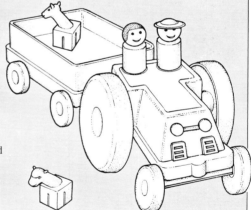

Tractor and trailer: driver and passenger bounce up and down as they go along. The animals can be removed from the trailer and replaced, along with the rails. Combined value of pull-along and shape fitting toy.

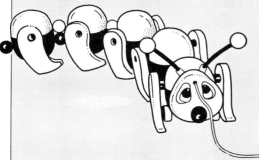

Pull-alongs encourage the toddler to refine control over her body: looking around to watch the creature as she walks requires a special, if basic, form of balance. This 'clatterpillar' has the added fascination of moving in wave-motion, and with a delightful clattering noise – which announces the child's presence.

598 Dependency

See 529. Because so many women nowadays have full or part-time jobs, more and more come to raising a family having experienced a high degree of independence, emotional and financial. Indeed, they may not realize just how much independence they enjoyed until they find themselves at home with the baby. It may be disillusioning to discover how much emotional independence was a result of financial independence.

You may, as a result, feel that you have lost status and security – a feeling of loss not helped by the child's constant demands. You cannot go anywhere or do anything without taking the baby or making arrangements for her care.

Don't be too depressed: it is not surprising that you feel this way, since society's view that women are dependent upon men is still strong. A woman's independence has still to be won. All your life, this conditioning has been rubbing off on you, and you may indeed question whether your feeling of independence had any firm basis when it vanished with the pay packet.

In any event, the time has probably come for a reappraisal of roles. In a family, the web of dependence and independence can be so complex as to defy analysis.

You have lost independence, but you have gained, in some senses, a new hold over your partner. He has lost independence too: because he alone must provide – at any rate for a while – he must play safe at work; he feels heavier ties of responsibility than ever before. But in other ways, you have both gained, there is a new depth in your relationship, a new depth in your life. It is part of your nature as a woman to be loved and needed by your family and that instinct is now being fulfilled. The price of this fulfillment may be your hard-won sense of independence; but everything has a price.

599 Learning the steps

A baby who can rely on the comfort of her parents is prepared to go out into the world and explore.

A man who can rely on the emotional support of his mother, and later his wife, has a firm base from which he can got out to conquer the world.

A woman who can rely on the emotional support of a man is likewise independent.

But if she cannot, losing economic independence as well (598) can make life impossibly hard for a woman confined to a nuclear family. Learning the steps of the new dance of dependence and independence is often like going through puberty all over again, with perhaps more at stake. See 601.

600 A model of care

What is really excellent childcare? First, I think it is putting oneself in the baby's place: adjusting what one gives to meet the baby's desires. Men and women are both capable of doing this, but what follows is intended especially as a model for men:

Babies signal what they need: excellent, sensitive carers interpret those signals and give promptly and appropriately. If they cannot give, they offer an alternative: offer, not force. You wait for the baby to accept. You take note of the early communication between baby and mother. You communicate your intentions, then move into the baby with the baby's permission.

You need not be especially good with babies or children, but you are probably good with people; you have empathy, and sympathy.

An insensitive father gears all interactions to his own wishes and moods. If he does happen to note a baby communicating her needs, he tends either to ignore them, or to respond as if he knows better. He is, perhaps, afraid to become too involved; he is, perhaps, used to being in charge.

As one might expect, children lucky enough to have a sensitive, caring father, cry less, are happier and more secure.

Children who are picked up and cuddled frequently are happier and more secure than those who are not and, surprisingly, cuddling a child in the early months makes it much easier to leave her later on.

601 Father's choice?

"We need to get that into the post tonight, do you think you can stay on a bit?" He could, of course, say "Sorry I have to get home to bath the baby." But babies can wait; the contract cannot. "He is an important client, could you take him for a drink?" It means missing her bed time, leaving supper and bath for his partner; but if he refuses? "Sorry, I have theatre tickets for tonight", may be more

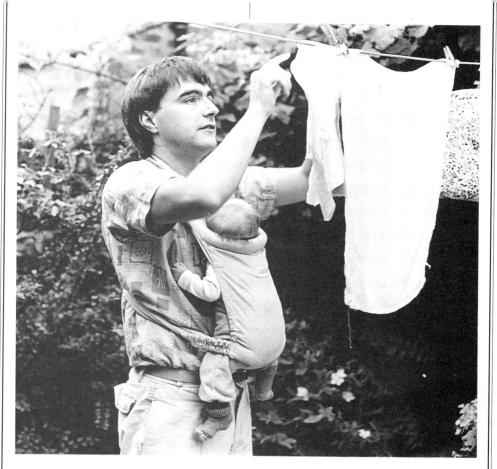

acceptable than "The children will miss their story." To suppose that it is easy for a man to tread the tightrope between family and work obligations is to be entirely naïve.

A working mother has the advantage of being expected to be responsible for children. She can say "I'll check with my sitter to see if she can stay on for half an hour", then come back and say "Sorry, she can't tonight. But I could get in earlier tomorrow".

Despite the fact that many mothers continue to work, and thus many men should be contributing their fair share of childcare, and indeed that more and more fathers want to make a commitment to rearing their children, there is often a lack of understanding in the workplace.

Corporate loyalty and long working hours are again a virtue, as they were in pre-war years. Staying until the job is done is the essence of professionalism. To climb the ladder and reap the economic rewards both partners may want for their family means being willing to put the company first. The pressures are not just intense, they are incompatible. See 666.

602 Starting solid food

Sucking at the breast is a pleasurable, comforting activity for a baby. Why deprive her of it? Babies thrive as well on breast milk as on formula milk for the first nine months of life.

When should you start her on solids? She is telling you she is ready when she starts putting things into her mouth; when she enjoys exploring like this it is time to make food one of the things she discovers. If you try to put food in sooner, you will find that her tongue tends to push it out; you end up pushing the spoon to the back of her throat in order to force the food down.

Other signs that she is ready for solid foods:

• Wanting extra breast feeds.
• Cutting the time between breast feeds.

She should in principle, indeed in practice, be able to feed herself before you wean her. Of course, it would be very messy, and rather wasteful, to let her do so all the time.

603 How to feed

Spoon feeding is an important social occasion, the talking and coaxing it involves are an important component of early parent-child interaction. If you find it a battle ground, you are probably trying too soon. Wait a little.

If you are really worried about your baby not having enough to eat, get one of those all-embracing baby aprons, and put her in a chair with a clean tray. Cover the floor, cover yourself and have plenty of tissues ready to mop up spills. Put piles of food on the tray and let her try to feed herself. Don't interfere; leave her to it. It will be very, very messy, but she will almost certainly get a taste for solid food. It is an activity for just before bath time, but not if you are dressed up to go out.

An advantage to leaving even small babies to feed themselves is that they do not overeat. If feeding has become a social game, it is always tempting to give the baby another spoonful; always tempting for her to carry on the 'conversation' by opening her mouth even if she is already full.

Some babies dislike the feel of a spoon in their mouths. If you have tried both metal and plastic spoons without success, try giving her food from your finger. Obviously, you need to wash your hands thoroughly first.

604 First feed

Imagine you are fixed to a chair, bib on. Someone comes up to you with a spoon. "Down the little red lane", she says as she forces a spoonful into your mouth. "Chuff, chuff, chuff" as the next spoonful comes along. You look away as the telephone rings and in goes a spoonful you had not expected and perhaps did not want. Spit it out, and it is scraped from your face and put back.

Maybe, after you have spat it out for the sixth time, she will get your message; maybe she will get annoyed, make you feel bad. Maybe she will give up. It can be delightful, yes; it can also be a time of stress.

Babies are not fools. Immature they may be, but they do know what they like, and how much they need; see 606.

I always started feeding with packets of dried food (not cereals) or tins. Lovingly prepared meals are for when you are sure she will not spit it all out. Cooking a meal

for three spoonfuls is a labour of love. You can purée a little apple or a few frozen carrots, but is this so very nourishing? Home-cooked food can be better, and may make you feel like a good mother, but there are almost certainly better ways to spend your time when you have small children than cooking for them in the first weeks of solid feeding.

605 First meals

Avoid cereals other than rice in the early weeks. Cereals are rich in carbohydrates (which babies can largely do without) and gluten (which some babies find difficult to digest). Avoid adding sugar and salt. Puréed vegetables or fruit, tinned mixed dinners, or baby rice are perfectly adequate. Sweet puddings will only encourage a sweet tooth and may stop your baby eating savoury foods.

As long as you avoid sweet foods, she will do the same.

606 When a baby knows best

An experiment was conducted in which babies were allowed to choose whatever they liked to eat from a range of wholesome foods placed in front of them. There were eggs, cereals, vegetables, fruits, milk and cod liver oil and they just helped themselves.

Sometimes they drank large amounts of cod liver oil; sometimes they ate three eggs a day; but soon, every single baby settled into a well-balanced diet of its own accord. None of them was ever sick.

607 But can you be sure?

Your baby is growing, but it really is not essential that she balances her food budget every single day. Few of us do. Becoming obsessional about her food is the surest way to unbalance her diet – she will pick up your anxiety and almost certainly become a finicky eater. While she still has plenty of milk in her diet, she will be getting plenty of protein, but in any event, she needs only a tiny amount of protein in her diet. If you are worried about its vitamin content, you can always give her a supplement. Obesity is more of a problem than malnutrition.

Opposite: It should be a relaxing, happy time: if it starts to be a battleground, see 603.

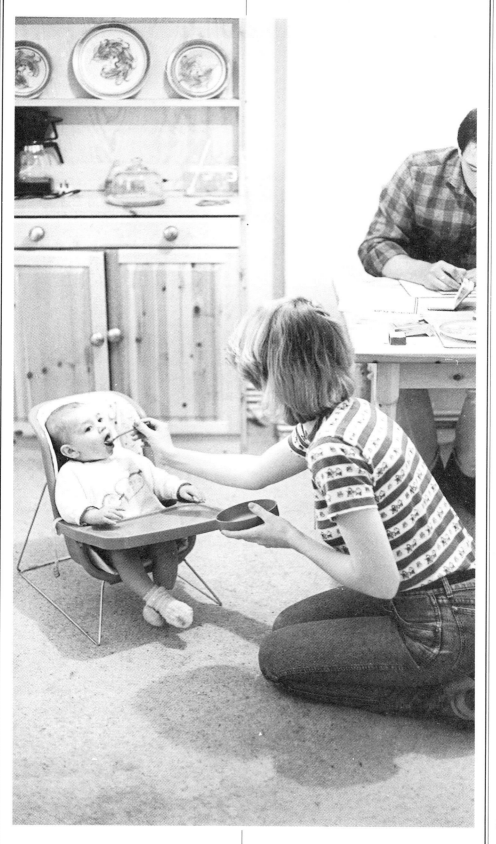

243

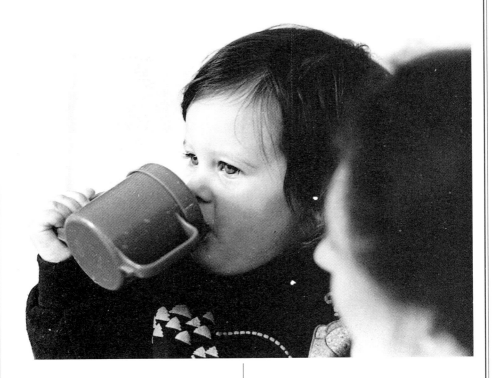

608 Homemade food is good because:

• It can be cheaper. (It can also cost more if you make too much.)
• You accustom your baby to your kind of food.
• You control the amount of sugar and salt.
• It contains no preservatives.

But:
• It is not automatically nutritious.
• You may be more upset if she spits it out.
• You can become obsessional about her diet.
• It is bad practice to reheat a little bit of yesterday's supper. If bacteria are developing in it, the heat will heighten their activity.

609 Packet food is good because:

• It is cheaper if you have to cook for a baby separately; if, for instance, you take your main meal in the evening.
• It is almost effortless to prepare, and there is little heartache if you throw it away.

But:
• It sometimes has added sugar, cereal thickener and salt. Check the label.
• It can be bland; possibly not a fitting introduction to the sort of food you eat as a family.
• It does not easily introduce different textures. Second stage lumpy foods are not always as acceptable to babies as mashed home-produced foods.

610 Cow's milk

By the time your baby is six months old and taking solids, you can replace formula and breast milk with cow's milk. Cow's milk should, of course, be pasturized or sterilized before it is given. A breast-fed baby can have cow's milk with her cereal and she may drink it from a cup.

But just because you are switching to cow's milk does not mean you can get haphazard about sterilizing her bottle. Bottles are sterilized because milk is such an excellent breeding ground for bacteria. It may seem odd to keep on sterilizing her bottle and teat when she is crawling around the floor, but it is wise.

Teats are difficult to get perfectly clean.

244

611 Weaning on to a cup

It is not necessary to replace the breast with a bottle: a baby can be weaned straight from breast to cup if it is done gradually. I introduced a cup to give fruit juice or water between feeds at about four months.

Most babies will drink a little from a sucking cup or beaker at this age, and certainly by about six months you should start introducing your baby to a cup, gradually reducing the number of bottle or breast feeds. A baby taking four feeds a day will be receiving most of her protein, and nearly all of her calories, from milk. As she takes more solids, she will need fewer calories from milk.

You should, however, ensure that she has enough fluid, and that her milk intake is not suddenly reduced. Babies drink slowly from cups, and will often take no more than a few ounces in this way at first. A special feeding cup may give you some idea of how much fluid she is taking. If she has a favourite meal, or a 'good' time of day, this is the best time to introduce the cup, otherwise start with the lunch-time meal.

If she is not very keen, a number of short drinks interspersed with the solids may be the better approach. Alternatively, give the solids first and then try her with the cup. In either case, you should finish with the breast or bottle. You will soon find that she is taking little from the breast, and that you can drop this feed entirely.

In this way you can gradually replace her day-time feeds with the cup.

You will find that your breasts are rather full for a day or two, but milk production will soon adjust to the reduced demand.

Once she has replaced day-time feeds, you may find it easy to replace the early morning feed with a morning drink, especially if you make this a ritual in which you all have a drink together. By the time she is seven or eight months old, she will probably want only breast feeding at her bed time. She will probably still want this until she is about a year old, as much for comfort as anything else.

612 Cups

There is a variety of special cups to choose from. Beakers or sucking cups with spouts are probably easiest because she can take the fluid either in a dribble, or by sucking. Angled cups are best for teaching her to drink from the real thing:

failing this, an old-fashioned teacup is better than a straight-sided mug.

Once she is drinking, she will probably try to take the cup from you; let her. In this way she will soon learn to drink by herself.

A day's food at six months
- First feed: breast or bottle.
- Breakfast: coddled egg with breadcrumbs; milk from a cup.
- Lunch: puréed vegetable and meat (four to five spoonfuls); fruit pure. A drink of milk or fruit juice.
- Afternoon tea: yoghurt, cream cheese sandwich or cereal with added cheese; milk from a cup.
- Dinner: breast or bottle.

A day's food at four months
- First and second feeds: breast or bottle.
- Third feed: one breast, or half the bottle, then one or two spoonfuls of tinned dinner, puréed fruit or vegetable. Finish the breast or bottle.
- Fourth and fifth feeds: breast or bottle.

---

613 Preparing food

- Check that there are no unwanted bits in the food, such as pieces of apple core in stewed apple. This applies especially if you use a blender rather than a sieve.
- Start by thinning the food with milk or water to the consistency your baby prefers. Gradually make it more solid; by seven months, her food should be only slightly sloppy.
- Steam, rather than boil, vegetables and fruit so that they retain the vitamins.
- Don't reheat – it can be dangerous; see 608.
- Don't add sugar or salt. Sugar will encourage obesity, salt puts a strain on a baby's kidneys.
- Don't cook tinned dinners for too long: it destroys the vitamins.

614 Obese babies

Everyone has fat storage cells just under the skin; in many of us, they do indeed store fat.

A baby's cell content grows rapidly in the first year, after which few new cells are added. By overfeeding her in the first year, you can encourage her to lay down too many fat cells. She will start to look plump, but the real damage will only be evident when she later puts on weight. Her plentiful fat cells will puff up – ooze – with fat. The potential is created for her to become an overweight adult.

615 Avoiding obesity

• Don't force food on her. If she is hungry, she will eat.
• Remember, she may eat to please you.
• Don't add sugar and avoid giving too much cereal.
• Don't reward her with sweets, or praise too highly if she empties her plate.
• Don't fob her off with a biscuit or chocolate drop when she wants your attention.
• Don't delude yourself by saying she is just bonny. She is fat.

616 If she is fat

• Let her feed herself: it will take a long time and it will make a mess, but she is unlikely to overeat.
• Play and talk at meal times – distract her from eating.
• Cut down her fat, sugar and carbohydrate intake.
• Ban chocolate and sweets from the house or ration her to one sweet in the morning.
• Replace puddings with fruit pure.
• Encourage her to be more active. Get her a walker if she shows no signs of crawling. Make her sit rather than lie. See 697.

617 A baby's world

To start with, she is most concerned about where things are; at two months she begins to concern herself with what things are. She starts looking not at movement and the edges of objects but at the details, the curves, the colours and the parts that make up the whole. She begins to look back and forth, taking in the whole object, where before she fixed on one part of it.

This is almost certainly because the visual cortex, the outer layer of the brain at the back of her head, comes into play.

Another development at about two months is her new interest in things which are moderately novel. Why moderately novel? Because if they were completely novel, she would have no basis for understanding them. If, on the other hand, they were completely familiar, she would have nothing to learn. By being interested in the moderately novel, she can gradually build up a best guess at the nature of the world around her. By three months, she has switched from captive to active, from having her attention captured by movement and sound to paying attention to things on which she chooses to focus.

618 Object concept

A baby has to learn at least three fundamental truths about the objects in her world:

• That they remain the same, even when they look different; that they have constancy.
• That objects continue to exist even when she cannot see or feel them any longer: that they have permanence.
• That objects retain their unique quality from one encounter to the next: that they have identity.

Object constancy means that she will perceive you as being exactly the same whether you are sitting in the chair or are walking towards the door.

Object permanence means that she will know you still exist even when you walk out of the room.

Object identity means she knows you are the same mother when you walk back in again.

It seems that she learns all this in the first two years of life.

619 Object constancy: seeing is believing

The eye is not like a camera; the world we see not at all like a photograph. As you sit reading, you hold a book. It is rectangular in shape with parallel sides. But is it? Unless you are looking directly at it, unlikely as you read, the image of the book perceived by your eye is actually a trapezoid shape: the top is narrower than the bottom because it is farther away. Do babies make these adjustments? Do they see the breast as the breast, whatever the angle?

By two to three months, they may do, but it is not certain that they can before this. If I, an adult, look at you standing next to me, you will fill my field of view. If I look at you across the room, I see tables and chairs as well. You should appear smaller, but you don't. I adjust your perceived size because I take into account how far away you are. When, by contrast, we cannot accurately judge distance, things look small, as from an aeroplane. At two to three months, babies also start to make this type of adjustment, but they probably cannot do it in the first weeks.

620 Object identity

This is not present at birth: you are new every morning, and out of sight is out of mind.

Object identity seems to develop at about five months. If you show a baby of four months a reflection of her mother in a mirror, she is delighted. If you show her five such reflections she is even more delighted. But at around 22-24 weeks, infants begin to be extremely upset with multiple mothers, which suggests that at this age they at least know that there should be only one mother. It is uncertain that they know anything else has an identity at this age, but by about seven or eight months, they do seem to: by then they may be wary of strangers and upset by moving away from the familiarity of home. Holidays can be a nightmare with a seven-month-old.

But although your baby has begun to learn, it is only a beginning. She will be six or seven years old before she is completely sure about all aspects of object identity.

621 Object permanence

This also takes a long time to develop. At three months, she has only the most rudimentary ideas of permanence. If she is playing with your sieve and you take it away, she will not mind as long as you give her something else. It is as if the sieve does not exist. At this age it is quite easy to leave a baby all day, she will not be in the least perturbed as long as she has a substitute carer.

If she drops a toy, she does not look for it; if you cover a toy, she will look the other way, unconcerned.

It seems as if she has no idea that objects continue to exist when she cannot see them; except perhaps for one little bit of evidence.

If you show her a toy and then cover it up, she will not show much interest. But if you take away the toy and then lift the cloth, she will look suprised, as if she expected the toy still to be there. But did she expect that toy? It seems not. If you show her a little train chuffing back and forth through a tunnel, she will watch quite happily as it goes into the tunnel, and will then look to the other side of the tunnel, waiting for it to emerge. It looks as if she is waiting for the train. But if a car comes out of the tunnel, rather than the train, she will not look at all surprised.

So, the stage she has reached is not perhaps one of understanding that objects have a separate existence of their own, but of knowing that something should be there, or should happen. See 726.

622 Immunization

This serves two separate purposes. It protects your child, and it aims eventually to eradicate disease. If no one can catch a disease, it will eventually die out – as small pox now has.

So long as everyone else has their child immunized, your child is to a large extent protected. If, however, the rate of immunization falls, the disease can take hold again – as whooping cough has tended to do in recent years.

Immunization gives protection against a whole range of diseases; a child may be given several injections, or they may be combined into a single injection.

Immunization works with diseases such as measles, whooping cough, Rubella and polio, which you can catch only once. The injection introduces a small number of actual 'germs' of the disease. They are specially prepared in a weakened form, sufficiently strong to fool the immune system into thinking the disease is present, but not enough to produce symptoms. The immune system reacts by building up specific antibodies and antitoxins to the disease. Next time the virus or bacterium tries to attack, the body can repel the invader.

The exact timing of immunization varies from country to country, but the programme usually begins at three to four months.

Some immunizations (measles is one) need to be given only once. Others, such as polio, need several doses before immunity is built up.

623 Immunization programme

The first immunization, a triple one, gives immunity against diphtheria, tetanus and whooping cough. Three doses are given in the first, by injection, and a final one just before starting school. A polio immunization is given at the same time.

A second triplet (measles, Rubella and mumps) is being introduced. In the U.K., this will be given in place of the present measles immunization in the second year. Tuberculosis immunization is normally given when a child is about 13 years old.

624 Reactions

After the triple immunization, children may become feverish, and the site of the injection can become red and sore. Very occasionally, there is a more serious reaction; see 625. Further routine reactions are a high-pitched scream, and a high fever which may last for two days or more.

If your baby's temperature starts to rise, sponge her with a tepid, damp sponge or put her into a lukewarm bath (below blood heat, but not cold) to lower her temperature.

625 Convulsions

This is the most serious and alarming reaction produced by immunization. Young children are much more prone to convulsions than adults, especially if they develop a high fever; indeed, most fits in small children are produced by fever. They may look alarming, but they are never fatal. The fever irritates the parts of the brain that control the muscles and the child twitches violently and uncontrollably. She will become unconscious. An unconscious child breathes in a noisy, strange manner, something like snoring.

A convulsion lasts no more than a few minutes, although it can seem like a lifetime; after, she will sleep.

626 If she has convulsions...

There is no need to panic: see the first aid procedures under **Convulsions** in the **medical section**.

627 Whooping cough immunization

There is an extremely small risk that a child will suffer a severe reaction to whooping cough immunization. In 1975, there were almost 9,000 cases of whooping cough in Britain, and 12 deaths, most of these babies. That makes a one in

750 chance of dying from the disease.

In the previous year, 50,000 children were immunized against whooping cough; 40 of these (one in 1,250) had a severe reaction, but not one of them showed any signs of permanent brain damage. The risk of permanent brain damage on these figures is less than one in 50,000.

So there is a much greater risk from the disease itself than from immunization against it.

There is added risk from the immunization if:

- A baby has already had convulsions.
- There is a history of epilepsy in the family.
- There is a family history of convulsions in childhood.
- If the first immunization produced a severe reaction.
- If the child has a fever, a cold, or is ill at the time of immunization.
- If the child happens to be taking a medicine or medicines, let whoever gives the immunization know that your baby is receiving medication.

---

628 Social baby

Between three and six months, she becomes a social baby. When you look at her, she looks directly back at you, her face brightens, her eyes widen and she beams. She may seem enraptured with you, her mouth will move as if to talk, she snuggles up to you, she starts to lift herself as you reach down to pick her up. Does she know your face? Probably not. But she may know you by your smell, voice, touch and face. She is everyone's friend: she will smile her toothless smile at anyone willing to engage in the interaction.

At about five months she begins to be more selective: her memory improves, she begins to realize that some faces are familiar and to smile more readily at them.

Once she can tell who she knows, she can, of course, tell who she does not know. Between five and eight months she will reach a stage when she is no longer an outgoing, smiling baby. She will start to scream when someone strange talks to her and will no longer happily take part in games of social interaction such as 'pass the parcel'. Eye contact with a strange face becomes enormously threatening, and she will turn away rather than look.

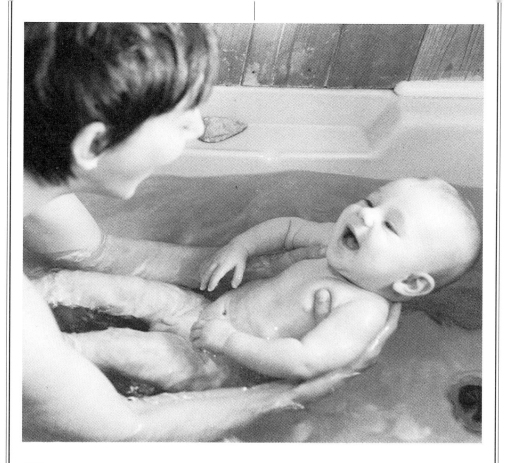

629 Making the world go round

As she moves into her second three months she begins to show she loves you. She woos you, and you in turn woo her. Some babies show their feelings more readily than others, as some people do. If she seems withdrawn, don't be tempted to jiggle, bounce, or tickle a response out of her: you may only frighten her. Wait for her openings and respond gently. Some babies are boistrous and outgoing at this age, some are shy. At the other extreme, an excitable baby may need to be calmed down, to be given soothing treatment as well as rough and tumble.

Babies feel for anyone who takes care of them. At this age it is not individuals who count, but how closely you mesh to her needs. If you find it hard to watch her showing just as much love to her grandfather or some baby sitter as she does to you, remember she will not give less to you because she gives to others. Just as parents can love three or four children, so she can love three or four carers.

Giving and taking love from a number of different people can only enrich her.

630 Sustained interactions

As she grows, so does her capacity to sustain interaction. At first, the times when you are finely tuned to each other are fleeting, but by six months she should be able to 'talk' to you for five or ten minutes at a stretch. If this is difficult for her, you may find singing games and playing together with toys helps this gradual progression. You should also try to stand outside yourself and watch whether you are not overwhelming her. Another small social milestone in these early months is when she learns to sustain interaction through a distraction: to look up as a car passes, and then back to you.

631 Thinking

At first, a baby's interactions with the world are automatic. However, she can change as the result of experience: for example, she can adapt how she sucks depending on whether she is breast or bottle fed. Slowly, she begins to realize that she can make things happen, and she enjoys this new power. As she begins to make things happen, she also becomes more systematic in the way she explores the world. But not until she is about four months does she start to distinguish between herself and the rest of the world.

632 Balancing needs

No one is a good parent all the time, or even perhaps most of the time. We are all sometimes withdrawn and depressed, subdued, over-stimulating and bossy. Our motives for having children are always mixed. No one has a child just for the child's own sake. We all indulge in fantasies about how her life might be and this is natural. The only danger is in not recognizing that they are fantasies – no more real than the dream you had at 13 of marrying a pop star or being a Nobel prize winner.

At the opposite extreme, perhaps, is the parent who sees the baby as a doll. Toys are fun to play with, but when you are tired of them, you can leave them on the shelf. They make no demands. It is hard in the months of waiting for the birth not to think in terms of the fun and delight that your baby will bring. In the early weeks it is sometimes hard to think beyond the demands.

All of us manipulate people to meet our needs: listen to conversations until we have heard what we want to hear, then change the subject so that we are at the centre of it.

It is easy to manipulate a small baby in this way: to give her love when she does what we want, and switch off when she behaves like a tiresome baby; to dress her up and show her off like a new doll, and then get upset when she is sick and cries too much. It is natural to have ambition for our children, and to expect them to bring pleasure. The danger comes only if you indulge your desires at her expense. The more often you stand back and ask yourself whether you are over-emphasizing what you want from your child, the better. You might gain a useful perspective on this by looking back at how your parents treated you: are you making the same successful moves? The same mistakes?

633 Questions

If you feel uncomfortable with your baby, discover why:

• Do you over-stimulate her in order to hide some anxiety about your relationship with her? For example, that she is not interested in you?
• Do you worry that she will love someone else more?
• Do you try to avoid seeing her as a person because you fear closeness?
• Do you, perhaps, envy the carefree and easy way she goes out to other people?

These early months are when you set the patterns of love and dependency for most of childhood; when you mould her social interactions with yourselves, and through you with others. It is probably easier to see mistakes now, and to make adjustments, than it will be in three or four years time.

634 Patience

A successful employee is decisive; he or she makes and accepts deadlines, has clear goals, and performs tasks in an efficient way. If it is to be ready by ten, it will be.

For a baby, the world could not be more different.

Finish by ten? A deadline for chewing the rattle, completing the feed, going to sleep? To anyone used to managing others at work, sitting back and watching a child play is painful. Letting her try again and again to put the square peg in the oblong hole can drive you mad. But it is through repetition that she learns. Somehow, you must acquire the same patience all over again; some find this much harder than others. If you find yourself despairing at not only the monotony but at your own impatience, remind yourself that in your busy life a complete change of pace can be good for you; relaxation can exist simply in change.

634 Security's foundations

It is easy to see that the toy moves when she hits it; easy to understand cause and effect in a world of objects. The social and emotional world is more complex. Perhaps that is why babies tune into it so firmly.

It needs practice to understand people. Unlike the brick she bangs on the tray of her high chair, which always produces a certain sensation in her hand, you do not always respond to her warmly and lovingly.

Looked at in terms of cause and effect, it is easy to see why a baby who gets a

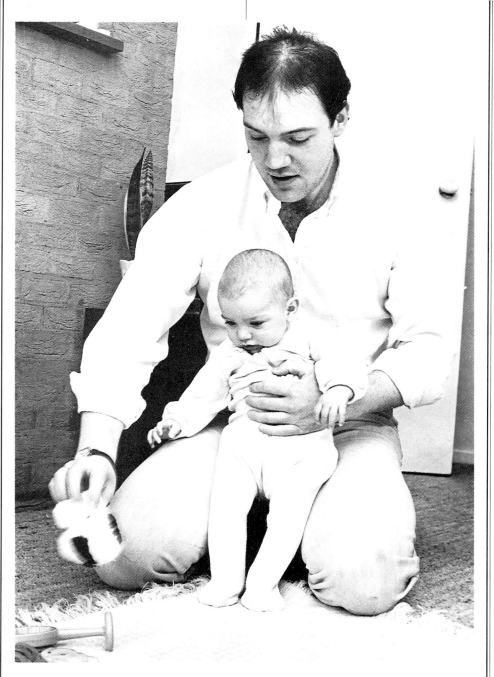

prompt response to her cries is calmer in her second year. Her emotional world has been consistent, and a consistent world is easier to understand. She is able to build her mental model of people gradually. To begin with she can fit them into a simple 'best guess': that they, like other things in her life, are influenced by what she does. They respond if she smiles, they pick her up if she is unhappy. Once this is firmly established, she can build in the complexities. She can begin to tune into

you, to understand that when you are looking sad, there is little point in expecting a reply.

635 Cooing and babbling

At about one month, babies begin to coo. The say something like "uuu", often with a gurgle. They say it when they seem happy and in 'conversations' with you; they say it more often if you talk to them. In the first

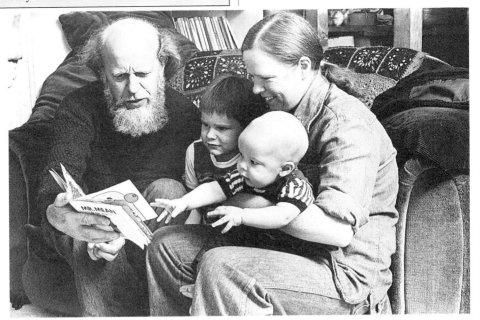

months, this, and a sort of gurgle, are their only sounds other than crying.

By the time they reach four months, most babies – even deaf babies – have started to babble. Babbling continues to build up over the next few months, reaching a peak at between nine and 12 months, when she may begin to say her first real words. For some babies babbling is replaced by this early language, for others the two go hand in hand for a while.

636 The universal tongue

A child babbles a wide variety of speech sounds. Some of those sounds will be made in the language that she hears around her, some will not. The clicks used in many African languages are produced by babies all over the world in these early months. Some of the sounds she hears around her will only be produced at certain times, if at all. She may, for example, start by saying "Gagaga" and "Kaga", but then both 'g' and 'k' sounds will virtually disappear for a while – even though in English they are common.

Since all children, all over the world, go through the same sequence of early sounds, we can assume that in the beginning it is not influenced by the language spoken around them. Indeed, deaf children make exactly the same sequence of sounds. It seems as if early

babbling has most to do with maturation of the vocal chords.

This does not mean that you cannot encourage your baby to babble. The more you talk to her the more she babbles. But say "Dada" or "Mama" all morning, and she will still persist in saying "Gaga" or "Googoo".

637 Sounds in sequence

All babies start with the sounds formed at the back of the mouth; the gutteral consonant sounds 'g', 'k'; then they develop the vowels which are formed in the middle of the mouth like 'a'. Then the focus shifts forwards again to the sounds made by the teeth and lips – 'b', 'd' and 'p'. At first they make the sounds alone: 'g-g'; then in combination: 'gaga'; and finally mixed up in a jargon 'paba boo dingga'.

638 Babble to word

One theory of how children come to speak suggests that parents pick on the sounds they want to hear their children say and slowly shape them into words. So that when she says "D-d", you say to her "Yes, there's dada"; or when she says "Dada", you say it straight back. Perhaps you just smile, or start paying attention when you hear a sound rather like a word. Or perhaps she, knowing all about cause and effect (630), says it again to get your attention.

Another theory suggests that she associates those who care for her with all sorts of good and comforting things and so tries to be like them. In the process, her random babbles slowly transform into real words.

There is some truth in both theories. Children are mimics, they do like to be like us. Just watch a three-year-old, and you will learn a good deal about yourself, some of which you might not want to know.

Listen carefully, and you will hear your baby raise the pitch of her voice as she talks to her mother, and drop it as she talks to her father. Listen to the intonation of her babbling as she approaches her first birthday: it is like speech.

But the mimicking theory cannot be the whole truth because, if it were, we should be able to adjust the sounds she makes by our smiles and cuddles; and we cannot.

Even at nine to ten months, when many babies are almost ready to say their first word, adults cannot get them to incorporate new sounds into their babbling. Your efforts will get her to babble more and more, but she will babble what she babbles regardless of what you say.

It is only as she begins to form her first words that she begins to pick up differences in sounds peculiar to her own language.

639 Hearing sounds

Children can hear before they are born and seem ready to tune into langue even in the first hours of life. Which is just as well when you think how complex the task is. To understand words she has to hear them, to match them to meaning and then reproduce them. Not just at random, but in meaningful sentences.

The differences between words are often slight: bit, kit, fit, hit, lit, mitt: they differ only in the initial sound. Bit and bat only in the middle sound; bill, bit and bin only in the last sounds. But even this is not as simple to pick up as it seems. Although it often sounds as if we are changing only the middle or the end of a word, when we analyse the speech sounds we see that often a great deal more has actually been changed. The 'i' sound in pin is not the same as the 'i' sound in pill. These subtle little sounds that make up words must be recognized by the child in order to understand and produce language.

All languages have different sets of little sounds properly called phonemes. In English, the sound 'p' can be said like the 'p' in spit, with very little breath, or like the 'p' in pit which has rather more. Say the words against the back of your hand if you don't believe they are different. Now try 'stop' and 'top', 'skit' and 'kit'. In Arabic and Hindi, the same basic phoneme is rendered different again by the amount of breath used. And we make distinctions in English that other languages do not: 'z' and 's' are not distinguished in Spanish, nor 'r' and 'l' in Japanese.

640 Adapted for speech

It may be a difficult task, but it seems that children do come well prepared to tackle it. In the first weeks of life they will suck at a dummy if it is rigged up to switch on a little burst of speech, but not if it switches on instrumental music. They move in time with speech. In the first months, a baby's earliest and simplest sounds activate the parts of the brain that we know are involved with speech in adults.

One way of changing the phonemes (639) is to vary the time between making a noise with the vocal chords and moving the lips. With 'b' the vocal chords vibrate just as the lips open; but in 'p' they open a fraction of a second earlier. It is a difference of 40 milliseconds, but even in a baby's first weeks she can make this distinction. The interesting thing is that if you delay the onset of the voice beyond 40 milliseconds it still sounds like 'p' both to us and to her.

Babies can hear language, even its fine details, long before they can produce it, just as most children will understand words well before they can say them.

641 First books

When is the best time to start her with books? – As soon as you can prop her on your knee and hold a book in front of her. Children like pictures and seem to be able to tell the difference beween a picture and the real thing in the first weeks.

Pictures of familiar household objects and of animals are always favourites. At this age, she will be happy to see the same book over and over again. The physical closeness and the interaction between you are as important as the book's content. It is never too young to learn that reading is fun. If she is not interested, don't worry: wait a month and show it to her again.

Six to Nine Months

642 Six months old

You put her on the floor; she rolls on to her tummy and tries to do push-ups. Rolling and squirming, she gradually moves across the room. When you pick her up to put her coat on, she beams and babbles at you. You hand her a rattle and she holds it with a rudimentary power grip, her thumb beginning to move around in opposition to her fingers. She sits in her push chair, delighted to watch the world go by, beaming at everyone she meets. She is vocal and noisy; laughs and gurgles. Loves splashing in the bath. She puts everything into her mouth. She may have a tooth. Almost certainly, she is taking solid food and sleeps less by day, and more by night. She is more fun, and less trouble.

643 Developing bond

Before she forms an attachment to you she must know you, which takes time. So she begins life by behaving in a way that will attach you to her: see 518. This you might call phase one: she is concerned merely to keep someone near her. Phase two is perhaps summed up as smiling more when she sees her carers a little less fully at strangers. She recognizes you when she sees you but does not yet remember you when you walk out of the room. Phase three, at about six or seven months, is distinguished by a sudden demarcation. She learns who you are. Out of sight is no longer out of mind – for you at least. She can remember you, and therefore wants you, even when she cannot see you. Now her attachment behaviour changes from smiling and crying to clinging and moving near.

She begins to use this 'most important person' as a safe base, a point of reassurance while she investigates the possibility that the rest of the world does not disappear when she looks away.

644 Fear of strangers

This is the first reliable evidence that she knows you, even when she is not looking at you.

645 The first 'working mothers'

See 572. In 1799, Johann Oberlin opened the first nursery in Alsace. It was to care for children left alone while their mothers worked in the fields. Today, nursery

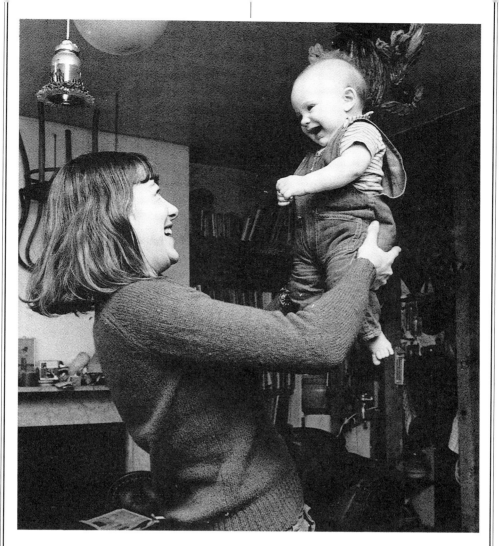

provision is still extensive in France, where 85 per cent of children attend *école maternelle*.

There is nothing new about a mother who wants, or needs to work, sharing child care with a surrogate. But how does it affect the baby?

646 The kibbutz

The founders of these communities sought to dismantle the traditional family unit with its close mother-infant ties. To this end, children were, and are, raised communally from the age of six weeks, when they leave their parents' house for the baby house.

There they stay with a group of some six other infants. Their mothers spend about four hours a day with them – they are encouraged to breast feed; but from six weeks, the mother returns to work part-time and the child is left in the care of a *metapelet* and assistants. After the first year, the mother spends about two hours a day with her child; it is, however, two hours of undivided attention in a family group.

At about 15 months, the children move to the toddler house (with their *metapelet*) and, from there, later move on at intervals through further houses, sharing two, three or even four *metapelets* during childhood but always staying with the same group of children.

How do these children fare? There is no evidence that they grow up to be emotionally disturbed, either as children or as young adults. In fact, they seem to be less, not more, neurotic than family-reared children. They are just as intelligent. In short, they come to no emotional or intellectual harm.

But neither are they immune from emotional problems. Statistics show they are as likely as any other young adult to be emotionally disturbed.

The Bruderhof community in the U.S.A. are a Christian group who rear their children along similar lines to the Israeli kibbutz. These children, however, receive their schooling outside the community, going to local high schools and away to college.

Again, they are not emotionally disturbed, nor unintelligent (most go to college) and more than 75 per cent choose to return to the community after they have finished their education.

647 Options for the working mother

In principle, there are several arrangements you can make. In practice, many women have little choice but to take what is readily available.

The major choices (with some restrictions on availability in some countries) are:

- A babysitter, mother's help, 'au pair' or trained nanny who will look after your child in your home.
- A child minder who will look after your child in her home (often with other children).
- A day care nursery or crèche in which a group of children are cared for communally.

Each type of care has its advantages and disadvantages.

648 A trained nanny

The nanny tends to be regarded as a uniquely British institution, but of course she is not. Perhaps the most interesting historical point about nannies is the extent to which they took over childcare; their charges visited their parents for perhaps an hour each day. Among the middle and upper classes of Europe and America, children, until the Second World War, really were to a great extent neither heard nor seen by their parents.

For today's working mother, it does not have to be like that, even if you do hire a genuine nanny with a qualification in childcare. The arrangement is much less formal; nannies generally (but by no means universally) are no longer

domestics on 24-hour duty but professional individuals who expect to share childcare with the parents. They rarely work seven days a week, nor even 12 hours a day. The perennial nanny problem is no longer 'Is she kind to the children behind our backs?' but 'Can she collaborate successfully?'

Nannies normally (but not always) live in. Sometimes it is possible to share them with another mother. The major duty is obviously childcare, but this may include cooking for the child, keeping her toys in order, and washing and ironing for the child, but not, usually, housework or cooking for the family. All things are, however, negotiable.

A mother's help, or babysitter, is unqualified, but apart from that is employed on much the same basis as a nanny. In practice she may be expected to do rather more housework.

649 Nannies, for and against

Advantages of live-in help:
- Your child stays in her own home.
- You don't have to deliver or collect at a specific time.
- Living as an extended family may seem more natural for your child.

Disadvantages:
- Expense.
- Nannies are not all stimulating, loving or competent.
- They are unsupervised.
- They often don't stay for very long.
- You have to share your home, unless you compromise by having someone come to your home each day, but that is expensive compared with live-in-help.

650 Childminders, for and against

These are often women with small children or women whose children are at school. They look after children in their own homes, and are experienced but rarely trained.

Advantages:
- Other mothers use the facility; there is supervision.
- They are cheaper than live-in nannies.
- Your child will have the company of other children.

Disadvantages:
- Childminders will not normally take a child who is sick.

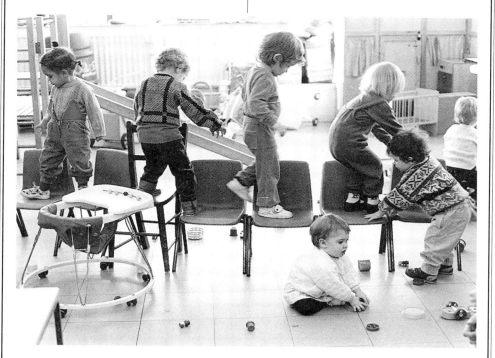

- You have to deliver the baby before you leave for work and collect her each evening.
- She does not get taken out so much as by a nanny.
- Sometimes childminders' homes get crowded when their own children come home from school.

651 Day care nurseries

These are usually regulated by the local social services or health authority, and the staff are usually trained. A few take children from birth, or soon after; others only take children from the age of two.

Advantages:
- Your child may be able to stay at the same centre all through her pre-school years.
- Playmates and stimulation for older children.

Disadvantages:
- Unless subsidized by the state or employer, good day care is expensive.
- Sick children may not attend.
- You may feel your child needs more individual attention, especially when she is learning to talk.
- You have to deliver and collect your child.
- She may not get taken on outings and visits.

652 Which?

A child's needs do not remain constant throughout the pre-school years. At six months, she needs love and cuddles. At 18 months talk, outings and plenty of individual attention. At four years she needs friends, space, activities, games and equipment.

In the first two years, a day care crèche may be less suitable (unless the ratio of babies to carers is low) than a childminder or babysitter. An untrained babysitter who is ready to cuddle and sing may be ideal at this stage; later, a day care centre can provide more stimulation and company for a child. Over a 12-year period I tried every system. My eldest son started with a childminder and moved to full-time day care just before he was three. My two younger children started with a mother's help, progressed to a live-in nanny, who became a daily nanny and finally a shared nanny. The individuals doing the caring always seemed to me to be more important than the actual system of care.

I always tried to provide some continuity between myself and the carer, with someone whose attitude to children was similar to my own. I was lucky to be able to provide this. It is as well to be aware of the fact that not all substitute carers do the job because they like children.

Nor do they necessarily provide children with a stimulating environment. It is wise to run a few spot checks on what goes on after you leave the house, or the baby. Anyone upset by your checking is probably unsuitable anyway.

653 Day care – questions you must ask

Visit day care centres and childminders in your area and talk to people who have previously employed any babysitter you are considering. If possible, visit the children who are currently in their care; they are the best guide. Ask yourself:

● As you go into the home or the nursery, does it feel good – relaxed and happy?
● Are the babies and children generally happy? If the care is good, the children will reflect it. If you are uncertain, make another snap visit. Bored children are bored. Withdrawn children probably neglected. Constant fighting is another bad sign. Anywhere that deals with children will occasionally be chaotic, but two or three visits should give you a fairly good idea.
● Were you and your baby made welcome

when you visited to inspect? Were you greeted warmly as you came in? Do you feel they will be pleased to see your child when you bring her each morning?
● Are the children clean? Are the premises clean? If the place looks unhygienic, it is not suitable for a young baby.
● Are there books, toys, play materials and places to rest? This last may not be necessary for your baby, but it reflects an attitude to childcare which your baby needs.
● Is there enough space for her to find a quiet corner away from other children? To ride a bike?
● Do the staff seem to understand children? To know enough about caring?
● Are the children well supervised? Does the childminder give you her complete attention, or does she break off from talking to respond to a child?
● Is it safe? Can you see any dangers for a crawling baby?
● Do the carers enjoy talking to the children?
● Is it haphazard, or is there some sort of routine?
● Are the children always herded into groups, or are they treated as individuals?
● Will you be able to talk to someone there about your child's progress and special needs?

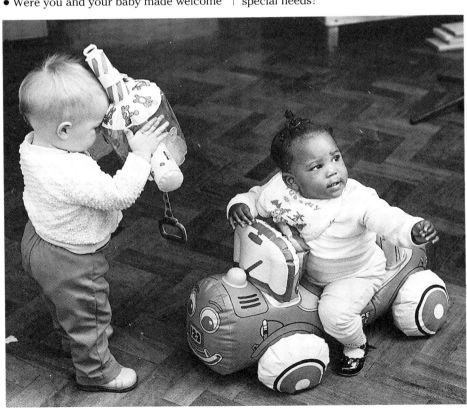

654 Should you, shouldn't you, go back to work?

Having read 645-653, are you still unsure about whether, or when, you should go back to work?

When actually faced with the choice, or the necessity, of going back to work, deep-seated doubts and fears will probably surface.

This is ultimately a personal matter, one that only you can decide in the light of your own needs and those of your family. What follows in 655-663 is an attempt to look at the underlying issues, and to advise and reassure, no more. To help you consider, for example, how the child is likely to thrive in your absence, outside the family, and at what stage it is best, from the child's point of view, for you to return to work.

655 Do babies need mothers?

Yes. Mothers should look after babies. Any woman who decides to go back to work when her child is tiny has somewhere in the back of her mind a nagging feeling that the baby might feel abandoned, might not learn to love, or be as bright as she could be if she stayed at home.

It is natural to think in this way. Many of the things that women with children have fought for in recent years, such as going into hospital with their children, and maternity and paternity leave, are based on the assumption that the bond between child and parent is important. The importance attached to pre-school education, to reading and playing with children in the early years, and to buying them stimulating toys, tells us again and again that parents have a key role in educating their children, especially in the first years of life.

If motherhood is so vital, leaving your baby in order to go out to work must be wrong. Or is it?

656 Essentials

First let us look at the evidence that suggests mothers are irreplaceble.

In *Child Care and the Growth of Love*, one of the most influential childcare books since the Second World War, John Bowlby presents evidence that early separation from their mothers produces lasting emotional disturbance in children, especially if separation occurs before they are five years old.

Bowlby noted what happened to children when their parents left them in hospital. When first left, the children protested: they cried and were very angry. After about a week, the children would become quiet, as if they had entered a period of despair, wimpering intermittently until finally they appeared to become detached. Then they became quite cheerful, appearing not to care.

This sequence seemed to be the same whether the children were in hospital for a prolonged period or they were entering an orphanage.

On the basis of this evidence, Bowlby hypothesized that all children are acutely distressed when separated from their mothers, and that progression from protest, through despair to becoming detached is characteristic of all children.

657 Fixation

Why did the children despair? Bowlby felt it was because all young children need to form an essential attachment to their mother in the early weeks and months of life. Without the attachment, their security evaporates and they despair.

Bowlby backed up his view by noting parallel situations in the animal kingdom. He noted that for many animals there was a sensitive period in development during which the young animal became attached to its mother. Moreover, if the bond did not develop properly at the appointed period, it never would.

What is more, and this is the difficult bit for women who want to work during the first five years of their child's life, Bowlby suggests that children who don't experience a warm and *continuing* attachment may well fail to develop healthy relationships with others in later life:

Motherlove in infancy is as important for mental health as are vitamins and proteins for physical health.

658 Conflicting evidence

For the working mother rushing home to feed her children on fast food, this is indeed a guilt-provoking statement. Bowlby's theory means that it is no use saying "It won't matter just this once"; leaving a child can, according to Bowlby, scar for life.

For 20 years or so after *Child Care and the Growth of Love* appeared, it was indeed argued that separation, even for as little as two weeks, does lasting harm. The early research seemed to point this way.

But, the early research was flawed. Later, rather better, work points to a different conclusion.

For example, Michael Rutter, in his book *Maternal Deprivation Reassessed*, gives the results of a study of large numbers of children who had been separated from their parents during this crucial period. He reviewed their emotional stability at 11 and found that for most of them there was no lasting harm.

Why then did Bowlby reach a different conclusion?

The results were different because they came from looking at different children. There are many reasons why a child might be separated from her parents: grave illness, death of the parents, mother in prison; indeed these were some of the groups in the studies from which Bowlby drew his conclusions. Other reasons for separation could include drug addiction, mental illness or alcoholism.

In some of the cases – recurring mental illness of the mother, for example – one might expect problems over and above separation to persist through childhood.

In other cases, children in the studies had returned to a secure and loving home.

When Rutter separated these two groups, he found that the only children with long-term problems were those who had more than simply a period of maternal deprivation with which to contend.

659 Multiple attachments

It is, in any case, jumping to conclusions to accept that bonds cannot be formed outside working hours. I worked full time, with no more than eight weeks off after each birth, with all my three babies. I am closely attached to my children, as they are to me. They are as loving, happy and secure as those of their friends whose mothers do not work. But they are not, nor have they ever, been exclusively attached to me. They are attached to their father, the nanny who looked after them when they were small, to each other, to their grandmothers, and to various other relatives and friends. Like most other children who live within families, they are attached not only to their family, but also to their home, their beds, their comfort objects. I am not – nor ever have I been – the sole basis for their security.

Should this worry me? Certainly not. Research which has looked at normal children in normal families suggests that most children have more than one attachment: within three months of starting to form attachments, 59 per cent of babies in the survey had formed more than one; by the time they were 18 months this had risen to 87 per cent. Multiple attachments are normal and, what is more, the strongest attachments are not necessarily made to those people with whom children spend the longest hours. They attach most strongly to those who love them most intently, who can stimulate and give undivided attention.

What evidence there is on the value of multiple attachments suggests that they do nothing but good – and could anyone who really knows children expect otherwise? Indeed, research suggests that exclusive attachment may be less than ideal. Some of the children who where exclusively attached to their mothers in one study were still being nasty to younger siblings six years later.

There are 168 hours in a week. A 40-hour week and ten hours of travelling to and from work still leaves 118 hours of childcare. Take out 70 to 80 hours for sleeping, and there is still plenty of time to form close and loving attachments.

660 Timing

Nevertheless, if you are going back to work, it is perhaps worth keeping some of Bowlby's findings in mind. The observation that a nine-month-old baby will protest at your absence is real. Leaving a child with a stranger at a time when she is newly able to recognize a stranger is bound to cause trouble. She will scream and howl, and it is not easy to walk away from this morning after morning. It is hard to imagine her happy in your absence when you can still hear her screams as you leave the door.

At two, three, even at four months, you are very much out of her mind as soon as you disappear. She will beam at you when you return without any knowledge that you have been away all day. By the time she knows you are not around, your absence will be a natural part of her daily routine.

661 Grudge?

But can a child love you less, in revenge for leaving her?

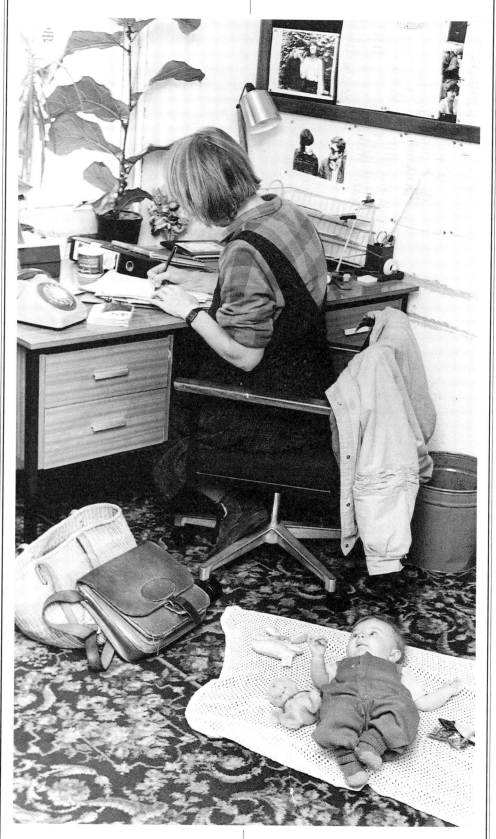

A baby does not have a pocketful of love which she divides between those who care for her; she just loves. Do you love your partner less because you have a child? Babies cry when their mothers leave them at home just as angrily as they do when they are left in day care, and babies in day care are just as attached to their mothers. They do not prefer the carers, they prefer their mothers.

662 Will she suffer?

Of course she could. Put her into over-crowded and unregulated day care with rapidly changing staff, leave her with an unloving and clumsy carer, and she might. But bad mothers harm children too, and it is possible to find an adequate subsitute for yourself.

663 Will you suffer?

It is hard work caring for a child and doing a job. It is only possible if you live within your physical and emotional means. Strain is reduced if you can:

• Allow the housework to slide, or get someone else to do it.
• Eat take-aways or convenience food,
• Buy clothes that do not need ironing.
• Have a washing machine, drier, dish washer, and self-cleaning oven.
Accept that it is impossible to:
• Prepare a gourmet meal every night.
• Keep the house spotless.
• Pay all the bills on time.
• Look your best all the time.
• Keep fit.
• Read everything worth reading.
• See all the latest films.

Indeed, to be the sort of companion, colleague and mother who always provides stimulating conversation, along with perfection; to provide cakes for the school bazaar and serve on the parent-teacher committee; to be the wife who comforts, stimulates, amuses and excites. But then, at the end of the day, who really wants or needs superwoman? Who could live with her? Who could ever grow up in her shadow? My children see me as I am, as I see them. It makes us human; it keeps us close.

The show goes on out there in the world. Here, at home, this is our show. This week we have eaten baked potatoes three nights running, and had take-aways on two other nights; there have been no clean socks (again); we have forgotten music practice; and a bed-time story was missed because of a writing deadline.

But our lives are fun. I know they are happy. However haphazard the care is at times, I am happy working. I am like countless other women, not certain (much as I love my children) that I would be happy otherwise.

An unhappy and depressed mother is the least successful of all mothers, and a woman who wants to work but cannot is often depressed.

664 Time budgets

In a house with babies and/or young children, the following jobs have to be done:

• Child supervision and care: this is shift work which can be divided into four shifts: early morning, day time, evening and night time. The job is rather different on each shift. With tiny children, it is a full-time, full- attention job when they are awake, but it can be shared with other jobs when they sleep.
• Feeding children, including preparation of food and washing-up. With small children this is a particularly time-consuming job.
• Bathing/dressing children.
• Clearing up after children.
• Playing, talking, educating and entertaining children.
• Taking children on outings and visits.
• Ferrying children to school, swimming lessons, music classes.
• Cleaning the house.
• Occasional heavy cleaning of the house.
• Decorating.
• Shopping.
• Menu planning.
• Cooking.
• Secretarial duties, paying bills, making appointments, answering letters, booking holidays.
• Entertaining your friends.
• Clothes care: washing, ironing, mending.
• Gardening.
• House and car maintainance
• Recreation.

665 Who?

Some of these jobs can be delegated to others – if you can afford it. But the catch with children is, of course, that often you have neither the time to do everything yourself, nor the money to get others to do it for you.

Some jobs can be left undone, or be minimally done: gardening, entertaining and decorating.

Some can be covered by machines: washing and dish washing.

Some can be cut to a minimum: house cleaning, (learn to avert your eyes); ironing (only absolute essentials); shopping (in one fell swoop); cooking (convenience foods *are* convenient).

But this still leaves an enormous amount of work – so much that the final item in 664, recreation, is almost always the first casualty. If you are working because the income is essential for your survival, there will be very little you can delegate.

666 Division of labour

See 601. I believe that the issue of how the hard work of childcare is shared is the single biggest obstacle to happy relationships after the arrival of children. Not only the feminist movement, but changing economic circumstances – with women making larger and larger contributions to family finances – have made it so.

It saddens me how rarely I meet a family where everyone seems happy with the division of labour. So many couples seem to be off balance, half co-operating when they ought to be closest.

Women who feel they do more than their share of the hard work blame, of course, male attitudes. They have a partner who, typically, was never brought up to consider helping with children – or anything about the house – as either his duty or, indeed, manly. He maintains that his job exhausts him; that with long working hours he needs total relaxation at weekends in order to preserve his sanity. He feels that changing nappies or soothing a crying baby emasculates him; he is embarassed to be seen doing such things by his male friends (although it has always fascinated me to note that many an unhelpful man often has a close friend who is the opposite).

This is the man who 'plays consort': he does not know how to stack the dishwasher or how to operate the washing machine. When he does make a few token gestures at intervals over a weekend, he thinks he is pulling his weight.

Just how pervasive is 'playing consort' you can gauge from the statistics in 667.

667 A father's role

In 1981 a Canadian survey found that if both parents worked full-time, duties were divided as follows:

● **Cooking:**
40 per cent of men said they often cooked.
36 per cent said they occasionally did.
80 per cent of women often did.
14 per cent occasionally did.

● **Housework:**
40 per cent of men said they often did housework.
41 per cent of men said they sometimes did.
91 per cent of women often did.
9 per cent of women sometimes did.

● **Car and house maintenance:**
42 per cent of men maintained the house or car.
46 per cent of men sometimes did this.
13 per cent of women often did maintenance.
27 per cent of women sometimes did.

● **Childcare:**
51 per cent of men often looked after children.
29 per cent of men sometimes did.
72 per cent of women often looked after children.
19 per cent of women sometimes did.

● **Play with children:**
27 per cent of men often played with their children.
42 per cent of men sometimes played with their children.
35 per cent of women often played with their children.
39 per cent of women sometimes played with them.

In a similar study carried out in Britain in 1983:

● 80 per cent of men with full-time working wives did less than half of the household tasks.
● Women spent on average 1.6 hours longer with children every day than their partners did.
● 72 per cent of women took the child to the child minder.
● 69 per cent took time off work for sick children.
● When the child cried in the night, 9 per cent of fathers and 60 per cent of women got up to see to their children; only a third of couples shared this chore.

See also 819 and 820.

In spite of this, only 36 per cent of women were critical of their men's role, and even these criticisms were muted. Most women had not discussed, or only briefly discussed, the sharing of childcare and household duties before returning to work.

668 A share of the blame

The female counterpart of the man who plays consort (666) is the woman with 'working mother syndrome'. Because she feels guilty about working, she tries doubly hard to provide 'full cover' of first-class childcare and a well-run home. She is the superwoman who tries to do everything and in the process exhausts not only herself but her partner: these are the couples you hear saying "We never relax". When the going gets rough, she complains bitterly; her partner takes no notice because, well, "She sometimes gets like this".

She never discussed with her partner, before the baby came, what the division of labour might be; she vaguely expects him to help, and when he does not, snaps out orders unpredictably: "Couldn't you just change a nappy this once?" Because of her inconsistency, he thinks she is merely a capricious female to be ignored, resisted or humoured.

It is odd, given the current climate of sexual equality, that statistics (667) highlight how few women bother to discuss how the responsibilities might be shared. It seems odd, too, that women should *expect* men to become competently domesticated overnight after thousands of years of conditioning to be the opposite; and, indeed, when many women still bring up their own sons to be just the same as their fathers.

All too many women fail to understand that it does not come naturally for men to contribute to childcare or household chores; that change will not happen overnight; that it must be managed with tact and diplomacy.

669 Is there a solution?

I believe so, but it would be poor advice to give a concrete model for all families – not just because they are all different but because it is such a personal matter and because circumstances are so different.

My personal ideal is this, assuming both partners do full-time jobs: that the housework and childcare is shared equally – literally so: each partner does the equivalent of 3½ evenings a week, one day at weekends, and alternate nights.

But the point is really that couples should work out the division of labour *together,* without reference to anyone else, or to any received wisdom, according to their own feelings and needs. They should give this discussion as much thought and care as any major decision in life – from getting married, to buying a house or deciding to have children.

But it is not enough just to 'work out some arrangement'. The spirit of negotiation is the key. You need to say what you expect of each other and then be prepared, on both sides, to settle for less than your original expectations.

Having done this, there is still one more essential: taking responsibility. It is no use, having agreed to dress the children on a Saturday morning, for a man to call his partner all the way up from the kitchen, where she is preparing breakfast, because he does not know which clothes the children should wear. One must know the job and do it without constant demands for help. Likewise, she must resist the temptation to be the helpless little woman when the car breaks down. Rather than bother him at the office, she should know the necessary steps to have the car removed and repaired.

If you can resolve this fundamental conflict, I believe you will get more from your children and your partner than you ever imagined possible. It is hard to find families where the division of labour has been well worked out, and in many ways it is bad advice to suggest that you look for them: your family must be yours, and comparisons in this respect are invidious.

But I would say this: in none of the families where I have noticed a happy and fair division of labour is the man in any sense lessened as a man; nor, for that matter, is the woman especially powerful. Both he and she 'wear the pants'; he dominates in some areas, she in others. There are arguments, just as in any relationship, but they rarely cause the kind of grinding despair which arises with so many couples where one or other partner is being exploited.

670 Will boys be boys?

Boys are aggressive, competitive and tough.

Girls are gentle, supportive, receptive

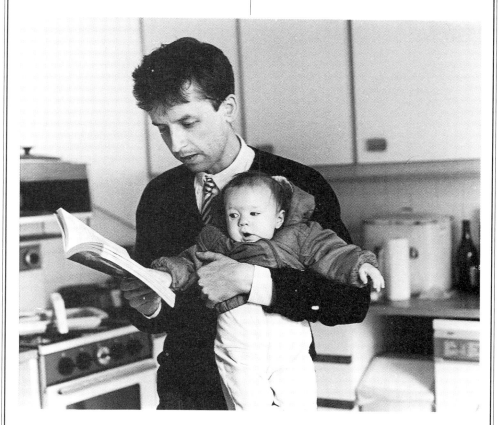

and understanding.

Stereotypes, of course. But how far do we still try to make our children fit them?

671 Welcome?

In most surveys, baby boys are still preferred to baby girls: almost twice as many parents say they would like their first-born to be a son. When a son is born, more than 90 per cent are satisfied with the outcome; only 56 per cent are satisfied with daughters.

Boys often carry a father's name, girls rarely a mother's. Parents give boys conventional, popular names and boys are happier with these; girls are more likely to bear fanciful names.

672 Prejudice. . .

How do parents see children of different sexes? The surveys show that parents see boys as bigger and tougher than girls; girls as gentle and soft; women call boys 'little devils', say they are strong, with minds of their own. They call their daughters pretty, placid, cute and self-possessed. In one study, fathers (who had not been present at the birth), looked at their babies through a window and described them in ways appropriate to the sex. It goes further: daughters are held close, stroked and talked to more often. They are retrieved soooner if they crawl away. Boys are tickled harder, thrown in the air more, and, when they crawl away, are allowed to go further before parents retrieve them.

Apparently, apes behave in exactly the same way, so parents are probably not merely reflecting cultural expectations. Which suggests that the way we treat boys and girls may reflect genuine differences in the child.

We know that girls learn to speak sooner than boys and are more sensitive to touch. Do parents encourage the process by talking to, and cuddling little girls more, and do little girls help this along by showing that these activities give them most pleasure? Who takes the cue from whom?

Modern psychology has no final answers. The only certainty is that babies mould parents' behaviour to their needs. And that what this moulding may do is gradually widen the gap between girls and boys; baby boys and baby girls may start similar, but together we make them different.

Teeth

Some have a first tooth at birth, but five to six months is most usual. It usually takes about two years for the complete set of 20 first (milk) teeth; there are 32 in the second, adult set. The order in which milk teeth arrive is fairly standard.

1 The top two incisors
2 Upper side teeth (also incisors)
3 Lower side incisors
4 First upper back teeth (molars)
5 First lower molars
6 Upper eye teeth (canines)
7 Lower eye teeth
8 Lower second molars
9 Upper second molars

Dental care

Teeth are important: you only have two sets to last a lifetime. Without teeth it is not only difficult to eat properly, but also to form words.

You need to look after them even before you can see them. The first milk teeth are developing throughout the last seven months of pregnancy, the second set as soon as the first are in place.

● The first stage of tooth care is a healthy diet in pregnancy. Avoid tetracycline antibiotics in early pregnancy as they can harm tooth development.
● Make sure she has plenty of calcium (milk, cheese, yoghurt) and vitamin D (liver, egg yolk, dairy products and fish liver oils).
● Sugar is the great enemy of the teeth. Try not to give your child a sweet tooth. Wean her on to savouries. A first child will not know about sweets, cola, ice cream or biscuits and cakes unless you teach her. You can postpone for up to three years the evil day when she learns about them from others.
● Don't dip her dummy into anything sweet.
● Don't let her go to sleep with a bottle of sweet juice in her mouth.
● Sweets that are eaten quickly are less damaging than sweets that are sucked over long periods.
● Start cleaning teeth even before they become visible. Wipe the gums with a little toothpaste on a gauze pad after meals. This removes food deposits and gets her used to the idea of cleaning teeth. She may protest at first.
● Although wiping is sufficient, you may like to give her a soft toothbrush at about ten months. Let her copy you as you clean your teeth. Make it fun.
● It does not matter how children brush teeth, as long as they brush them. Up-and-down or side-to-side brushing can both remove plaque. Toddlers and young children will find side-to-side brushing easiest; many will do no more than chew at a toothbrush; but chewing flouride toothpaste is good for

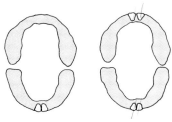

Lower front teeth are always first, usually followed by upper front.

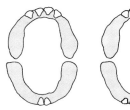

Next appear the upper side teeth, followed by the lower side teeth.

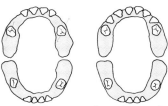

The upper molars come through next, then the lower molars, followed by the upper eye teeth on each side.

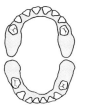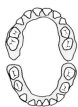

Lastly, the lower eye teeth and the second molars appear, first in lower, then in upper jaw.

the teeth anyway. More sophisticated techniques for brushing teeth really need not be learned until later, if at all, according to some dentists.
● Brushing teeth after every meal or snack can be counter-productive if it makes tooth brushing seem like a punishment.
● Unless your water supply contains fluoride, you should give children between the ages of

two and 12 daily fluoride tablets. This has been proved to significantly reduce tooth decay. Fluoride-containing toothpaste helps too.

Moulding the face

The first teeth help the face to develop. She does not need them for chewing – she uses her gums. The early teeth are, in fact, for biting, not for chewing. Without solid food to 'gum' and without the breast or bottle to suck, her jaw would do little work. Without work, it may not develop properly.

• Breast feeding is hard work, so is bottle feeding if the teat has a small hole.
• Let her chew as soon as she can. She will naturally use her mouth to explore. Make sure that some of the toys she explores this way are good to suck and 'gum'.
• Introduce her to solid food, such as peas, carrots and little sandwiches as soon as she starts taking toys to her mouth at five or six months.

The second teeth

It may seem early to start worrying about the second teeth before the first are in place, but caring for the first set ensures that the second are sound and come through in the right place. If a tooth is removed, it leaves a gap into which neighbouring teeth can slide. When the second teeth come, they use the first as position guides; missing first teeth can lead to second teeth out of place.

Teething

You can see your baby's teeth as little white patches beneath the skin. As they begin to push through, they will form small pale bumps on the gum.

Practically everything that goes wrong for babies in the first two years is blamed on teething.

Teething does *not* cause fever, temper tantrums, diarrhoea, sickness or convulsions. These all have other causes which should not be swept aside because you think 'She is just cutting a tooth'. Babies do get ill, and illness can get out of hand quickly. However, teething can make babies uncomfortable and out of sorts. It may soothe her if you:

• Rub her gums gently with your finger.
• Give her something to 'gum' (see under 'Moulding the face'). teething rings, raw carrots, hard rusks or a special cooling ring.
• Rub her gums gently with a little piece of ice. When your fingers feel cold, so will her gums. This can, however, be overdone: babies have been known to get frostbite on their gums. The same goes for teething rings kept in the freezer. Keep them there by all means, but let them warm up slightly before giving them to her. It may be safer to keep them in the fridge.

• Don't use teething powders or medicines. Used over four or five days for each tooth, they expose the child to much more medication than is ideal.
• Teething gels containing local anaesthetics may be useful if she is having difficulty settling to sleep; but their effect does not last long.
• If she feels out of sorts, it is comforting to be kept warm and to be cuddled. Going out shopping in a pram or buggy in a cold north wind will make her miserable. She will be happier snuggled up to you in her papoose.
• Don't give aspirin to a baby. Nor should you give paracetamol syrup too readily, unless she is very unhappy.

Breast feeding once she has a tooth
Easy. She cannot bite until she has both top and bottom teeth. If she does bite, tell her to stop in no uncertain terms. It usually works.

Sweets

You can delay sweet eating – see 'Dental care' – but it is difficult to ban it. Banning sweets is like banning guns: it can turn the forbidden fruit into an obsession. Every supermarket trip can be become a nightmare.

Sweets which can be eaten quickly are better than those which take time to chew, so some health food bars are probably worse for teeth than chocolate drops. Sugar is the ingredient that causes tooth decay whether it comes in raisins, yoghurt, fruit juice, honey or sugar lumps.

Control is usually better than an outright ban. An early morning sweet is special, and can be rapidly followed by a session with the tooth brush. Put the sweet in a special place, together with something interesting for her to discover when she wakes. It may set a routine which gives you a few more minutes in bed.

673 Sex-appropriate toys

In view of 672, it is naïve to expect that the gap between the sexes will be reduced by, for example, keeping dolls away from girls. Indeed, toys have probably never been as sex-stereotyped as they are today. Sixty years ago, boys and girls shared toys and games such as skipping ropes, hoops, tops, five stones and marbles far more than they do today. Toy museums suggest that the young middle class child, boy or girl, of the 1920s might typically have possessed a Noah's Ark with wooden animals, a rocking horse, a hobby horse, some building bricks, and mechanical toys that could be wound up to perform tricks. None was aimed exclusively at one sex or the other; the only truly sex-stereotyped toys were dolls, dolls' prams and dolls' houses. True, there are dolls for boys in today's toy shops, but they are exclusively 'macho'.

Is this because most people are happy to let boys be boys? Or because a vocal minority has concentrated on trying to rid society of female stereotypes, rather than concentrating on 'sexist' boys' toys?

I suspect the answers to these questions matter less than the fact that the gap between the sexes is gradually closing. Not much that you can do while raising your children will accelerate the process – if that is your ideal.

We have, after all, reached a stage where men cook, clean and iron sheets; where even the most macho man is no longer embarrassed to be seen holding his daughter's hand.

674 Span of attention

A tiny baby is practically incapable of concentrating. Move something away, and she forgets about it.

During the second half of her first year, you will become more and more aware that her span of attention is increasing. This comes out in little things like her ability to look up at you, smile, and then go back to a game.

Adults have an attention span of about seven items: we can 'hold' seven numbers, seven names or seven sentences in our minds. A child of five can manage about four. Just now, she is beginning to get a span of one or two.

Until you can 'hold' in your mind something you no longer hear or see, you cannot understand speech; you cannot realize that anything in the world has any permanence, including yourself.

675 'Me'

It follows from 674 that a tiny baby has no sense of 'me'. To know 'me', you must know what is 'not me'. But understanding 'me' is more than simply understanding that you are not part of your cot, or of your mother. You have to understand that you are a continuing event. Once a baby does this, she begins to be able to recognize herself in a mirror. She no longer reaches out at the mirror, but at herself. This may happen surprisingly late – perhaps well after her first birthday.

You can monitor her progress by sitting her in front of a mirror from time to time. Does she smile at herself yet? Does she pat herself in the mirror? Can she recognize you in the mirror? Does she turn around and look at you?

676 Copy cat

Babies learn by practising over and over again, and by copying. It is quite an achievement. She has to watch what you do, hold a picture of it in her mind, then plan a set of movements to match that picture. She can do it in the first few weeks of life, then she forgets. Only at six months does she begin to be able to copy again.

When she does, she starts taking cues. The singing games you play with her now should include those in which she can participate, following a lead from you:

> Pat-a-cake, Pat-a-cake, baker's man,
> Bake me a cake, as fast as you can.

(Clapping her hands together as you say it.)

She will now begin to to wave "Bye bye" and to respond to gambits such as "Arms up like a big soldier" as you undress her, or "Splash" as she plays in the bath.

Later you can get additional value out of action rhymes by playing them in front of a mirror.

677 Expanding memory

As her span of attention (674) develops, so do other aspects of her memory. She will remember people and places; get upset if she cannot sleep in her own cot, or if you wear a hat or sunglasses. By nine months, you may feel that she remembers a game

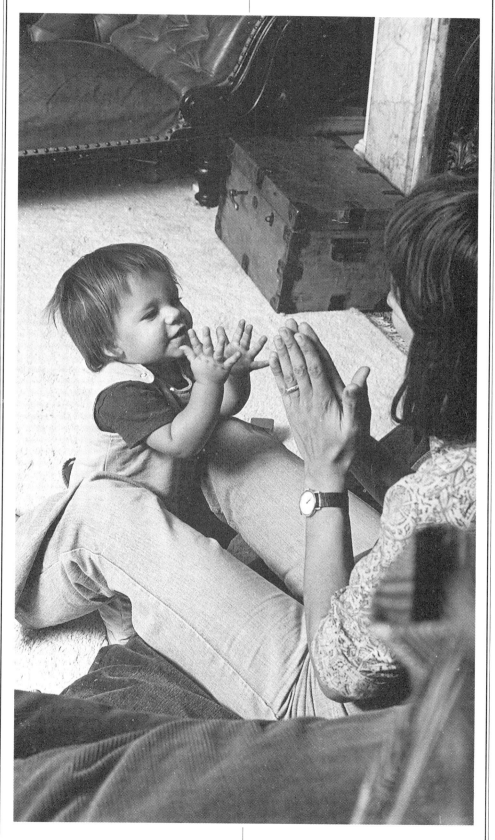

you played yesterday; and it is probably not your imagination.

678 More about sleep

Babies need less sleep as the weeks pass and often take more of it by night. However, they rarely change their underlying habits. A baby who has slept little in her first half year is unlikely to become a sound sleeper as her first birthday approaches or, indeed, her seventh. Only puberty seems to alter the basic pattern. Most babies sleep for less than 13 hours in 24 by their first birthday, some for as little as eight or nine.

The pattern of a baby's sleep at one year can likewise be predicted by her pattern in the first months of life. Long sleeps in the first weeks mean she will now sleep longer at night. In other words, wakeful babies don't suddenly reform, they just sleep for longer stretches.

By the second half of her first year, she will sleep when she needs sleep.

At first, little will break her pattern of waking and sleeping, but towards her first birthday you will find that a strange place, tension and excitement can unsettle.

679 Bed time

If there is a universal problem with children of this age, it is their refusal to go to bed. She may be tired, indeed she may be over-tired and close to tears, but she still will not settle or relax.

Often, teething or going on holiday produces the initial upset, but however it starts, the disruption continues long after the apparent cause is removed. The root of the trouble is her new attachment to you. She now misses you when she is alone in her cot; she no longer feels relaxed and secure when you are absent. Sit with her and she is happy and relaxed; as soon as you creep to the door, she starts to scream. You can busy yourself around the room, but she will keep herself awake screaming each time you make for the door, beaming every time you return.

She will keep it up, having by this stage of the evening far more patience than you.

680 Remedies

About 15 per cent of children are still wakeful at the age of two, and there are no

solutions to the problem. These ploys are, however, worth trying:

• A familiar bed-time routine: bath time, getting into night clothes and then coming down for a quiet time with the family, including a story, perhaps, or a go in the rocking chair.
• Don't try to put her to bed at six if she is obviously not tired. She may go readily if you leave her until seven or eight o'clock.
• Try moving the cot to a room closer to where you spend the evening. When my eldest son was small we had an upstairs sitting room; after his cot was moved from our bedroom into the room next to the sitting room, he miraculously started to make much less fuss about bed time.
• Rituals: "Goodnight mummy, daddy, pussy, room, stairs, pictures, toys. . . Hello teddy. Oh, Teddy's gone to sleep." Then sing a song. The nightly repetition is familiar, reassuring.
• A comfort object, blanket, toy or bottle, can offer the security she needs when alone.
• Sucking a dummy, a thumb or a bottle can also give comfort. It will not harm the teeth unless you fill the bottle with milk or sweet juice. It may not look attractive, but principles have to be pretty important if they are to undermine a child's happiness and a good night's sleep for her parents.
• Rocking her to sleep on your lap may become a chore, but it may also be easier than going up and down to her room all evening.
• Gently calming her down in stages before bed may help; certainly you should avoid exciting her before bed time by tickling or other rowdy games.

681 And if these fail?

You can leave her to cry. But cry she will, and her aversion to bed time may grow.

Actually, leaving some babies to cry does work, but others habitually scream for an hour or two every night, even after months of being left. There is no disguising the fact that this is a dilemma. You can pick her up and bring her downstairs, whereupon she may well learn that you will come and pick her up every night, then cry every night until you do.

Or you can go and comfort her in her room as often as it takes, refusing to let her downstairs. But that can take most of the evening.

The way you solve the problem, or learn to live with it, depends on how much you value your evenings free of small children.

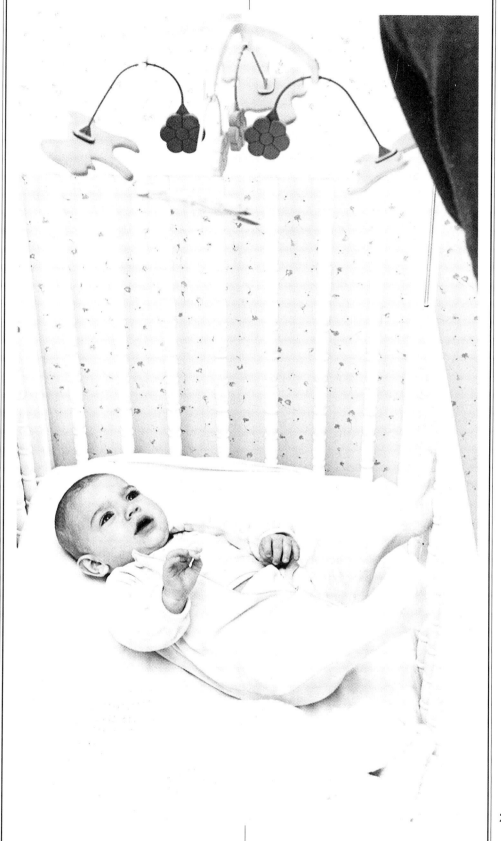

Encouraging her to sit

By the time she is six months old, she will be well in control of the upper part of her body. Sit her firmly on her bottom with her legs spread out and lean her slightly forward and she will sit, probably just for a moment. Until she has more control over the bottom half of her body, she cannot balance.

She will topple easily, even when she first sits independently. Surround her with cushions. It will take her about a month to find her balance; at first she will help herself by leaning forwards on to her arms. Once she has the knack, she is theoretically in a position to sit and play with her toys. In practice, she cannot yet adjust her balance rapidly enough to stay upright while reaching or turning.

The Ganda tribe of Uganda dig little holes into which they wedge their babies' bottoms at this age. An alternative is to wedge her bare bottom into a potty. I remember coming home one day to find a childminder had planted my eldest son in this way. At not quite six months, he was sitting upright in front of the T.V., eating a stick of salami. I was horrified; he, of course, was delighted. The childminder was right: he loved to sit and watch the world from this position. He never toppled over. Once your baby starts to sit, even for a short period, you may find that she is much less content to lie, and tries to lift her head and shoulders from the floor. If you offer your hands, she will probably pull herself up into a sitting position.

Sitting

• Start encouraging her to use her back at about two months, sitting her up whenever you can. At first, she will need plenty of support, but gradually the support can lighten as she brings her back under control.
• By four months she will probably only need you to hold her hands when she sits. She may be somewhat rounded, but her back will straighten over the next month.
• As soon as she can sit for a moment, you can use a harness to sit her upright in her pram. Put plenty of toys in front of her and a pillow behind, so that she does not hurt herself if she flops backwards.
• Once she starts to balance better, remove some of the supporting cushions.
• Once she begins to sit, she will also begin to pull herself up into a sitting position. She will now always need strapping into her chair or pram. It is not safe to leave her unstrapped, even for a moment. Light weight baby chairs become particularly unstable once she reaches this stage, as can a light carry cot.

Games to encourage

Many traditional action rhymes that parents play with children at this age are valuable as learning aids. They teach them to balance, and indeed much more. They teach them to predict and remember at a time when memory is developing; and to use pre-language.

These two can claim to be universal favourites:

'Leg over'

Cross your legs at knee level. Sit the baby in the crook of the upper foot, support her back with the foot and hold on to her arms. Lift the leg up and down as you say:
  "Leg over, leg over,
  The dog went to Dover,
  When he came to a style. . .

Now pause, catch her eye, and uncross your legs, sweeping her upwards, saying
  Up he went over."
To start again (she will probably ask you to do so in an early example of pre-language), cross your legs again, saying Leg over as you do so.

'This is the way. . .'

The baby sits facing you on your knee. You say:
  "This is the way the lady rides,
  Trit-trot, trit-trot, trit-trot."
– Mimicking a walking motion with your knees as you do so.

Then you say:
  "This is the way the gentleman rides,
  Gallup, Gallup, Gallup,"
– Mimicking a galloping motion as you do so.

Finally you say:
  "This is the way the old man rides,
  Hobble. . .dee, Hobble. . .dee. . .
  and down in a ditch."
– Tipping her gently off your knee on to the floor, holding her all the while.

Pre-language

Both the action rhymes in the panel encourage a baby not only to balance, but to start communicating. You may find that she tries to bounce as she sits on your knee, or lifts herself as you pause before going over.

Holding her arms up when she wants to be picked up is another common way of letting you know what she wants.

To my daughter I used to sing "The wheels of the bus went round and round" rotating my hands as I did so. Her younger brother, only nine months, used this action every time he saw a bus. By nine months or so, she may use a number of these pre-language signals, and by her first birthday she will develop many more.

Jean Piaget

This Swiss scientist is famous for his pioneering work on child development. He asked children about the world, their beliefs and their understanding of it. Asked them, in fact, the questions they often ask us: "Why does the sun shine?" "Does it hurt a flower when you pick it?"

He developed a theory that logical thinking develops in steps: that up to two years, babies have one scheme (a sort of best guess about how the world is constructed) and that from two to seven years they have a second, more elaborate scheme, and that only from about seven years do they begin to think with adult logic.

Children, he believed, are not like empty suitcases waiting to be packed with knowledge. They are more like empty filing cabinets. At first, they organize all the information in one way, but as they begin to understand it better, they try a more sophisticated filing system. But right from the start, their knowledge is all put into some sort of context: they actively construct their understanding of the world by interacting with it.

They begin to learn how objects look by watching, they modify these ideas by exploring, they change them by finding what objects do.

Suppose you look at a broom without touching it. You could see the red handle and the black bristles, but you would not know how it felt, or that the bristles were flexible until you had explored it. So your initial idea of a broom would change when you felt it.

Now, given a new broom, you could begin to understand it much sooner. You might expect the bristles to be soft, even before you touch them.

In the first months of life, this is how your baby behaves. The baby sees the broom in terms of a handle (good to suck) and bristles (good to feel). When she starts using the broom to sweep floors, her view of it will change radically. Handle length, bristle colour, even shape are no longer important. That it can sweep makes it what it is.

Crawling

- At birth, she will crawl as a reflex action: this soon disappears as she uncurls over the first weeks.
- By about four months, she will lie on her tummy and raise her head and her feet at the same time.
- By about six months she can get into a crawling position. She will probably rock in this position for up to a month.
- By seven months she may be reaching out with one arm.
- By eight months she begins to crawl, slowly at first, but soon at speed.

Once she crawls, you may wonder why you ever encouraged it. She can now empty book shelves and cupboards, clear coffee tables, eat, rip, and chew the newspaper. But encourage her you probably still do, for she must pass through this phase, like any other. You can:

- Sit in front of her and call her to you.
- Put something just out of reach, and challenge her to crawl to it.
- Crawl around with her.

It is best to put her on the carpet. Rugs and slippery floors are difficult for her. If she is wearing a dress, tuck it into her pants. Understand if she gets frustrated. Give her the toy which she cannot quite reach, don't make her wait for ever.

Safety for the semi-mobile child

A crawling baby should not be left alone. Many potential dangers, from glass ornaments to poisonous plants, are obvious but you cannot predict every eventuality.

Steps will be crawled down; corners bumped into; furniture pulled over. Rearrange the room, if necessary, so that she does not bump into sharp corners. Ensure that anything she might pull herself up on will not topple over.

My elder son once pulled a small cabinet full of glasses over. We were lucky: he was so shocked by the crash that he sat still screaming among a sea of broken glass.

- Keep a gate on the stairs, and across doorways of any room which has not been baby-proofed.
- Guard all fires, and radiators if they get very hot.
- Take her to the door or phone when you have to answer it. Or invest in a play pen to pop her into at such moments.
- Pick up everything small enough to swallow, and put it out of reach.
- Cover electric points with safety plugs.
- Allow nothing breakable within three feet of the floor.
- Don't leave wires trailing, especially wires to electric kettles.
- Keep poisons in high cupboards.
- Move all the dangerous chemicals from the cupboard under the sink, or fit a lock or child proof catch.
- Check that none of the plants she can reach are dangerous.
- Check that she cannot crawl through the banisters on the landing.
- Keep cups of tea and coffee on a high shelf or table.
- Put away table cloths for a year or so. She can easily pull everything on top of her if she tries to use the cloth to pull herself up.
- Keep drawers closed. If a child pulls up and leans forwards, the drawer can close on her fingers.
- Watch for children's fingers on the hinged side of the door.
- Swinging doors are lethal to babies.
- Wedge doors open.
- Wedge books into bookcases with folded newspaper.

Nine to 12 Months

682 Baby into child

Although the changes are gradual, between nine months and a year she begins to shed her babyhood. It is hard to pinpoint, but perhaps the most important indications are her obviously developing mobility; the increasingly independent way she handles objects, plays and investigates the world; and the gradual abandoning of special baby foods for a normal diet. But, above all, there is the emergence of communication and her understanding of the world about her. There is, too, an emergence of planning and intention. At first you could say she knows what she likes, now you can begin to say she knows what she wants. Somewhere between nine months and two-and-a-half, she changes from a baby into a child.

The threads of development, physical, perceptual and intellectual, make a complex weave. Development progresses slowly and in some ways steadily, yet it gives the impression of travelling in stages.

683 Tea time, ten months

Her mother is trying to prepare the evening meal, she is sitting in her high chair. She has a cup of juice, a dish of small sandwiches and some chopped banana. There is a spoon but she is more inclined to use her fingers. She takes a piece of banana and, holding it out, drops it. She looks over the side of the chair at the banana on the floor, watches for a while, but when nothing happens, loses interest.

Next she takes her cup and shakes some of the juice on to the tray. She swirls the juice around with her fingers, watching the patterns she makes. Her mother says "No" and the baby, looking up to her, smiles. Watching her mother carefully, she drops the cup over the edge of her chair. Her mother rewards her attention with a smile and a "Naughty baby" before picking up the cup. It is, of course, quickly dropped again.

This is the child-baby in the last three months of her first year.

684 Hormones and growth

The rate of growth and physical maturation between birth and puberty is largely controlled by growth hormones released by the pituitary gland in the brain, just above the roof of the mouth.

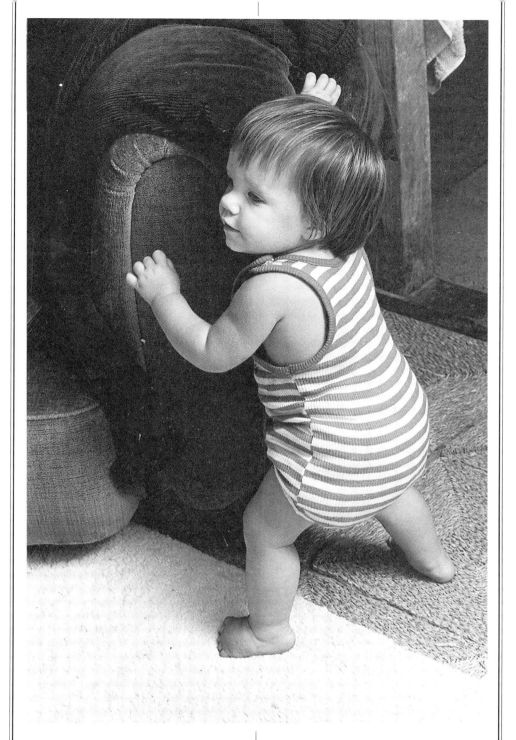

More of the hormone is released by night than by day.

A second hormone, thyroxine, released by the thyroid gland, is also involved. It affects brain development and overall rate of growth. Large quantities are released during the first two years, and then at a lower, steadier level until maturity.

In middle childhood (at about eight years) the sex hormones (testosterone in boys and oestrogen in girls) are released in low levels, but enough to cause slight physical changes. Boys become a little broader in the shoulder, girls in the hips.

275

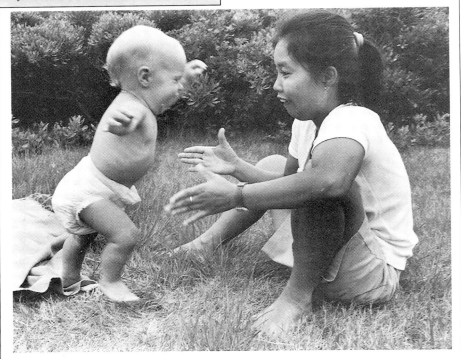

Walking sequence

• A newborn baby, held with the sole of one foot on the floor, will step out with the other in high steps.

• At about eight weeks she will raise her head as you hold her in a standing position.

• By 36 weeks she can pull herself up and remain standing as long as she supports herself.

• By 48 weeks she can walk forwards if both hands are held.

• By one year she can walk if you hold one hand.

• By 13 months she will walk alone.

• By 18 months she can walk upstairs and down again.

• By two she can run, walk backwards and pick things up from a stooping position.

• By 2½ she can balance on her toes.

• By three she can balance on one leg.

• By four she walks downstairs using alternate legs. Left, right, step by step.

• By five she can skip on both feet.

Standing

Just as her muscle control moved down her back to her hips enabling her to sit, so it moves down her legs to her feet so that she can stand. Until she has control of all these muscles, she will be unable to make the minute adjustments necessary for balancing. To practise, she will pull herself up and stand propped against the furniture.

Gradually she will exert control over her legs; before walking unaided, she will practise stepping out while still holding a prop.

• By about 12 weeks she will stand with her head erect if you support her.

• By about 24 weeks she will make jumping movements as you support her. A baby bouncer will encourage this.

• By about 28 weeks she will dance on your knee when you hold her up.

• By about 32 weeks she may walk if you give support under her arms.

• By about 34 weeks she can take her full weight on her feet.

• By about 36 weeks she may pull herself up into a standing position.

• By about 48 weeks she may be cruising around the furniture.

• By about 52 weeks she will use her arms only for balance, supporting herself as she stands.

• By about 54 weeks she may stand alone for a moment.

• By about 56 weeks she may be able to stand unaided.

Cruising

Once she has gained enough confidence to stand while holding on with one hand, she will start to cruise around the furniture. At first she uses it for support, later only for balance. Often she can stand, or even take a step or two without holding on. Almost without realizing it, she is walking.

Encouragement

• Bare feet are best for balancing.
• Don't rush her. She will learn. Sustain her confidence by helping her to avoid accidents. Don't polish the floors, and remove loose rugs.
• Safety: She may now be able to reach window sills: remove breakable objects. If you have low plate glass windows, keep them dirty or put stickers on them; the same applies to glass doors: it is surprising how many babies walk into them. Check if they are made of safety glass and consider replacing them if they are not.
– Check cables. Could she pull the TV over?
– Make sure the furniture stands firmly. Rocking chairs can be dangerous at the cruising stage (toes become trapped under rockers), loose bookshelves and unstable cupboards are potentially lethal, as is anything with a sharp edge. She will fall. Look for anything she could cut her head on as she topples.
– A table with a central leg can be dangerous too: she may not realize at first that she cannot walk underneath it.

• Arrange furniture so that she can progress down one side of a room and across to the other. Once her balance is good, move the furniture props apart so that she needs to stretch out between them. In due course, increase the distance until she has to take an unsupported step.
• Opening your arms and calling her to you will accelerate the process, but only by a few weeks. She will walk when she is ready: identical twins usually walk within days of each other.

Early walking

Typically, she will waddle along with her feet wide apart and her arms up and slightly forwards for balance. She will often set off in a straight line, unable to swerve or to stop. If she deviates, she falls. But in practice, these 'first walks' vary. Some babies launch themselves even before they can stand and walk at speed from place to place. They need speed to keep their balance; as soon as they stop, they sit down. Others step out slowly and deliberately only after they have stood for some weeks. These are the toddlers you feel sure could walk if only they had the confidence to try. Clearly, the motivation to walk varies. If a baby is an efficient crawler, she may well stay cruising and crawling for a long time. A child who has never crawled has only one way to cross a gap in the furniture, on her feet.

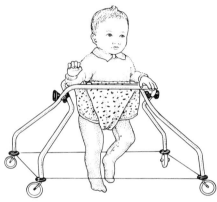

Baby walkers

Some have trays, some built-in toys to amuse a child. This is a good idea because it is not easy to explore from a walker, since the wide base prevents her getting close enough to touch things. True, she can see the world from a walker, but at this stage she is not a looking baby, she is a feeling, handling baby. Walkers are useful, but not all the time.

A child who is an efficient crawler probably does not need a baby walker, but if she is otherwise immobile, it will give her a sense of independence and great pleasure, especially if she is slow to sit.

Once cruising, a 'toddle truck' is ideal. There are two varieties: those that are open like a small trolley, and those that she can later sit on to ride. Either will give hours of pleasure over the next year.

At this stage she can toddle behind it, dropping to explore and then hitching herself up again as she sets off to a new spot. Later she can ride it or use the trolley to move her toys from one side of the room to the other. See also 684.

685 No hurry

Standing, cruising and walking cannot be accomplished until a baby is physically ready or until she has sufficient motivation and confidence. The dates given in the illustration feature on page are average. If your baby or toddler takes longer than the average, you should not fear some long-term physical inferiority. If she has been slow reaching other milestones, she will also be slow to walk. Her body matures at a steady rate. It is unlikely to speed up suddenly just because her first birthday is approaching. Many children are more than a year old before they pull themselves into a standing position. If she has a couple of bad falls, she may take time re-build her confidence. She also needs to be motivated.

New-found mobility means your baby no longer has to sit and wait for you to bring the world to her. She can discover a vast amount about it that she could not learn before: things can be found in cupboards and inside boxes; there are two or more routes to the same place. As she moves around objects, she gets more and more experience of their permanence (621), and she learns about depth and distance.

As she goes from one room to another, she learns about the identity of objects, too. With mobility comes a noticeable surge of mental development.

686 Gripping

The switch from holding to power grip is gradual; it starts at about five months and is usually complete by the end of the first year.

A baby begins by slowly moving her thumb into opposition, so that at first the thumb does little more than hold things in place. From this basis she uses her fingers in an independent fashion. It takes a great deal of practice to manage a variety of objects; moving things between floor and mouth is often the motivation which provides the practice.

About now she will develop a pincer grip too: thumb and forefinger are opposed. Its purpose is holding small light objects as opposed to longer, heavier ones, for which the pincer grip is reserved. These two essential grips are the basis of all manual skills, and the period in which she learns them is one almost solely of absorption with objects.

687 Touching

Some time before she reaches nine months, your baby will also have started to touch and to stroke with her whole hand. She will run her hand along the carpet, stroke the satin binding of her blanket, and feel the fur of her soft toys.

It is now that she will love a toy telephone. She can poke her finger into the dial (push-button models are useless for babies) and listen to the noise it makes as it turns. She will be poking her fingers into every small hole, and yet another new round of baby-proofing is required.

688 Both hands

• Two hands can make identical motions – for example, coming together to hold a big ball.
• Two hands can do different things: one hand can pass something to the other.
• Two hands can work together: one hand can hold while the other turns.

689 From hand to hand

Even the most rudimentary kind of letting an object go enables a baby to pass things from hand to hand. At first she uses her hand for storage. She takes one object, and when offered another, will transfer the first to the other hand before reaching out to take the second. It is now only a short step to realizing that objects can be used to make things happen. She cannot quite reach the brick with her hand but, holding a stick, she can. This, like the other steps, is important because once she realizes that objects (and people) can work for her, she has to start figuring out how to make this happen. She has, in fact, to learn how to communicate her intentions.

690 Dropping

As her hands become skilled at picking things up, she also develops the skill of putting things down.

In the beginning, she let go purely by chance. Now she begins to let go on purpose. At first she simply opens her hand and lets the toy roll out: not a sophisticated response, but nonetheless intentional. Ask her to give you the toy and she will, or at least she will try. It is easiest if she is sitting in her high chair. She can put her hand on to the tray and use this stimulus to help open her fingers.

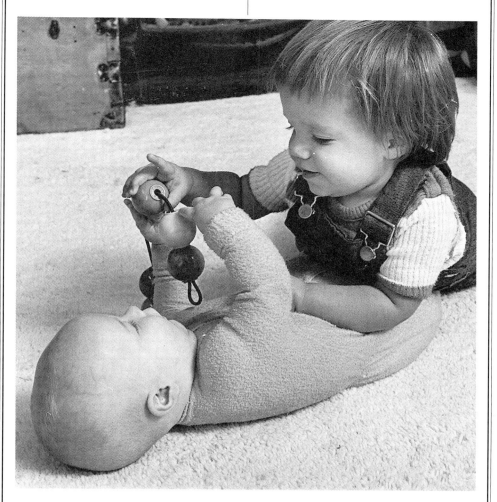

Dropping is a classic – and tiresome – baby game. She wants it to go on and on, long after you have given up. The only way to practise is, after all, to practise. You can make life easier for yourself by:

• Putting a cardboard box on either side of her chair: at least this will collect most of the objects for you to return to the tray.
• Tying the objects to the tray or to her pram with wool. She may learn to pull them back up herself.
• Letting her play the game at a table: she can then drop and pick up by herself.

As she looks at you, asking you without words to pick up the fallen object, you will realize that the game is about more than practising letting go, it is about communication.

691 Left or right?

When she holds with one hand and works with the other, which hand does the holding? Which the work?

For most of us, it is the left hand that holds and the right that works, since most of us are right-handed.

Early on, many babies seem to show a preference for the left hand (sucking this one perhaps more often than the right), but when it comes to working with one hand while steadying with the other (around the first birthday), most will choose the right hand for working.

It is usually not absolute at this stage and many babies swop hands for a while. It is important that you don't try to pressurize your baby into using one hand rather than the other. She has to make up her own mind.

Left-handedness runs in families. If both parents are left-handed, they have about a one in four chance of having a left-handed baby. Even if one identical twin is left-handed, the other is as likely to be right-handed as left. If parents are both right-handed, there is a one in ten chance that their baby will be left-handed.

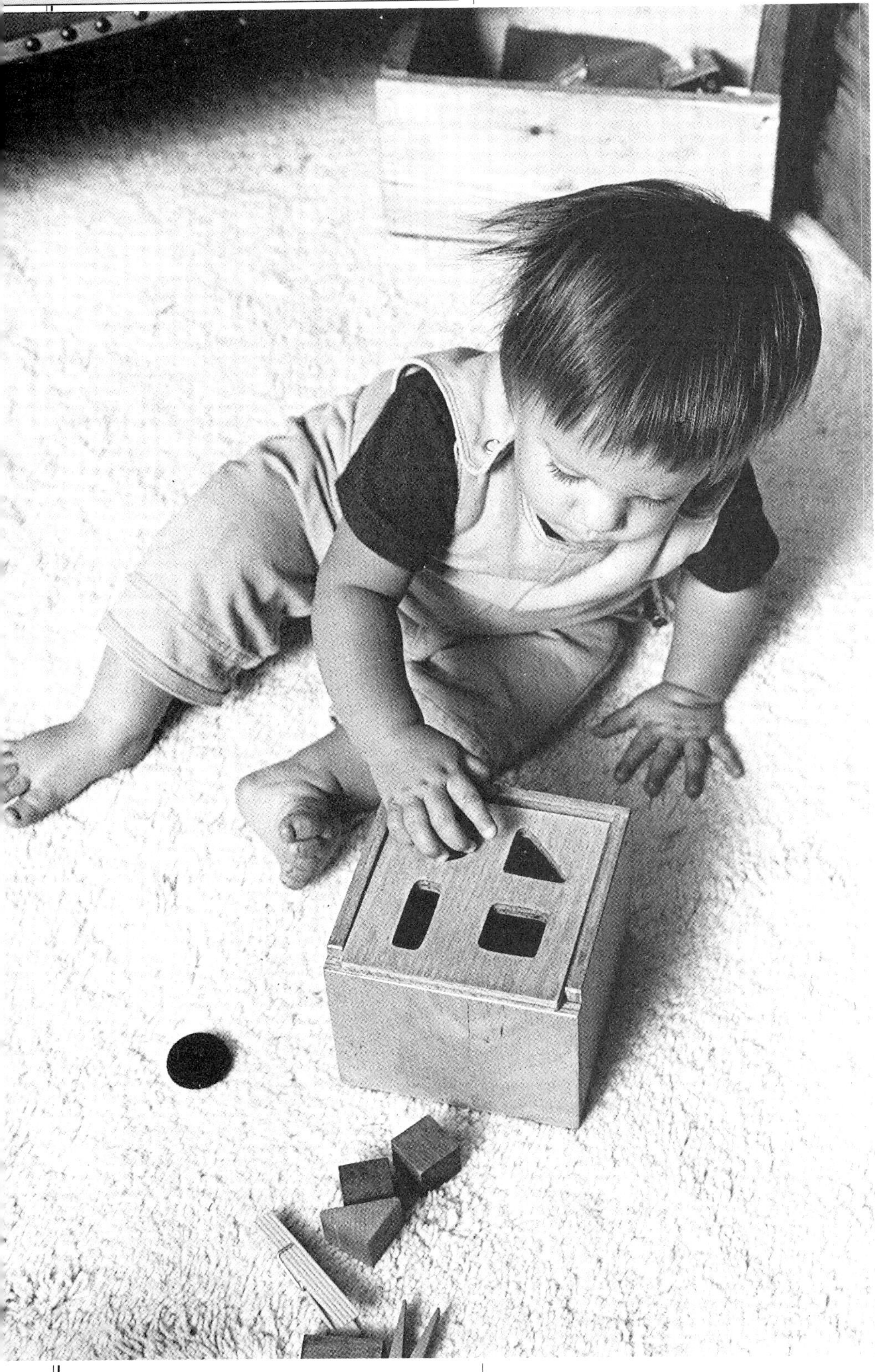

692 Origins of handedness

Why are some children left-handed? It is easier to say why not, than why. The left-hand side of the brain controls the right-hand side of the body, and vice versa. For most people, the left-hand side is dominant, so it stands to reason that most of us are right-handed. Or does it? Actually, it does not, because although it is true that almost everybody who is right-handed is (as it were) left-brained, not all who are left-handed are right-brained. In fact most of them are left-brained too.

So why is your baby left-handed? Despite many fancy theories, no one is sure. A genetic component is probably involved, but it is not a simple matter. Why people clasp hands, or fold their arms in a different order, are also poorly understood.

693 Hand toys

Because of her new manual skills (686-688), at around nine months your baby will now expect toys and household objects to behave more interestingly than before. She will want things she can bang, drop, move along, look through and turn over; things small enough to pass between her hands or to pick up with a pincer movement; things to put into a trolley or drop from a high chair; things to roll, to poke and to prod.

• A wooden spoon and a set of cheap saucepans may be banged like drums, stacked, nested, and later be used to carry around treasures and cook pretend meals.
• A ball can be rolled back and forth, or away, out of sight, behind the settee.
• She can now turn the pages of a book.
• Things to press, or a box for posting different shapes, become popular, as do a variety of kitchen utensils: boxes, pots, containers, cardboard boxes, empty washing-up liquid bottles; yoghurt pots on a string to pull along; things to hold that are hard, soft, fat and thin.

She will need plenty of bath toys, too: cups, sieves, things that float and things that sink; sponges to squeeze, flannels to drip and a teapot from which to pour water.

It is also scribbling time: provide a fat crayon and some newspaper.

694 Last bottle feed

My three children all had bottles until they were at least three, my daughter giving hers up with great difficulty when she started school. For the younger two, the bottle became a comforter. For the older one, a toy puppet only replaced the bottle as comforter when he was about two. Clearly, I have little expertise on this topic.

Weaning from the breast and bottle to the cup was not the problem. With all three children, I managed this quite easily by the time they were eight months old. The difficulty came in trying to deprive them of the small night-time comfort feed: I managed to wean them from the breast by nine months, but only by replacing it with a bottle.

I then weaned them from a full bottle (even a partly full bottle) to an empty one (better for teeth) but not from the teat itself. All this happened, as it does for most babies, at about nine or ten months.

To overcome the problem, try:

• Cutting the morning and evening bottle or breast at about six months, leaving the breakfast or teatime feed as the last feed of the day. That way a baby is less likely to use the breast or the bottle for comfort. Let her suck a baby beaker in the cot if this makes life easier. At the same time, make a positive effort to introduce other potential comforters (soft toys, soft silky pillow slips, a lambskin).
• Wean her from the breast to a cup: never let her know about bottles. Let your partner put her to bed during the period in which you try to wean her. She will probably need to suck something until about nine or ten months.
• Be firm: she has to give up the bottle sooner or later; it is always going to be hard.
• Replace the last feed with a last ritual – see 680.
• Try to avoid comfort sucking right from the start, since a baby who sucks for comfort will always be difficult to wean. This means never letting her suck because she is unhappy, has fallen over, or is cutting a tooth; never letting her walk around with her bottle, or allowing her to hold it in her mouth as she plays: not impossible but you must be consistent.

695 Diet

If your baby's diet is primarily milk, it will give her most of the nutrients she needs. But as she switches away from milk, you should monitor her diet more carefully. The box on page 282 provides a yardstick against which you can check.

696 Eating with the family

As she grows, it is fun to let your baby eat with the family, even if she is not yet always sharing your meal. At nine months she may well begin to feed herself, although you may still want to help her some of the time. If your family eating area (or dining room) has a carpet, it is worth investing in a sheet of plastic to put under her chair, particularly when she reaches the dropping stage.

697 Fun food

Children like to play with food: to pile mashed potatoes in a mound, to wobble jelly, to chase peas around the plate and to throw things on to the floor.

No matter that you have spent time preparing it; no matter that it is wasteful; accept her games and she is less likely to persist. Meal times cannot be avoided, and it pays dividends to do everything you can to prevent them becoming tension-ridden. If she sits and plays with her rice, you can at least get on with your conversation.

By her first birthday she should:
- Weigh about 16 lb (7.25 kg).
- Eat about 800 calories per day.
- Have about 20 g of protein per day.

Her typical daily diet should come from the following five sources:
- One egg or 2 oz (57 g) of meat or fish, or the equivalent protein intake if she is vegetarian.
- One pint (0.5 litre) of milk, or ½ oz (14 g) of cheese, or half a carton of yoghurt.
- One slice of wholemeal bread or 3 oz (85 g) of pulses (peas, lentils, beans) or 2 oz (57 g) of nuts, or a small helping of breakfast cereal.
- One piece of fresh fruit, 2 oz (57 g) of vegetables (some raw) and a small protion of salad.
- Half an ounce (14 g) of butter or margarine.

A typical day's meals might be:
- An early morning drink of fruit juice.
- Cereal with milk, banana.
- Chopped fish, potatoes, peas, yoghurt, fruit juice.
- Cheese on toast with tomatoes and a milk drink.

A healthy diet at one year plus

A healthy diet is one which remains balanced over time. She will select her own well-balanced diet if you offer the basic essentials.

- Proteins: fish, meat, peanut butter, eggs, hamburgers, cheese, liver, peas, beans. Proteins are also found in bread, potatoes, grains, lentils, nuts, brewer's yeast and soya products.
- Fats, found in cheese, butter and milk.
- Carbohydrates, found in bread, flour, cereal, root vegetables; also in sugary cakes and biscuits, though she does not need to take them in a sweetened form.
- Minerals: calcium, found in milk; iron in liver and egg yolk. Most other minerals are only needed in tiny quantities. A normal diet will provide all that she needs; if you are worried buy a tablet-form supplement.
- **Vitamins:** if she is taking milk, eggs, vegetables, fruit and meat, she has all the vitamins she needs. But what if she refuses all fruit but oranges? Or lives basically on baked beans and milk?

Vitamin and mineral supplements can set the mind at rest for a small weekly outlay. Needed or not, they can reduce tension at meal times: if you know she does not really

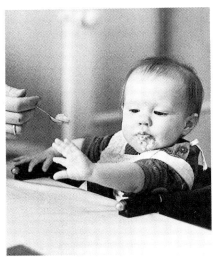

need her spinach, you can relax when she refuses it. It is often said that the old Irish subsistence diet of potatoes mashed with milk and butter, together with a little soda bread and cabbage, provided a near perfect diet for raising children. Keep this in mind. Her needs are basic.

698 Feeding equipment

The best equipment for feeding babies is made from plastic such as melamine or polypropylene.

- She will need a beaker with a lid (especially if she likes to walk around with it or if she likes to have a drink in the bedroom in the morning). She should be able to drink from a normal cup by the time she is a year old.
- Bowls with suction bases, or which keep food warm, are useful for the baby who feeds herself. Those with pictures on the bottom can encourage her to leave a clean plate.
- She cannot yet manage a knife and fork, and plastic spoons, and fingers, are the best utensils.
- A high chair enables her to sit close to you at meal times. If you have space, look out for a seat that can convert a normal dining chair into a baby chair, or for a seat which clamps on to a table. These last two come into their own when you are away from home, but for everyday use they are not as practical as a high chair which supports the baby firmly in a seated position.

   Some children start to eat much better once they sit with the rest of the family; fussing over food may be a way of attracting attention.
- She will also need a bib: the plastic ones are ugly, but practical.

699 More about obesity

See 614-616. If your baby is more than 20 per cent above the average weight (see chart) she is obese. Where are you going wrong?

- Does she eat 'empty calories' – sweets, biscuits, chocolate, ice cream, lollipops and cakes?
- Does she eat much fried or fatty food – chips, crisps and creamy cakes?
- Is she allowed many snacks?
- Does she overeat? Does she go on eating as long as you keep giving her food?
- Does she eat because she is tense or upset?
- Does she eat to please you?
- Do you like her plump?
- Does she get exercise?
- Do you comfort her with food?
- Do you reward her with food?

700 Dangers of obesity

- Slow physical development. She cannot easily pull herself up, climb or run.
- Difficulty in playing boistrously.
- Teasing.
- Mechanical disorders of the hips, legs and feet.

701 Like child, like adult?

There are many more obese adults than obese children, so keeping her slim now is no guarantee that she will not put on weight as an adult. Most obese children, on the other hand, do grow up to be obese adults. In some studies it has been shown that eight out of ten fat children become fat adults.

702 Causes of obesity

- The first factor – the inherited tendency – you can do nothing about. Only about seven per cent of normal-weight parents have fat children, but if both parents are obese, 80 per cent of their children will be obese.
- A second factor is diet during the first two years of life (and also during adolescence). These are the two periods when fat cells are laid down; see 614.
- The third factor is exercise. Obese children simply don't move as much or as quickly as normal children. In one study, normal-weight girls were found to be moving about 90 per cent of the time, while the fat girls moved about only 50 per cent of the time. The fat ones tended to be much more placid and easy going. They also lost weight when encouraged to run about.

703 Mechanism of obesity

First, a baby inherits a tendency to put on weight, together with a placid, easy-going temperament. As a result, she moves about less and spends more time sitting. She eats everything that is given, partly because she is so easy-going, partly because she is happy to sit in her chair at meal times.

704 Body build and personality

In men (the research has not yet looked at women) there seems to be a relationship between body build and personality. Does it apply to tiny children? Nobody knows. The classic endomorph is soft and round, aggressive and assertive; the classic ectomorph is long and thin, considerate and thoughtful; the mesomorphs are muscular, self-confident leaders.

705 Diarrhoea

Diarrhoea is caused by eating contaminated food, or by bacteria ('germs') on dirty hands, cooking utensils or dish cloths. If there is recurrent diarrhoea in the family, it is wise to sterilize the baby's spoons and to wash your hands thoroughly before preparing her meals.

Diarrhoea is potentially dangerous at this age. See entry in **medical section**.

Shortage of mineral elements
Shortage of mineral elements should not be a major worry since a balanced diet contains them all in abundance; see page 282. If your baby does lack essential minerals, the outcome may be:

• Too little sodium (salt): cramp. Excess salt is more likely; it can cause kidney damage and high blood pressure.
• Too little iron: anaemia.
• Too little iodine: goitre.
• Too little calcium: softening (and weakening) of the bones.

Vitamin deficiency
• Vitamin A: skin and visual disorders, lower resistance to infection.
• Vitamin B: general poor health, berri-berri or pellagra.
• Vitamin C: growth retardation, scurvy.
• Vitamin D: rickets.

---

706 Is she ill?

If a baby is active and alert, eats and sleeps well and seems to be growing and developing at a normal rate, she is well. Obvious? Yes, but even the fittest and most robust baby has the occasional day when she just feels ill without particularly obvious symptoms, and this is when you begin to worry about sinister underlying causes.

Few babies get through their first year without colds, earache or stomach upsets.

She may indeed have recurrent problems such as asthma or ear infections in the first year. Some babies have endless colds. If she is in contact with other children, at a day care centre, or if she has school-age brothers and sisters, she will catch more than her fair share of infections in her first year.

Most minor ailments can, of course, be dealt with at home, but the two essential cautions are: never ignore fever in a baby – her temperature can get alarmingly high; and never ignore sickness.

707 Signs of illness

You know that doctors are trained to recognize serious illness, while you are not, but it is still possible to doubt whether one should call in medical help.

I suspect the best approach is to trust your intuition. You know your baby, and you know when she is out of sorts.

If you think she is ill, she almost certainly is. A temperature, a runny nose or spots will often confirm your suspicions, but first signs can be just as useful: a boisterous child becoming quiet; a happy child becoming miserable; a baby who normally sleeps at night becoming wakeful.

A well child is: active and usually happy; curious and ready to explore; spends much of her waking time playing; responds eagerly to your invitations to play; may wake and demand attention but be easily comforted.

A sick child is: listless; miserable and unhappy; apathetic; loses interest in play; goes off her food (or, if feeding is a battleground, may suddenly accept food); cries fretfully, dozes and whimpers; screams with obvious pain.

None of these is actually a reason for desperate anxiety or reason to see a doctor urgently – though a visit to the surgery may be needed in a few hours time. Remember, you should always be able to get advice from a doctor over the telephone.

Safety, cars and cots
If you take a baby in a car, carry-cot restrainer straps are essential. The specially moulded safety lie-back seat, though expensive, is however the ideal – designed to give maximum protection in case of an accident. Early models, without handles, are perhaps a little awkward to carry.

If you buy a second-hand cot, check that the paint is lead-free. If in doubt, strip and re-paint.

Medical emergencies

Remember a baby can become ill quickly.

Call the doctor, or rush the baby/child to hospital, if:
- She is unconscious. This is more serious in a baby than in an older child – the brain is likely to be at a more critical stage of development.
- Has a fit.
- Vomits on and off for more than four hours.
- If a fontanelle bulges.
- If a fontanelle sinks in. This is a sign she is severely dehydrated.
- She goes blue for more than a few moments.
- Bleeds from a cut, or anywhere else, for more than a few mintues. A baby has little blood, so prolonged heavy bleeding is extremely dangerous.
- If you suspect that she is very ill.

Eight good reasons for telephoning the doctor for advice:
- She seems to be in pain.
- She cries when you touch her tummy.
- She cries when you touch her ears.
- She is unusually thirsty.
- Passes much wind and cries when she does so.
- Her tummy seems tender and she is vomiting. All babies vomit occasionally, and if she is happy and hungry immediately afterwards, she is probably well; if she is not, or the vomiting persists, you need advice.
- She gets diarrhoea; all babies have the occasional greenish, foul-smelling motion. If it persists, you need advice.
- She has difficulty breathing. All babies get colds, and some wheeze when they do. If she wheezes without any sign of a cold, seek help.

It is safe to wait until morning if:
- She develops lumps in the neck or groin or tummy; these are swollen glands.
- She has a discharge from the ear without pain.

  See **medical section**.

But she was ill
Most parents have the disconcerting experience of calling the doctor to their home only to find that the baby is perfectly happy by the time he arrives. It happens all the time, and doctors are used to it. Babies and children recover much faster than adults.

Sick baby, basic needs
Besides the prescribed medicine, she will benefit from:

- Extra drinks.
- Extra cuddles.
- Company.
- Singing, soothing and rocking.
- Old, undemanding toys.

A sick baby does not need:
- To stay in bed.
- An over-heated room.
- Feeding up.
- To be left alone.
- New toys which she does not yet understand.

Hospital
During the first five years of life, 15 out of every hundred babies or children go into hospital at least once. The principal reasons for admission are:

- Poisoning, mostly from helping themselves to medicines or cleaning fluids.
- Infections, particularly those producing wheezing, diarrhoea and vomiting.
- Surgical problems, especially for congenital malformations of the heart, intestines or other organs; also for broken bones and ruptures.
- Accidents.
- Asthma.

  See also **medical section**.
  It is taken for granted that the mother will accompany the baby or child. It is natural for the baby or child to be frightened and afraid, and if she has never been alone before, now is not the time to leave her.

The Second Year

708 At one year

You baby will be cruising around the furniture, maybe taking her first steps. Finding a toy cup on the floor, she lifts it to her lips as if to drink. When she sees a dog she points with her finger and says "Ow-ow" over and over again.

She will crawl up to other babies and look at them; she may even hold out a toy. She is just beginning to relate to other children.

She is a little more independent: she will crawl out of one room to explore another, feed herself and drink from her cup. Sometimes, she is pleasantly co-operative, helping as you dress and change her. Sometimes she is less so, rushing away as you try to change her nappy. Sometimes she will fight you as you try to put on mittens and hat.

She communicates with a few words, but there are many more sounds and gestures. She loves outings, enjoys swings and slides, her bath, even swimming.

She is no longer a baby, but not yet a child. She still wants you to feed her, to be with her, to follow her around.

709 Physical shape

Once she gets up off all fours you may notice all sorts of shortcomings: fallen arches, bow legs, a pot belly and the absence of a neck. These are all normal at this age, and yet by the end of her second year she will have the physical shape of a child (though it may take longer to lose her pot belly). Now her head is still relatively large, and her legs short, but as she becomes more mobile her legs will grow faster.

710 Feeding

By the age of one she should be able to eat much the same food as you. Simply mash or cut up the food into small pieces for her. She may like fairly solid pieces of food, such as carrots, meat and peas, in a separate dish to eat with her fingers while you help her to eat more liquid food with a spoon. She is probably now trying to eat with her own spoon, though not efficiently.

She still does not much like highly spiced or peppery food, but may enjoy strong flavours such as those of blue cheese, brie, olives and garlic.

As before, she needs a sound, mixed diet: meat, fish, cheese, eggs, vegetables, grains and fruits. She still needs milk for calcium; a pint a day satisfies all her needs and you will almost certainly be providing this in cereal, chocolate drinks, milk pudding, yoghurt, custard and so on.

711 Messy, fussy eaters

Do try and distinguish between your worries about her diet and the frustration of seeing your lovingly prepared food thrown all over the floor. Malnutrition is a rare problem in the developed world. (The first sign of malnutrition is not a pot belly but extreme lethargy: if she races around between meals, she must be getting enough food.) If you are uneasy, supplement her meals with plenty of milk, and with vitamin drops.

If she eats well at breakfast, make this her main meal; there is no reason why babies should have their major meal in the middle of the day. But above all, relax. It is no use expecting her to behave in an adult manner, and table manners can be learned later. Let her mix whatever she will, eat in what order she chooses and with what implements she desires. Let her get down when she has finished. If she does not eat, she will get hungry; when she is hungry, she will eat.

If she wants to eat only sweet things, it usually makes sense to try and a way around the issue. While it is true that a sweet tooth will undermine her natural ability to select a balanced diet, you can make good by creating a 'sweet' diet around, say, nourishing egg custard with apple, plus a slice of wholemeal bread with honey, macaroni pudding made with wholewheat pasta, raisins and chopped nuts. Sugar does not kill off goodness.

Don't take much trouble preparing her food if she is fussy, since it is likely to make you tense.

Make allowances for her likes and dislikes. If you find a food she adores, give it to her repeatedly. Make a big batch and freeze it: spaghetti Bolognese for lunch seven days a week will do no harm.

712 Junk food

It need not be all empty calories. There is nothing wrong with serving pizza, hot dogs, hamburgers or ice cream. They are all respectable sources of protein and other essential nutrients, just as good in many instances as the 'nutritious' meals you prepare. Even crisps are a source of vegetable protein. Snack-style meals can make a balanced diet: try apple sauce cake, or banana bread made with wholemeal flour, carrot cake or Bakewell tart with a piece of fruit or a little raw vegetable. She will, however, need to clean her teeth after these, and you will need to watch that the level of sugar and fat does not make her obese.

713 Only snacks?

Feeding your baby mainly on snacks can help you all to relax at meal times, and once she sees feeding as a time for shared pleasure rather than tension, she may want to eat in a less babyish fashion.

If eating between meals suits her better than at meal times, so be it. A carrot eaten while she sits on the floor playing has exactly the same food value (even more if raw) as a carrot on a plate.

Of course, not all snacks are good. Sweets have little food value.

714 Self at around one year

As your baby moves from babyhood to childhood, it is easy to see the advances she makes phyically, less so the leaps in emotional and social development.

One of the great strides she makes about now is in stringing together little pieces of behaviour. When her father comes in, she looks up, puts down her toys and toddles over to him. She smiles and lifts her arms to be picked up, giving him a cuddle. She might even say "Dada". She shows her emotions in a more organized fashion than a few months ago. Love is expressed with tenderness, hugs, kisses and obvious delight in seeing you. She may even pat you if you hurt yourself. She will show anger too: run away, hide and sulk, throw her plate of cabbage on the floor, hit her brother. Disappointment will be expressed with looks that can break your heart. Do you have to leave? Fears and anxieties are also expressed with desperation. She refuses vehemently to enter a room that frightens her, to go on an escalator, or be left with a stranger. She has no shame, no guilt, and as yet, no empathy. She will not see your point of view. Only when she has a clear sense of self, at about 18 months, can she start to manage this.

715 Thinking and feeling

Many of a baby's emerging intellectual skills are applied to her emotions. A child

Comforters

Getting attached to a comforter often starts between six and nine months; at much the same time, in fact, that she becomes attached to people. It may be a small soft toy, a bit of blanket or cloth, a dummy or a bottle.

The attachment can be strong, and useful. Once she has her comforter, she may find it much easier to settle into her cot at night. Indeed, you may find that she starts to sleep through the night. When she begins to wake, she can reach for the comforter, and, thus reassured, may fall back to sleep.

It is not a sign of insecurity to need a bit of blanket. On the contary, it is often a sign of independence. She has found her own way of feeling secure. Comfort objects are usually soft, probably because mothers and other carers are soft.

In a famous experiment where baby monkeys were raised without mothers, it was found that they were happier if they clung to cloth 'mothers'. Two such mothers were placed side by side, one covered in cloth, the other made of wire. The wire one had the feeding bottle. The baby monkeys clung to the cloth and contorted themselves into all sorts of precarious positions to feed from the wire mother without letting go of the cloth.

The problem with a comforter starts if it becomes essential for sleep. At some point, she will inevitably lose it. My eldest son was attatched to a Paddington Bear puppet which went everywhere with us. One summer we arrived in London from Montreal without it. I spent the whole day in a haze (having not slept for 24 hours). I rang every shop in the area to find a replacement.

The one I eventually found was reluctantly accepted after we had washed it a few times.

If she becomes attached a blanket, it is probably worth cutting it up into two or three pieces, so you have a reserve in case of accidents. Put a spare section into her cot for a night or two before you wash the current comforter. It may pick up something of the required smell.

who can learn that hitting the drum makes a noise can learn that being happy makes others happy.

716 Together

She is scribbling with crayons; you are too busy to catch her eye or look at her work. She throws it on the floor in a temper; she has caught your attention.

She has learned, you might say, to respond to your unreasonable behaviour with her own. This is perfectly healthy: she needs to learn a whole range of behaviour in order to thrive. She does it not only by gut response, but by copying: her close emotional ties with you make this natural,

a pleasure. She now sits with a book 'reading', just like you, shakes her head like you, and later she will say things exactly as she hears you say them (often swearing to herself in a way which makes you cringe).

She also begins to express her needs, perhaps by bringing you a book, or cuddling up on your lap when she feels sleepy. Once she begins to organize a course of action, she can find security merely by looking at you and smiling. Before, she needed to be picked up and cuddled, now it may be enough to look at you and know that you would pick her up if necessary. This is a big step along the road to independence. Later still, simply knowing that you will support her can give security, even when you are absent.

717 First word

What does she say first? A child's first 50 words usually include the important people in her life. Mummy, Daddy, her favourite foods, banana, milk, apple; often it is her own baby-word for food such as num-num or nana. There are also the objects she likes to see: cars, tractors, cows, cats; and things that happen every day: going to the shops or having baths. And there are the words she uses when she wants something: more, all gone, up, down, wee-wee.

718 All-purpose words

Calling the milkman Daddy is more than a joke, it is typical of the way she uses words. For many children the word dog may initially include cats and cows. She probably over-extends words because she starts by labelling just one aspect of an object. In forming a concept such as car, labelled with the correct word, she has to ignore variables such as colour and size (toy cars are cars, after all) and even movement – parked cars are still cars. To make sense of objects, she must not be too precise. Except for people's names, the words she hears are general, and her own words will follow suit. Later she will gradually fine down the meaning.

719 The motive to talk

What parent can resist the early words of a child? Pointing a finger at an object and saying the word is almost bound to start social interaction. Soon simple words are also used to express needs: want, look, bye-bye, more, down.

720 Tandem

She may well recycle much of her non-verbal communication in harness with these early words. She lifts her arms and whines to be picked up; attempts to undo her straps and shouts to be put down from her chair.

721 Understanding and producing

To say a word, a child must not only understand it but physically produce it. Most children's understanding is ahead of their production skill. Occasionally, they understand very many more words than they can produce. These are the children to whom you can say "Bring me the pink pig from the red drawer" – and they will do so, before being able to utter a word. You will hear it endlessly remarked that Einstein said nothing before he was two; the reason was delayed physical ability to produce words rather than tardy intellectual development.

722 Helping language

Language is part of living. Early language is learned against a background of living together; it is a way of sharing. When she points and says "Woof-woof" she is sharing her pleasure with you. If she hears little language, she will learn little. If she does not realize that talking is enjoyable, she will not be motivated to learn. The process is marvellously self-fulfilling: as she understands more, so her understanding of the world improves. As she knows more words, so she has a means of expanding her memory.

Talk should be part of all games and interactions.

● Books with attractive, clear pictures help her to name things.
● Games that fit actions to toys help her to differentiate: a penguin that pecks her tummy; a bear that jumps into her cot.
● Naming clothes and parts of the body is another speech game you can play as she sits on your knee. 'Where's my foot?' 'Where's Alice's toe?' Playing in front of the mirror makes it more fun.
● Say words after her, but don't correct her. If she says "Bu" for book, say "It is a book", never "No, book not bu."

If you praise her, she knows you like her to talk. If you always correct her, she may feel it is even too difficult to try.

723 Baby talk

"Never", I said. But like most parents I did. Doggies and woof-woofs were as much a part of my vocabulary as my children's. First words often repeat syllables: children love the rhythmic sounds; so doggy and bow-wow are more appealing than dog. There is absolutely no evidence that baby talk holds up language development. It always drops out naturally, returning only when a child wants to be a baby.

724 Not quite there

A child will set out to say a word, but does not always make it. Sometimes her words are far from precise, even when she knows what she means. 'Do' can be dog and also door, but she does not confuse dogs with doors. She simply cannot form the ends of words.

Most children simplify words. Spoon becomes poon, brush bush, smile mile. Clusters of sounds are among the last to be mastered by English-speaking children and some children still have difficulty with them at four or five.

Another common error is to make all the consonants the same: Doddy for dog and lolly for lorry.

She will often replace unvoiced sounds like 'p', 't', and 'k' with voiced sounds like 'b', 'd' and 'g'. So she says "Doe" for toe.

725 Memory stages

Earlier, your baby developed her memory through action and perceiving object permanence; now she begins to remember situations. When you put her bib on, she expects supper. But as language begins to come on tap, she can remember events in detail because she can talk about them in detail. Think how much of your own memory is based upon words.

726 Object permanence, nine to 18 months

See 621.

● By about nine months she will search under a cloth for a hidden toy, but she is still not sure it is there, even though she saw you hide it. She still treats the object she finds under the cloth as if it is new.

● By ten months she connects actions with objects: knocking over a pillow to reach a toy, for example.

● By 18 months she will understand that two objects can be in the same place if one is inside or under the other.

She will now begin to use pictures in her mind to guide her actions: images, words and actions stand for objects; she can begin to manipulate ideas. As this happens, she becomes more thoughtful and possibly ready to engage in the simpler forms of fantasy play.

But until she reaches seven she will not always be sure whether to believe her eyes or her mind.

727 Play

At all stages you will see her practising. She will enjoy putting little people into cars at one stage, hiding them behind doors at another. Bags, buckets and wheelbarrows are a delight just now because they help her to practise the ideas of inside and under. So do stacking cups, shape sorters and bricks: all classic toys for this age. She will also enjoy pushing things along and dragging things behind her.

Remember what it is that she has to learn and you are unlikely to go wrong when you select her birthday toys.

Peek-a-boo and hiding games can give her essential practice with all stages of learning about object permanence.

728 Physical co-ordination, 12-18 months

● At 13 months she should be able to draw with a crayon, place one brick on top of another and take off her shoes.

˙● By 15 to 18 months she should be able to stoop down to pick something off the floor.

● By 18 months she will build a tower of bricks three or four high, post a simple shape in a posting box, be skilled with a spoon, turn the pages of a book, undo a zip, pull off her socks and walk up and down stairs.

Safety for the mobile child·

Once she starts moving about the house, you will need to extend your child- proofing yet again. See box opposite.

● Once she can walk, she will also climb. Fit bars or locks to upstairs windows.
● Never leave her alone near water. A child can drown in a full bath someone has forgotten to empty.
● Keep all medicines in a locked cupboard.
● Keep all cleaning materials out of reach.
● Keep hiding places such as cupboards locked.
● Don't leave a toddler in the garden unsupervised.
● Make sure she cannot escape from the garden.
● Fill in garden pools until she is old enough to treat them sensibly.
● Make sure garden sheds and garages are locked.
● Make sure weedkiller and other garden poisons are out of reach, in case she does go into the shed.
● Don't leave fires unguarded.
● Make sure clothes are flame-resistant.
● Use the back burners on the cooker, and turn all pans so that the handles cannot be knocked.
● Be sure she cannot reach the kettle or the iron.
● Empty the kettle after use.
● Don't polish wooden floors so well that she will slip.
● Make sure rugs don't slip.
● Make sure she cannot lock herself in the W.C., bathroom, or any other room.
● Make sure she cannot open the front door.
● Never leave old fridges or freezers where she could climb inside.

729 Stairs – when semi-mobile

Until your child can safely manage the stairs it is obviously sensible to block them with a barrier. However, it is even safer, and less of a nuisance, to teach your toddler to negotiate stairs carefully. If she crawls, she will almost certainly climb stairs without any problem, and will also be able to come down safely if you show her how to turn around at the top and negotiate them backwards. Sit with her and help her to come down: move her feet

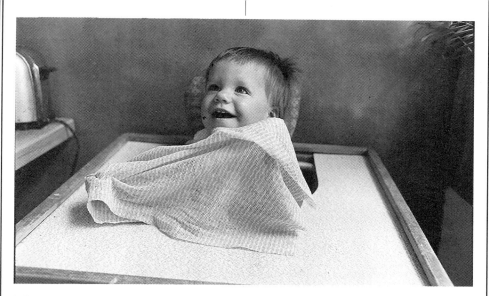

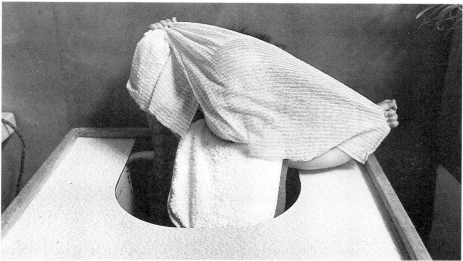

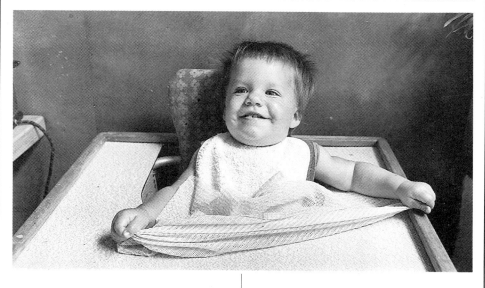

down one step at a time, following with her hands. Two or three lessons and she will be safe.

730 Stairs – walking

There is a difficult stage when she begins to walk up and down stairs, and this will need attention. Show her how to hold on to the banisters. It is still wise to block off the stairs with a gate in the morning if she is up before you.

A third difficult phase is when she learns to walk around carrying toys.
The weight, and the mental demand of carrying, undermines balance. Discourage her from taking toys on the stairs.

731 Friends

There comes a point in her relationships with other babies when she stops treating them like objects to explore and starts treating them like other babies. This is usually some time around her first birthday. After that she will happily play if not with another child, alongside him, and sometimes offer him a toy.

She will touch children, but quite gently: the action is more social than the exploratory touches of a baby of seven or eight months. She is likely to look the child in the face as she touches, and to run to another child and chatter and shout in excitement. She may even take the other child's hand.

But it is not all sweetness. She will snatch and get angry if something is taken from her. She may even hit out and bite in a deliberate, angry way.

Sometimes she feels good towards her peers, and sometimes she feels bad. The main point is that she feels.

732 Shared play

Toys can serve to focus two children's attention on the same idea, and to suggest co-operation with the other child. If both children have played with their parents, they may begin a rudimentary form of shared play with toys quite early in their first year.

However, they only look at each other fleetingly; the social moments are but moments. Children of the same age don't fully interact in play until they have passed their second birthday.

733 Outings

It is often in the excitement of an outing that your baby will find the new word that has been forming: it is so much easier to learn when you are excited; so much easier to notice details. Think how you feel when you first arrive at a delightful new spot on holiday. Picture books of the zoo or park will remind her of the experience and help her to remember.

734 Herself

By 12 or 13 months she will begin to emerge as a real individual. You saw the roots of this development in your baby's first year, but now her character will be sufficiently obvious to define it with a range of adjectives: bold, shy, friendly, withdrawn and so on. One of the clearest ways you can help is to admire her: show her that you like the way she is and value her unique qualities. As she tries out all her rapidly developing skills, your pride and admiration are reassurance. You will need to be a close observer, to follow her lead and read her intentions.

735 Over-excited

Children wind themselves up, frequently in the last half hour before bed time. "It will end in tears" you say, but calming them down takes real skill and a mixture of distraction and close interaction. "Come and read"; "Come and run your bath"; stay involved with her, especially if you have a new baby. She needs your attention just as much as the baby now. She can wander off from playing beneath your feet, but still needs to know that you are interested and involved in what she is doing. You will need to balance this need for support and security with her developing independence. In the long term, this independence will become her main source of security.

736 Goodbye to babyhood

If you have enjoyed your baby's total dependence, you may find it difficult to say goodbye to her babyhood.
• Do you find it difficult to let her be boss?
• Does her independence make you uncomfortable?
• Do you let her take the initiative?
• Does her curiosity about your body disturb you?

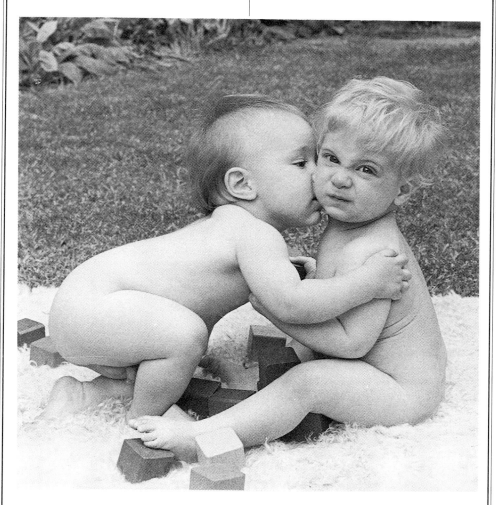

737 Crying

It is not always easy to offer support and security to an angry, crying child, and anger and tears are very much a part of the second year. As her awareness grows, so does her awareness of her limitations.

As she develops, she will spend less and less time in contact with you. Sometimes this will make her frightened. Perhaps she is on the far side of the room engrossed in play, looking up at intervals to get your reassuring smile. Suddenly she realizes you are no longer there: she wails. But sometimes her anxiety seems more fundamental than this. She becomes quiet and clinging.

The best way to deal with anxiety is of course by offering love and reassurance.If she is anxious when you are not there, it is unkind to nip out of the room when she is not looking. Let her know you are going, offer a hand if she wants to come with you or leave the door open for her to follow. As she builds up her understanding of language, tell her what you are doing, and mean what you say. If you say you are going to make a cup of tea, do so; don't settle down in the kitchen with the paper.

If she can trust you, she will be able to develop independence from you.

A child who has formed attatchments to a number of people (659) often feels less anxious than one who is securely attached to only one person.

738 Age gaps

People tend to hold firm and contradictory views on the best age gap between children. Parents say their offspring are good friends because they are so close in age, or that they fight and quarrel for exactly the same reason.

Some feel that for children to be companions they should be close enough in age to play together, others that the elder child should be old enough not to feel displaced.

In fact, the actual gap seems to be irrelevant. All children show great interest in a new baby, and all, whatever the age, show disturbances in behaviour once she arrives.

There is a difference in the way they react, but it reflects their age, not their underlying feelings.

A 15-month-old baby becomes miserable and clinging when her young sibling appears.

A three- or four-year-old will become difficult and demanding. If there is a very large age gap, the older child will often care for and teach the younger child in a way that does not happen when the gap is small.

In short, there is nothing to recommend any particular age gap. How well children get on together is mainly influenced by the sex and personalities of the children.

739 A second child

One child can easily join adults in a restaurant, on a visit to friends, or be dragged along on trips abroad. Two children is another matter. Because of the practical difficulties, a pair of children, or indeed several children, are not taken around with their parents as much as an only child.

There is also great intimacy and intensity in the relationship between brothers and sisters. They are friends, rivals, playmates and quarrellers. They understand each other in a way that it is difficult to understand anyone else. A relationship which outlasts that with their parents, partners and their own children.

The younger child may often begin to play imaginative games because an older sibling understands how to play with her. And through a sibling, a child can demonstrate great social understanding at an early age.

740 Only children

They don't suffer the trauma of seeing a small, demanding baby suddenly taking over their mother, but neither do they have a constant companion. Friends are, of course, essential to only children for they must learn to play with other children if they are to fit into the social world.

Play a game with any child and you tend to make allowances, letting her win. Other children don't do this: it is a hard lesson she will have to learn when she starts school, unless brothers and sisters have helped her make a start. Once she is old enough to socialize, at about 18 months, you should make an effort to introduce her to other children.

It is easy to over-indulge an only child. Other children in a family ensure than any one child is not always the centre of attention. The tendency to over-protect is exaggerated because it is quicker to do things for her. You need to remind yourself that if her life is too cushioned, she will probably cling, and that it may even sap her curiosity.

Adult company has its benefits. First children (who by definition spend some time as only children) are more intelligent and are more likely to succeed in all spheres of life. Great scientists, past and present, are predominantly first children, so are leading businessmen and politicians. Don't let anyone tell you that being an only child amounts to being handicapped. If the difficulties are overcome, balancing intimacy with plenty of stimulation from other children, she will have special strengths not shared by children of conventional families with more than one child.

741 At 15 months

Mobile, inquisitive, curious, increasingly independent; stringing together sequences of actions which give her behavour obvious purpose. You are beginning to feel she really knows what she wants. She understands much of what you say to her and will communicate with you in words (or sounds) as well as inactions.

742 Physical development

The brain is rapidly maturing. By 18 months, the motor areas (controlling movement) and the visual areas are virtually complete. She now experiments and explores with obvious intent, and this can take her farther and farther from you. She has moved into an expanding spiral of development. She will use her emotional attachments as a safe base from which to explore the world.

743 Original

Some time during her second year she will start to do things that no one has shown her. She puts a piece of bread on her head

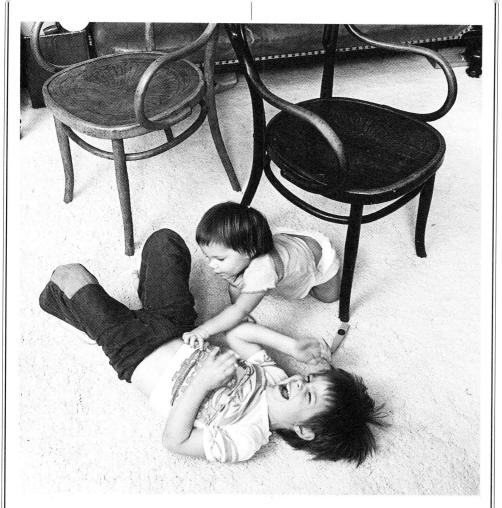

and laughs; or perhaps she puts a cup to a doll's lips; or puts on your shoes and picks up your bag. This is a small beginning which will grow to enormous and delightful proportions over the coming months.

744 Pretend play

It is rudimentary at first. She puts a cup to her lips even though there is no drink in it; she takes a toy drill to the wall as if to drill a hole. Pretending? Or simply imitating? Whichever it is, it demonstrates that she partially understands the object's use.

745 Self at around 18 months

She begins to be more curious about herself. She looks at her body with interest, at yours; at last she recognizes herself in the mirror or in photographs. She starts to use her name. Her knowledge

of her self comes partly from her knowledge of others. Chimps, who can also recognize themselves in a mirror, learn to do so only if they are raised with other chimps.

746 Accepting limits

As her understanding of word and gesture increases, so does your ability to control her behaviour. You can say "No". And she can now decide whether to obey or not.

747 Helping her organize her behaviour

• Before you read to her, ask her to fetch the book.
• Let her find her bib and take her spoon to the table.
• Let her carry her nightclothes to the bathroom at bed time.
• Wash a table together.

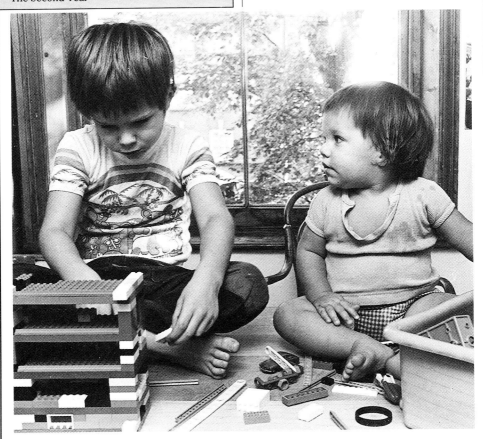

748 Emotion

She rages; she is overcome with delight; she is curious, loving, demanding and stubborn. In a rudimentary way, she is all the things adults can be, but she cannot always deal with these emotions because she cannot yet fully communicate what she needs to fulfill them. Frustration will enrage: toys will be inexplicably hurled to the floor; and she will be difficult for no obvious reason.

749 The role of play

Play is your baby's means of learning. Its repetitive nature is essential – her gains need to be consolidated by constant practice. Nature has made it fun: how could a child learn all she needs to know unless that process gave pleasure?

At present, she does not find work drudgery, and you can take advantage of this by involving her in all kinds of 'work' processes in the guise of play. Let her help you clean the car, water the plants in the garden, do the shopping; later she can help sort the washing, brush the floor and lay the table. This not only shows her how you work as a family, but gives her experience of carrying tasks through to the end – which is not always provided by pure play.

750 Books

At first she will want simple pictures to name, later more complex ones to explore. Then she can move on to the simple stories that relate to her own life.

As her understanding increases, she will want stories that reinforce her make-believe world. As time goes by (in the third to fifth years) pictures will become less important, for she will be able to make her own pictures in her mind.

You can use books to give a child an opening into the fantasy world of the mind, and to give her an opening into the reality of the world: as she grows up she will enjoy reference books as well as stories.

● By 14 months she will want increasingly

elaborate pictures.
- By 18 months she will enjoy books with flaps that lift to reveal pictures; and you may be able to start reading simple stories. Look for stories in which she can take part.
- By two she will be able to listen to more complex stories, but will still need pictures in support.
- By three she can listen to stories without pictures.

751 Messy play

Small children love mess, and naturally make plenty of it because they must explore everything that comes to hand.

What is safe?
- **Mud:** To be on the safe side, supervise her constantly – she should not, ideally, put it in her mouth, since in some parts of the world this can be dangerous.
- **Clay:** Supremely messy – although you think you have cleared it away, a thin film always remains. But it is a wonderful play material if you have a suitable place in which she can use it.
- **Play dough:** Much cleaner than clay, it can be used for much the same activities. Make it at home with flour, salt, water and a little oil.
- **Sand:** Wet and dry sand have interesting, contrasting properties. Always keep a sand pit covered, otherwise cats will use it as a litter tray.
- **Food:** Mashed potatoes and long strings of spaghetti can keep children busy for hours. (For added interest, put a few drops of food colouring into the water while the spaghetti is cooking.)

752 Single parent

Single parenthood has been blamed for many social ills, but don't be misled by the published reports unless they are the careful ones which compare like with like, for example children of married teachers with children of single-parent teachers. No real differences are found between these two groups, their children develop in exactly the same ways.

753 Social child, second to third years

- Between one and two, children spend more and more time looking at each other. They will play in parallel with children of

their own age, and can be drawn into play with an older sibling.
- By three, children are able to talk to each other, play elaborate games together.
- By three, also, children begin to prefer children of their own sex.
- By five they often have firm friends.

754 Friends without children

No longer can you give friends your undivided attention, something they may find hard to understand. Fascinating as your children are to you, to your friends they are just children. There is a sense in which the decision to have children (or not to have them) highlights essential differences between otherwise close friends. Don't be surprised if you find yourself drifting apart from childless women friends. If you are forewarned of the problem, you can often joke your way through it. It may be that for a while some friendships will go into something like cold storage – but with humour, and openess about the problem, there is surely no need for permanent rifts.

755 Identity

Watching people, and classifying them as big and small, fat and thin, nice and nasty and then placing herself in similar categories now gradually builds up a child's self-image – what psychologists call her categorical view of herself. Another important category is age. She will tell enquiriers that she is "three and a quarter" – as if the final three months were a life-and-death distinction. Another category she will comprehend early on is that of possessions. What she can do also forms part of her idea of self: she is a person who can ride a bike, climb the stairs; who cannot run as fast as the boy next door. As she starts to categorize herself in terms of her skills, she will become insistent that she does things by herself. "Me do it" will become household words. I suspect that this is more than a simple plea to practise skills. It is as if she must monitor the ever-changing boundaries of her skills.

Many of the frustrations children feel in this phase are part and parcel of the developing categorical self. Her insistence on putting on her own socks, her refusal to share her favourite toys, her tantrum when you give something of hers to her baby brother, are easier to understand if you know the underlying reasons.

This is just a beginning: her categorical self develops slowly over the years before she starts school and it is coloured by your support and belief. She is the child who can do all these things, or she is the child who can only do them badly.

756 'I'm a girl'

Gender is an important aspect of self. It is difficult to say exactly when a fundamental sense of gender starts to develop, but by the time children can answer questions on the subject, they certainly have an idea of what it is.

It has, however, been shown that even babies show more interest in other babies of the same sex. This is not simply because they tend to wear the same clothes: a girl will show unusual interest in another girl, even if she wears a blue suit; and she will be less interested in a boy in a pink dress. It is unclear what clues she uses to make the identification. Later, children use hair length, clothing and names to guide them much as adults do.

And when do children start to expect boys to be rough and girls to be gentle? The answer is, almost as soon as you can ask them the question.

Surveys have established that at two-and-a-half both boys and girls think girls play with dolls, help mummy and like to cook dinner and clean the house. They also think girls talk a good deal and never hit people.

Boys, they consider, like to play cars, help daddy, build things, and say "I'll hit you". You may, or may not not, find this depressing news. As I dropped my five-year-old at school one morning, he told me that "Daddies went to work, but mummies stayed at home". He seemed genuinely surprised when I pointed out that I was on my way to work. "I thought you were going to college", he said. That daddy also went to college had not occurred to him.

757 The importance of self

A child's view of herself underlies everything that she does. A child who believes that she cannot do something will behave very differently from one who believes she can. If she thinks she is hopeless at arithmetic, she may well end up being hopeless. She may, on the other hand, work away in great anxiety.

758 First words

In the first 50 words a child speaks:

● 51 per cent will be general nominals; that is, words a child uses for a class of objects like ball, car or cup.
● Next will come specific nominals; the names of people and animals. . .Mummy, Tom, Rover.
● Next (13 per cent) are action words, used to describe or accompany an action. Many are verbs such as go or look, but there are others, such as hi and bye-bye.
● Modifiers (9 per cent) refer to properties of objects: big, red, all gone, mine.
● Personal-social words account for another 8 per cent: words like please, yes and ouch.
● Function words, with only a grammatical use such as what or where take four per cent of her output.

So it is clear that early language is mainly about naming; moreover, about naming in an active way. Most of these early names are concerned with things the child can do. Looking at lists of early words, it is possible to get a picture of the child's day:

Dog, cat, duck, horse, mummy, daddy. Shoe, hat.
Milk, bottle, nana (banana), apple. book, ball, clock, light, key.

A day of outings, meals, getting dressed and play.

759 First meanings

Whatever words she chooses, she is soon using them in a variety of ways.

To greet the cat, she says "Puss" as she rushes towards the family pet.

"Puss" she also says as she points at a picture in her book; "Puss" she says again as the cat jumps out of her reach. This time she means 'Come back cat'.

She will make her meaning clear by the expression she uses, and the gestures that accompany her words. Although with most children a rising tone to "Puss" when they see a picture of a lynx may mean 'Is it a cat?', and a falling tone 'It is', some have a pattern of intonation that is all their own.

760 The role of grammar

However many words she knows, she cannot convey meaning without grammer, nor can she understand when others speak.

At simplest, this means understanding what word order conveys: man eats shark is different from shark eats man.

When children first begin to combine words, often in the second half of the second year, they don't make random combinations but maintain the normal word order of English. They usually say "Daddy hat", not "Hat daddy" and "Go park" not "Park go".

Their first simple sentences express actions:

"Me walk."
"Nana fall."
Possession:
"My hat."
"Mummy shoe."
They label:
"That shoe."
"That car."
They demand:
"More juice."
"Go car."
And they express the state of things:
"Mummy home."
"Apple gone."

Children learning different languages all express the same early ideas. The words are different, but children the world over, from Kenya to Japan, say the equivalant of "me walk", "my hat", "more juice" and "apple gone".

761 First sentences

These are simple forms of the ones she hears adults using, but she is not just copying. Sooner or later she will say something you know she has never heard you say.

She comes in from a walk and announces "I seed the sheeps" or "I runned home." An enchanting mistake; and it shows us that the child has an in-built abilityto construct sentences.

If you say to a four-year-old that a paperclip is a "Zug", then give her another and ask what she has got, she will answer "Zugs". Say to her "This teddy is zigging", then ask what he did, and she will say "He zigged."

Long before she has ever had a lesson in the structure and rules of English, she will practise using them. If the English language obeyed the rules as well as she does, she would always get it right. She listens, she extracts the rule, and she constructs.

762 'Motherese'

Its sentences are grammatically well formed, and fairly short. Its grammar is simple: plenty of questions, but few tenses. The pitch of voice is higher, the pace is slower, and there is more variation in pitch and speed than in ordinary speech. The vocabulary is small. Motherese tunes to the child: as her language expands, so does Motherese, moving ahead in step. There is seemingly endless repetition: "Where is Jenny's hat?" "Here is her hat." "Mummy's got the hat." "Put the hat on, Jenny."

How does motherese evolve? Because children mould us to it. We watch for signs she is understanding, repeat if we are unsure, move on a step when we are fairly certain that she does. We always look to see that she is still interested and taking her turn. If we rush ahead too fast, we lose her, and this means we have to start again. Recasting her sentences, expanding them into the correct grammatical forms, seems the right thing to do, and it is.

To practise early words there is nothing better than a picture book with simple, clear pictures. Wait until her language and ability to focus her attention on small areas of a picture improve before you begin to show her more complex scenes.

Once she can follow a simple story read to her. Show her you are pleased when she makes an effort to speak. Take your turn in conversations with her. Listen and let her feel she is telling you something important.

Games such as 'Here we go round the mulberry bush' and other action rhymes can be adapted for smaller children.

As she grows, you will need more to talk about. Outings, even bus journeys, can be mulled over together, especially if you have a book or photographs as a reminder.

Don't be afraid of long words. Children often like a 'party piece' – one long word they can say really well to impress.

As long as you wait to see that she is following, and keep your sentences short, don't be afraid to use language she may not fully understand.

763 Basic trust

Experiments have shown that if a child has no one she can trust:

- She will lie down for long periods at a time.
- She will have 'radar gaze': that is, she

will sweep the field of view without turning her head.
• She will have an expressionless face and poor muscle tone.
• She will feel cold.
• She will have pallid skin.
• She will be backward.

Basic trust is even more fundamental than security. A child who does not trust anyone does not trust herself. She does not explore, or use her body. In extreme cases, a child may even fail to grow.

A child who trusts you will learn to model her own behaviour on yours, will develop your values.

Some parents believe that it needs but a light hand to guide their child. That she will discover the world for herself, come what may, and do her share of right and wrong, regardless of how they try to direct her. For these parents, it follows that, as far as possible, a child should have her own way.

Such children are not always popular with other people. If she is used to having her own way, she will expect it at all times, and the world is not as indulgent as her parents.

Other parents believe that it is their duty to make clear to their child what they consider right and wrong, and how they expect her to behave. Their children are sometimes left little room for exercising initiative.

Others take the hardest line of all. They believe that, left to their own devices, children will break every rule. These parents feel they have to establish from the start that they are boss. The tight control is not much fun for parent or child, and tzhe children often grow up to be rebellious teenagers.

And there is another class of parents who are so overwhelmed by their own problems that they leave their children to bring themselves up. An inconsistent approach, day-in, day-out, leaves an erratic child, uncertain what to expect from anyone.

764 Tricky situations

What do you do if she plays in the lavatory bowl?

• Say "How exciting! Shall we get you a chair at the sink?"
• Say "No, dirty! We have to scrub your hands now."

• Say "Stop! My children don't play like that."
• Ignore or smack, depending on how you feel?

What if she empties flour and cocoa all over the kitchen floor?
What if she runs on to the road?
What if she wets her pants on the bus?
Draws all over the walls?
Climbs up the tree out of reach?

765 'Yes' and 'No'

In the early months and years, parents, I believe, should say "Yes" to babies, most of the time. It is these supportive 'Yeses' that build her trust; allow her to explore you and through you to know herself.

But occasionally, we all have to say "No". We also have to say "Keep away", "Stop", and "Don't touch" for her own safety.

How do you do it?

You can, of course, protect your child from all danger. Child-proof your house, move absolutely everything that could be damaged out of reach and leave it that way until she reaches the age of reason – about seven years.

Or you could demand that she fits in with you right from the start, learning from day one that some things should not be touched.

Although in the first instance you provide her with a heavenly world where all things are possible and no dangers exist, it cannot last long. The day must come when she is exposed to the unprotected radiator or stairs in someone else's house.

What is more, not teaching her the meaning of "No" can expose her to real danger. If she hurts herself too often she may lose faith in your ability to protect her. You have, in other words, to steer a course between the freedom you can give her as a baby by making her environment totally safe and the freedom you must give her as a child by letting her enter the largely unprotected world outside the home.

766 Discipline

Everyone has to learn discipline: all societies must have rules if they are to have freedoms. A child has to learn the limitations of your tolerance and the acceptable bounds of her behaviour.

For her own safety, she must learn that

the world is not always safe and that sometimes other people are better judges of that safety than she is. Before she is one, a child is unable to understand why she should not do something, except in the simplest possible terms. Even when her language is well developed, she will not understand moral issues, nor will she have a sense of conscience or a well-developed sense of guilt. To feel quilty requires a clear understanding of herself as a person. At two this is asking too much.

767 Crime and punishment

So what is the best way to teach a child discipline? In one study, researchers put children in a room full of wonderful toys. There was also a hamster in a box and the children were told to watch it the whole time because it was always escaping.

The children managed to concentrate on the cage for a while, but sooner or later were tempted away by the toys. As soon as they looked away, a trap door in the cage was opened and the hamster escaped. Soon after this, the researcher returned and asked what had become of him. How did the children respond? Did they confess? Did they insist they never looked away? Did they say someone else must have done it?

What the researchers actually found is of some interest to parents wondering how best to train their children.

If children had parents who regularly punished them for bad behaviour, they were the quickest to turn their backs on the hamster and go for the toys. What is more, they were the most likely to deny they had done so.

Children whose parents withdrew love and affection at bad behaviour did not fare well either.

The children who resisted temptation longest, and were most ready to own up, were those whose parents had used reason when disciplining them.

If she hits you on the head with a wooden spoon you can:

- Say "No!" and smack her hand.
- Get up and walk away from her.
- Say "Stop hitting me; it hurts."

Both theory, and practice, show that the last solution works best in the long run.

Of course, explaining in those terms is not easy if the child is small. But it can be tried. She is tuned to your tone of voice and your facial expression and, in her second year, can begin to respond to your mood. Looking hurt and telling her you will cry may be understood.

She will learn that if she hits it makes you sad; just as she learns that if she is happy, you are happy.

768 Why does it work?

Suppose you simply say "Naughty." She knows that you do not like naughty children, so she stops. She does not like you to see her being naughty. But unless she feels you can see her at all times, she may feel perfectly justified in carrying on being naughty when you cannot see. What is more, if she feels like being naughty (which all children sometimes do) she knows just what to do.

Suppose instead you smack her. She then learns that you will inflict pain if you catch her doing this. But it does not teach her why she should obey you. If she does it to avoid being hit, there is no reason to stop when you are not there to smack.

Suppose you say "I won't love you if you do that." Then she will learn that your love is fragile and unreliable: that it needs to be earned. This is a difficult concept for a small child who is trying to discover the rules of the world. It gives little security.

An explanation is a long-term solution. It gives a reason for behaving in a certain way which works even when you are not there to police her. You provide her with something akin to a conscience before she is able to develop one of her own accord.

However true all this may be, there is hardly a parent who can escape sometimes smacking a child in temper and, providing this happens against a background of an otherwise reasonable and consistent approach, there is surely no harm done to the child, and no reason for you to feel anything but regret. Having blown a fuse, you will feel better; that is the moment to explain to the child that you don't enjoy hurting her and that there is a reason for feeling so strongly about what has happened.

769 Saying "No" in the first year

In her first year, a child needs to develop a basic trust of the world. The only reason to say "No" is if something is unsafe. The easiest way is to say "No" immediately and remove the dangerous object or the child.

If, for example, she approaches a hot radiator you can say "No, hot. It hurts", taking her away. Do this every time she goes to the radiator. If she touches it and hurts herself, you simply say. "Hot, hurting radiator" and comfort her. There is no need to be angry or to chastise.

770 Saying "No" in the second year

As she becomes more capable of understanding your explanations, you should continue to set limits for her. Make it clear, for example, that she cannot use sharp scissors. But let her know when she is allowed blunt scissors that they are "special children's scissors" which cannot hurt her.

Later, when you introduce her to sharp knives, she may use them "because she is grown up".

If she has older brothers and sisters, you will of course use age and experience as explanations, which is perfectly reasonable.

771 Example

A child's natural tendency to imitate adult behaviour is especially strong as she approaches the end of her second year. Watch her doing the things that you do. This modelling can be a natural basis for her self-discipline. Which means that it is no use saying, "Do as I say, not as I do." You really need to set a good example and to be consistent, both in your praise and in the limits you set for her.

772 Frustration

As she becomes more mobile and enlarges her understanding of her world, she will want to exert far more power over it than she can realistically manage. Life will present conflicts, in some of which she must inevitably lose. Sometimes there is not time for her to walk beside the pushchair. If it will make you late picking an older child up from school, she has to stay strapped in. Sometimes she may not continue stamping in the puddle for another ten minutes; but sometimes she may.

In setting the limits, it is important to work out what is really important.

• It does not matter whether she wears the red socks or the pink ones; eats her toast before her cereal; does not eat cabbage; gets down from the table before

you have finished; takes her shoes off; gets her hands in her mashed potato; throws her bath toys out of the bath.

It does matter:
• If she runs away from you while you fold the pushchair to get on the bus.
• Pokes a screwdriver in the power points.
• Spoils her sister's games.
• Pulls your hair constantly.
It may matter:
• If she drinks from the drain.
• Eats berries off any type of tree or bush.
• Throws her sister's puzzle all over the bathroom.

773 Positive

Unacceptable behaviour can be controlled as easily by being positive as by being negative. If she wants to eat some dubious berries, suggest instead that she makes them into a bird cake. Embed them in a ball of lard and hang them from the branch of a tree so the birds can feed on them. Praising her for picking up the puzzle, for stroking your hair and cuddling her sister has to be the major part of her training. Learning what is right is as important as learning what is wrong.

774 She says "No"

• "No, nasty" – and she spits out the medicine.
• "No," and she spits out her peas.
• "No" and she runs away without a nappy.

Sometimes you cannot be consistent. She has to have medicine, but not the peas. Sometimes running off without a nappy can be a game; sometimes it cannot. You have to be very clear why it is, or it is not, today.

775 Tantrums

– Cries for help: even though she is crying "No" and "Go away", she is really saying 'I cannot cope.'

Suppose you have taken your child to visit a friend and she has played with a telephone all afternoon. It is time to go and she wants to take it home with her. You take it from her and she screws up her face and screams; lies on the floor and kicks. Nothing calms her. Eventually you pick her up unceremoniously and dump her, still screaming, in the car.

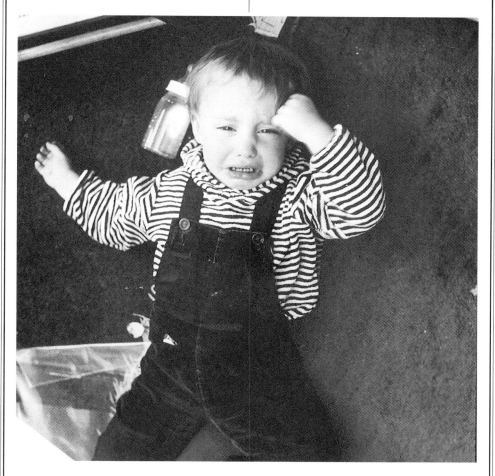

All toddlers have tantrums, some more than others. When a baby cries, you may not always know why, but you respond. When a child has a tantrum, your response cannot be nearly so simple.

You have to try to say two things at once: 'I understand you cannot cope' and 'No matter what, you cannot have your way.' It is no good saying, 'You don't want that telephone.' It is no good collapsing in tears. She needs to know that you are still strong. This is easier said than done, especially in the supermarket queue with everyone looking on.

776 Tantrums: an approach

● Acknowledge her feelings. Say you understand about being angry and afraid; about being small and not quite able to do things. Explain the problem: "Tom will be very unhappy if you take his telephone away."
● Try to find an alternative way of coping with the frustration and anger. Stamp away with her for a while, and tell the bricks how stupid they are to fall over.
● Try to distract her. It sometimes works, expecially if you feel a tantrum brewing and can get in just ahead.
● Don't give in after a tantrum has begun.
● Ignore her. Move the furniture out of the way and leave the room for a while.
● Don't bear grudges. Always make up when it is over, in fact, treat her with warmth and understanding when it subsides.
● Look for an underlying cause. Has she just started nursery school? Talk to her about this; perhaps you are pushing her too hard.
● Are you under stress and trying unsuccessfully to hide it from the child?
● Give her plenty of opportunities to let off steam: bikes, push cars, swimming, rolling down grassy banks, splashing with water sprinklers or garden hoses in summer, stamping in puddles in winter.
● In my first job, we had a frustration bin. All partially broken glassware was collected; when we got to breaking point we could fling it into the bin. See if you can find a similar activity for her.

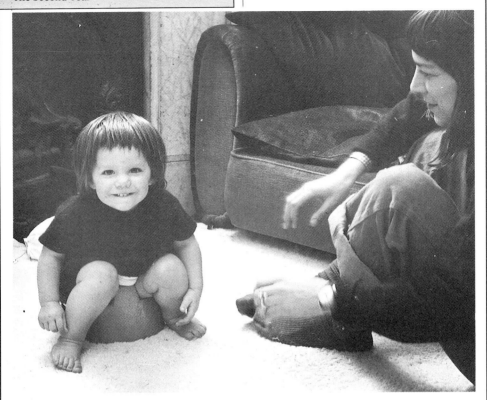

777 Potty training

You can lead a child to the pot but you cannot make her use it. At a year (or less) you might predict correctly that she has a bowel movement at eleven o'clock each morning, catch it and call her a clever girl. But she is not. She is just more predictable in some respects than in others.

Sit her there for long enough, and she is almost bound to pee. Later, when she has more control, she will sit for half an hour and then get up, leaving an empty pot.

However soon you start, she is unlikely to be completely reliable before she is three. However long she seems to need nappies, she is unlikely to need them day or night by the time she is ready for school. Be reassured: bladder and bowel control will come. Some time between about 21 months and her fourth birthday, she will be clean and dry, apart from the occasional accident.

Bowel training often happens before bladder control. A full rectum is easier to control than a full bladder for adults and children alike. By the age of 2½, 90 per cent of girls and 75 per cent of boys will be clean and dry by day. It may be another six months before they achieve night-time control.

Until the body has developed to the point where a child can physically control the muscles of the rectum and bladder, there is little point in expecting her to use a pot.

778 Saving nappies

Forty years ago, potty training began at six months, 20 years ago it started at 11 months, and today it usually begins at 20 months. When I asked my mother about this, she pointed out that 40 years ago she had no washing machine and no means of drying nappies except outside on the washing line. Disposable nappies did not exist, and nappy cleaning services were only available in large towns.

Today, saving nappies is not so much of an issue, and we have the luxury of being able to take into account some of the recent psychological findings about potty training. It is understood, for instance, to be an anxious time for a child; first-born children tend to get the worst of it and are slowest to learn. Parent and child are meeting a new challenge with no training to help them.

Surveys have established, too, that

mothers who are anxious about sex tend to start potty training sooner than mothers who have few sexual hang-ups.

Commonsense indicates that frustration at another wet nappy may be passed to the child just as easily as frustration at not using the pot. Both can make it more difficult to learn.

Or, to put it at its simplest, potty training can easily become a battle of wills; the potty itself can become a symbol of her stubborness and your frustration. She will win in the short term: she has no choice, but to 'win' – she does not have the control to perform for you. In the long term, you may both be losers, since there is a danger of break-down in the close relationship between parent and child. It is not worth it.

779 Anal personality

Early, anxiety-provoking potty training can cause children to retain excrement. Some psychologists believe that this has profound effects on the later personality: that as adults, such children will retain anxiety and emotion within them as they now do excrement; see 783. In order to understand this important theory, and the thinking associated with it, read 780-787.

780 Freud's theory

Freud viewed personality as a largely hidden or unconscious pattern of thought and emotion. He saw behaviour as driven by this unconscious energy, and he thought that the basic ingredients of personality are shaped by crucial childhood experiences.

He believed that personality consisted of three parts: the id, present at birth, and the centre of the libido; the insinctive life force which basically says 'I want it now, and I want it at all costs'. Which is, most parents will acknowledge, an excellent description of a baby in the first year of life.

This basic drive to get what she wants remains part of a child's personality, but because gratification can often be achieved more successfully by planning, talking or asking, rather than by simple demand, the child gradually transfers some energy from the id to the ego.

The ego operates in the real world and it directs us towards satisfying the demands of the id in a rational way. It is the part of the personality that plans, organizes and thinks. In the second year, a child functions with both id and ego.

Only later does the third aspect of personality emerge. This is the super-ego, which oversees both id and ego. It is a sort of moral watchdog which decides how things ought to be: a super-conscience, which we as parents form in our children. It is naturally the source of a great deal of anxiety.

Putting it very simply, the id says 'I want pleasure and I want it it now.'; the ego says 'Be realistic, you are living in fantasy land, this is the real world; I'll see how I can organize it for you.'; and the super-ego says 'You cannot do it that way, let me tell you how it ought to be done.' When conflicts arise between these different parts of personality the result is anxiety. Sometimes the ego is able to handle the anxiety, sometimes it cannot. If it cannot, we resort to defence mechanisms, automatic, unconscious strategies for reducing anxiety.

Defence mechanisms repress the anxiety, rationalize it, and redirect it elsewhere so that instead of dealing with anxiety we merely displace it. All this we do naturally and unconsciously. It is a normal mechanism, a way for the most part of protecting ourselves from everyday anxieties and worries. Only when taken to extremes can the process become neurotic illness.

781 Libido

Freud defined the libido as the motivater of all action; an instinctive source of sexual energy, but not sexual in the literal sense. When he describes the sexual desire of a child for a parent, he is not talking of sexual arousal and passion, more the possessiveness of love and affection. The pleasure of exchanged caresses comes, according to Freud, from the same source as the pleasure in sexual intercourse. But he does not imply that when the child cuddles up to the mother or sucks her breast, he becomes sexually aroused in the way that his father might. The arousal is pre-genital: it produces no erection or genital stimulation.

782 The oral stages

During their first two years, babies suck. The infant finds pleasure in having something in her mouth, be it a nipple, a thumb or a rattle. In this early, oral stage, she is not encumbered by ego or super-ego. She needs constant care because without the help of the ego she cannot organize gratification. She can only cry with rage if it does not come.

If a child's needs are not met or satisfaction is delayed, she will grow up to be pessimistic and mistrusting in adulthood. Freud would say she becomes fixated at this stage, unable to progress to a more mature level of control and organization.

The major problem for the individual fixated at this stage is the inability to love another as an individual. Love in later life is like the love of a baby. A love which does not really differentiate between oneself and the outside world. A tiny baby loves her mother as an extention of herself. An oral-fixated adult loves likewise.

783 The anal stage

The oral stage is followed by a shift in the source of major sensual pleasure to the anus. Sucking is still enjoyed, but anal stimulation is preferred. The child begins to feel pleasure from bowel movements and from holding excrement in the anus. This happens when she becomes capable of controlling her bowel movements.

Freud saw the anal phase as lasting from about two until four. It coincides with the period in which we train our children, praising them for becoming aware of just these feelings. Freud saw the child as loving her faeces, which is why she likes to look at them, play with them, and may even enjoy smearing the bathroom floor with them.

Freud saw difficulties at this stage as leading to problems later in life. Because the child loves and takes pleasure in holding back faeces, so in later life she may become over-possessive and over-retentive to the point of meaness. If parents have been too harsh in potty training, she may become harsh in her concepts of regularity: a slave to the clock, to having everything exactly so.

The ego begins to make its appearance in the anal stage.

784 The phallic stage

By the time she is about four, the area of most intense pleasure moves to the genital region. During this stage, children have intense emotional feelings which are directed at the parent of the opposite sex.

First she loved the breast, then her faeces, now she loves a person. It is partly her growing maturity that enables this.

785 Penis envy – in boys

As the source of gratification moves to the genitals, a boy finds his penis very small compared to his father's; a girl, of course, finds she has no penis at all.

The boy desires the mother, but finds his father a constant competitor, not only is he always in the mother's bed, but he has, to the dismay of his son, a much bigger penis.

This big, strong lover tells the small boy to stop clinging to his mother, and the boy feels fear that he will be blamed and even 'castrated' for desiring his mother. Lying in bed with his mother, he snuggles up to her in a childish sexual advance, which his mother refuses. Only by identifying with his father can the boy, in Freud's opinion, resolve this conflict.

786 Penis envy – in girls

For a girl, the situation is different. She longs for her father, but sees herself as an inadequate rival to her mother. Noticing she has no penis, she believes that it has been cut off in punishment for her desire to replace her mother. The girl imagines that the same thing has happened to her mother, and so, in time, resolves the conflict she feels by identifying with her mother who shares the affliction. She identifies with her in the hope that she, like her mother, will one day have a man of her own. In identifying with the parent of the same sex, the child has a model for later behaviour, a model which enables her to develop a super-ego. A conscience which will give her a strong desire to be 'good' and like her parent.

787 Not convinced?

I have never found the female side of this theory very convincing. If the girl sees herself as already punished (having had her penis cut off), it is not clear why she should wish to resolve the conflict with her mother. Is there any need to do so if punishment is not forthcoming? Nor am I convinced that a girl always sees her mother as a rival for her father's affections. The close tie between mother and child is there for many young girls as it is for their brothers. The jealousy is surely just as likely to be for the possession of the mother as the father.

788 Potty training: sure it is not too soon?

With Freudian thinking on child development in mind, you could, regardless of whether you agree with everything he says, do worse than reflect carefully on whether you and your child ae ready for potty training:

• Are you free from other stresses and strains?
• Will you keep your temper if accidents happen?
• Have you a few sets of quick-release clothes?
• Can you spare the time?
• If it does not work, will you rush her back into nappies?

If you have any doubts, wait. The longer you wait, the quicker it will be over. Many parents find that children are clean and dry within a week: it is just a matter of finding the right week.

789 Ready?

• Does she show signs that she wants to urinate or pass stools?
• Does she let you know if she has urinated or passed stools?
• Does she go at least two hours with a dry nappy?
• Can you ask her to do things?
• Does she know what you mean when you say "Wee-wee" or whatever phrase you use?
• Does she know that you use the lavatory?
• Can she pull her pants down?
• Can she sit on the pot or lavatory seat unassisted?

790 Steady?

She should be able to:
• Stand steadily.
• Balance when sitting.
• Walk forwards and backwards.
• Climb on to a bed and back down again.
• Sit down on the pot (or low chair) and get up by herself.

791 Go

• Let her know the family words: Say "Did you do a pee (or a poo)"? Use the same word and let everyone who is likely to change her know what it is. This is no time to confuse her with different names.
• Dress her in quick-release clothes, or leave her bottom bare if it is warm enough.
• Watch her carefully. She will often give a sign that she is having (or about to have) a bowel movement. Ask her if she is doing a poo, and suggest she uses the potty. Praise, do not scold. Something along the lines of "Are you doing a poo? That's a good girl. Why not sit on the potty?" When she sits, "There's a big girl."
• If you can catch her when she has just urinated it is worth pointing this out to her too. "Did you do a pee? That's a good girl."

The aim is to praise her for becoming aware, not for performing in the right place.
• Let her know that you know you need to use the lavatory: "Wait a minute, Mummy better do a pee before we go to the park."
• Try to get her to sit on the pot for a minute or two, or the lavatory seat if she prefers, before her bath, in the morning and before meals. But it should be her choice. If she will, praise her, otherwise forget it. Boys will probably prefer to stand up "like daddy".
• You now have all the pieces of the jigsaw. The next step is to try to put them together. Wait until you think she is ready to go, and suggest that she uses her potty.
• When she succeeds, praise her in no uncertain terms. Wipe her bottom (give her some paper too); don't rush to flush it away – let her help you to tip it out.
• Wash the pot.
• All wash your hands.
• Praise her if she tells you in advance that she wants the pot, even if she does not get there in time. Don't delay once she tells you; there will be little warning at first.
• Praise her if she tries to pull her pants down.

792 Softly, softly

• Don't force the pace. This is something she must achieve for herself, with your help.
• Don't scold or punish if she fails to perform. Tension will not make it any easier for her to gain control.
• Ignore mistakes. It may be hard if she has just peed all over the carpet or, worse still, someone else's carpet, but shouting helps no one except you.

- Don't overdo the praise. You may hand her a weapon to use against you.
- Don't get too emotionally involved. It is just bowel control.
- Don't compare. It is not her fault if she is a little slower than the girl next door.
- Girls are generally quicker than boys.
- Don't show disgust at the contents of the pot. She is likely to feel you do not want her to perform.
- Don't be surprised if she wants to look at what she has done, or even play with it.
- Don't be surprised if she takes a sudden interest in the lavatory. It is, after all, where you tip the precious contents of the pot. To her it is a good place.
- Never hold a child forcibly on a pot, it will make her tense and afraid.
- Teach her to wash her hands and wipe her bottom. You may need to do it for her as well, but let her try. A girl should be taught to wipe from front to back, in order to stop infections from the bowel entering the vagina. It does not matter how boys wipe themselves.
- Trainer pants may make things easier, especially if the child has developed some control.
- Many children like the feel of a warm, wet nappy. Trainer pants let the urine run down the legs which is less pleasant: the child soon gets cold and uncomfortable.
- It may be worth waiting for warmer weather to try trainer pants. Accidents in the garden are easier to deal with and children usually have fewer clothes to remove.
- For boys and girls, trousers without bibs are quicker to pull down. Dresses are even better.
- She may be frightened of falling into the lavatory bowl. Stay with her if she is nervous.
- Some children may like to use the lavatory with or without a child's seat because it makes them feel 'big'.

793 Dry at night
This comes last of all, often not until the child is at least two-and-a-half. Ten or 12 hours of sleep is a long time for a child to control her bladder.

The moment to leave the nappy off is when you find that it is dry most mornings. Once she has shed her night-time nappy you may need, however, to put her on the pot before you go to bed, and especially if she still sucks a bottle before going to sleep. If she uses a pot, you can

put it by her bed. Make sure there is enough light for her to see what she is doing. Be prepared for mistakes.
- Put a plastic cover on the mattress. If mistakes happen, it might be sensible to use an old cot sheet as a draw sheet. Under this put a small plastic sheet: see the illustration. If there is an accident, you have to remove only the small plastic sheet and the draw sheet during the night.
- Make it as easy as possible for her to use the pot. All-in-one zip-up suits are fine for babies in nappies, but are much too difficult to get off quickly at night.
- Don't get angry or upset when she wets the bed. Many children still have the occasional accident even after they have started school.

794 Late control
Some children don't gain control of bowel or bladder until well after their third birthday. You may find it reassuring to consult your doctor about this if she is still in nappies by day after her third birthday, or still in nappies during the night at five.

795 Moving on to the lavatory
Some children never use a pot, progressing straight to the lavatory. A special, fitting child seat will make this less daunting.

Most lavatory bowls are too high for a toddler unless there is something to help her up. She will need a step to reach the wash basin, too.

You can teach a boy to stand at the lavatory: encourage him to aim into the water, but be prepared for mistakes. His aim will not always be good, especially when he is in a hurry. Place a sheet of polythene on the floor behind the lavatory bowl and cover it with a towel.

796 Persistent bed wetting
Many children continue throughout childhood to wet the bed occasionally. It often happens because a child is sick, upset, or if there is a change in lifestyle: a new school or a new baby, perhaps. It is quite common for a child to regress to an earlier stage of bowel control in these circumstances.

Treat it in a matter-of-fact way. She will probably be upset and embarassed: there is no need to make her feel worse. She will grow out of it.

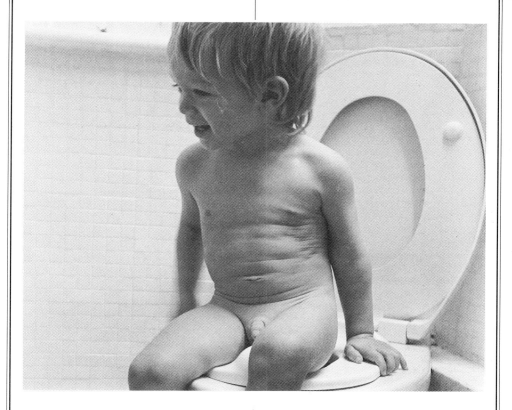

797 Letting off steam

It seems to be as necessary to a child as breathing or eating. Nursery school teachers often claim that the only thing to do after a wet weekend is to get out the bikes and let the children race about for half an hour. Only then are peaceful activities possible.

Developmental psychology has no certain theories on why explosive play is so necessary. It is the one universal form of play, seen not only in primates such as monkeys and apes but in all mammals: cats, dogs, even mice. Some suggest it is needed for normal social development (autistic children do not play like this), others for normal physical growth. A trip to the park, a boisterous time at the swimming pool, a game of wrestling on the floor, a few tickles or chasing her around the settee seem to be a necessary part of each day.

798 Graduating to a bed

Most children move from cot to bed during their second year. It gives them, of course, the freedom to get up and run about exactly when they want to.

Not only that, but they can also play or come and slip quietly into bed beside you.

799 No locks

Once she is in a bed, the only way to be sure of keeping a child in her room is to lock the door.

This is wrong; it is cruel to imprison a two-year-old. She has to learn to control her behaviour reasonably and this cannot be achieved by imposing barriers.

You may be able to teach a child to knock on your bedroom door, or to wait until you call her before coming into your room. If you lay out a little surprise in her room the night before, perhaps a drink and a game to play, you can delay the patter of tiny feet next morning.

If mornings without her are especially important to you, you will have to be firm but reasonable, taking her back to her room until it is time to get up.When the time comes, as it always should, make her very welcome.

Lying in bed listening to childrens' elaborate games of pretence is one of the joys of parenthood which will remain with me always.

800 Bed time

• Establish a routine: bed at the same time every night. But give children a warning so that games can be finished off. "Ten more

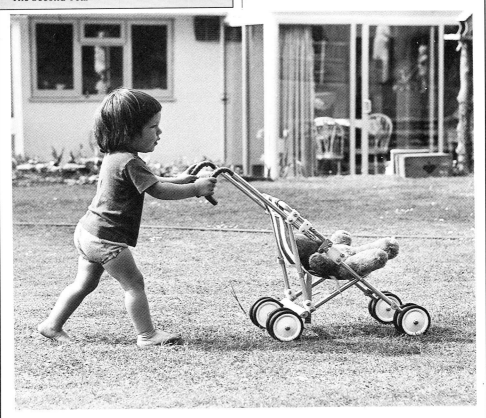

minutes", then "Five more minutes", then bed, 'ready or not'.

● The rule is about bed time, not sleep time. Let children look at books and play in their room until they are ready for sleep.
● Children are best sharing a bedroom when they are small, for they provide each other with company night and morning.
● A nightly ritual of a cuddle, a song and a chat about the day are important in developing a feeling of closeness and security before sleep. Later a child should have a story. Such rituals should continue until she is ready to give them up.
● Once she enjoys stories, listening to story-tapes (pre-recorded, or of you reading) can be very soothing, especially on long summer evenings.

801 Night fears

Many children are afraid of the dark. There is no reason why your child has to sleep in a pitch black room. A night light, a dimmer switch or leaving her door open and the landing light on make sense for a small child. This will enable her to see to get up in the night and come to you if she feels ill or afraid. She can also get a drink for herself or use her pot, and so can become independent more easily.

802 Nightmares

Nightmares will not begin until your child has imagination; until her language and memory are mature enough to hold fear. They will start at about three, a time when children develop many fears of monsters, snakes and spiders.

She will often treat her day-time fears with her own form of psychotherapy: pretend play. You will find her playing (and laughing) at monsters in the day, while at night she has fears and bad dreams.

It is not abnormal. If you had a phobia about going on buses, a psychiatrist would treat it in much the same way. You would be asked to think about (and later experience) buses while relaxing and feeling happy.

There is little you can do for a child in the grip of a nightmare except hold her and comfort her. Don't leave her until it is over.

If nightmares happen every night, and if she sleepwalks, you should take active steps to identify the source of the anxiety and reduce it. This is easier said than done, of course; the most practical way to tackle it is to find another parent who has had a similar problem.

Often, a child will push and hit out at you in a dream. Ignore what she says and does: it is not you she hits, or screams at.

When I was a child, my mother used to put a little cloth over my pillow to keep the 'nasty things' away after a night terror. I still remember the security and calmness it brought me, and it did the same for my own children. The cloth should be put on the pillow after the nightmare. It cannot, of course, really prevent a nightmare, but if the child is relaxed and happy going back to sleep, the night terror will not return.

803 Time for another?

Mothers who choose to have a small age gap between their children tend to say it is good to get nappies, broken nights and bottles out of the way as quickly as possible. But it is hard work while it lasts.

Your view of the ideal age gap between children may well spring from your own childhood, reflecting, perhaps, what did not happen as much as what did.

From the point of view of a mother's health, it is probably best to leave a couple of years before having another baby. This gives plenty of time for the uterus and vagina to get back into shape, and for the body to get back into balance after breast feeding.

A gap of under nine months, and there is a slightly higher chance of miscarriage, probably because the cervix dilates more easily, although no one is entirely sure why it is so.

How well you are able to cope physically with two children is another important consideration, and this is influenced by several factors. A child who is slow to walk and heavy to lift is obviously more tiring to cope with in late pregnancy. A wakeful toddler is also a disincentive to having another baby too soon. There is little point in hoping that the second baby will sleep better than the first: the odds are that he will not.

In a second pregnancy there is, statistically, less chance of morning sickness and of pre-eclampsia, but there is no guarantee of how you will feel in any pregnancy. See also 506-512.

804 At 21 months

She is walking down stairs holding the rail. You offer her a hand. She says "No" – it is one of her favourite words. She sits down on the bottom step, picks up a toy car and pushes it back and forth saying "Brmmm" to herself. She looks up at you and says "Car". Then, as if this reminds her, she gets up and walks into the kitchen where her sit-and-ride car is waiting. Sitting on it, she scoots rapidly around the room.

805 Small space

Before your first child reaches two, she will begin to feel the confinement of a small space, especially if you have no garden or nearby park. A small space can, however, be made more interesting:

- An obstacle course for a bike can be made by rearranging the furniture.
- Beds make occasional trampolines.
- Chase her around the sofa.
- Catch her as she jumps from the table.
- Let her a swing from a hook in the ceiling, or fix a swing in the doorway.
- Push her around in a cardboard box.
- Put a large sheet of polythene over the carpet for messy play with sand, water and playdough. Encourage her to paint. She will need only one colour at this age.

806 Readjustment

An active toddler can wind up even the calmest parent. Having tuned yourself to a dependent baby and learned to love her, it is not always easy to let go, to allow her new independence. You learned in her first year to mould your life around her so that there was a balance of caring for her and for yourselves. Now, to some extent, you begin this process all over again.

807 Assertiveness

A mind of her own; strong willed; a real charmer. It is what many of us want of our children, but in the short term it can be pretty hard to live with. As she pushes and demands, it is sometimes hard not to feel a little envy at how she gets her way. Would it not be good if life were so easy for you?

Well, you may not actually feel that, but certainly her brothers and sisters do. Teasing, taunting, over-stimulating her are ways of undermining that assertiveness when they have had enough of it.

See 506-512. If you get depressed at the inevitability of jealousy between your children, remind yourself that even as they are jealous, they can support each other. Your best and only means of combating jealousy is to foster this supportiveness; to accept the jealousy and to continue to love and support even the jealous child.

808 Over-control

As a child emerges from babyhood it is easy to over-mould her to be the person you want, or the person you wanted to be.

If you want her to be bright you may encourage her when she looks at books, and deny her desire to play with her doll. How many mothers say "I'm not going to buy her any girls' toys"?

It is possible to deny a child's individuality. Then, to break free from your bonds, she may refute all that you have hoped for her. Or she may go through life looking for someone or something that will take away that pressure.

An attitude of over-control may be a reflection of your own fears at her growing independence. Or it may be that you are just bossy. If you let her, she may rebel; or she may, perhaps, go through life waiting for others to take over.

If you are aware of being bossy, it makes sense consciously to practise giving her the lead. There should be times when you hold your tongue and sit on your hands while she works it out for herself. You might even encourage her to tell you not to interfere.

809 Fearful

Suddenly finding yourself in charge of a person with her own ideas awakens many emotions. You admire her, take pride in her independence, but at the same time may feel a little rejected and abandoned. The more intense the relationship, the more difficult it is to let go.

But the intensity cannot go on for ever if those involved are to be separate people. You have moved from the intense, inward-looking phase of being in love with your partner to a broader, more outward love, which is less blinkered, more accepting of each other as people. So also you must move from the intensity of that first parental love into acceptance of your child as a person.

Sometimes she will move too quickly for you. Must this delightfully straightforward love come to an end so soon? Of course, it does not cease but slowly changes. Your child still needs you, although the need is now different.

A sense of loss at her babyhood disappearing is natural, and she too may well feel it.

810 Over-protective?

Ask yourself how many times she has thrown you into panic today. If the answer is 'often', you are probably in danger of being over-protective. Maybe you should make a point of asking other parents what they think is normal. You need to match the level of protection to the child.

811 Your régime

Freedom or restriction: from now on, getting the balance right is one of the hardest things asked of you.

I suspect that you will make fewest mistakes if you remind yourself that since you are asking her to fit in with you, it is reasonable to fit in with her as well. It is unreasonable for her to play in the sink while you are cooking; it is unreasonable of you to expect her to stay quiet for two hours while you work.

Never doubt, though, that a child needs limits. Without them, she cannot learn to organize her behaviour. You do her no favours by being excessively liberal or excessively restricting. It does not matter if your régime is different from what you observe in other families, as long as you are striving for a balance. Children will develop under many different styles of management. Consistency is as important, or even more important, than the boundaries you set. Example is important too; see 771.

812 The terrible twos

They can hit you at any time between 18 months and three years.

"No": she will not wear that dress.

"No": she will not go in her pushchair.

"No": she will not hold your hand, wear a coat, clean her teeth.

But do they have to be terrible?

A child needs to experiment and play with *everything* she learns – that includes anger and belligerence. How else is she to learn control? How else is she to understand her emotions?

So much happens to her in this period. She becomes so much more independent, yet she is still also very dependent on her family. She becomes much more capable, physically and mentally, of doing things for herself and understanding what goes on around her. Yet she is still quite clumsy.

It is difficult to know when she needs your help, since she probably does not even know herself much of the time. She is experimenting with ways of seeing and feeling and it is not surprising that sometimes the experiment gets out of hand, that sometimes her concept of the world breaks down. At times she will need love and reassurance, the security of your embrace. But before accepting it, she may lie on the floor and kick in frustration.

813 Gardening

When really depressed about the terrible twos, you might try looking at this phase as weeds growing in a flowerbed. That the weeds grow at all reflects the richness of the soil – a richness which enables trees and shrubs to grow too. It is because she can grow that she can be frustrated. It is because you have fostered her security that she can reach out independently. It is because you have given her confidence that she sometimes reaches too far. It is because you have allowed her curiosity that she now has the confidence to test your patience. It is because you have set limits that she can now test them.

814 Parents disagree

If you are really close to someone you inevitably come into conflict.

Parents bring their own past histories into a marriage, and that includes their own experience of childcare. Maybe they agree with their parents' ideals, maybe they disagree violently, but they cannot help being influenced: two parents, two histories and perhaps two very different philosophies of child rearing.

Sometimes it is possible to compromise, sometimes it is possible to agree to differ, sometimes you each hold out for your own ideals. Pretending that disagreements will go away may in the end cause more problems than it solves, especially if the disagreements concern children.

Suppose you have a basic disagreement about smacking children. How do you solve it? You could agree to disagree, but where does that leave the child?

- With mummy smacking and daddy thinking it is a bad idea?
- With mummy smacking and daddy opting out of childcare?
- With one parent reluctantly fitting in with the other, but never talking about it?

Whatever you do, it can be harmful for the child:
- An inconsistent approach leaves the child not knowing how to respond, and with no model for her behaviour.
- A prolonged and unsolved disagreement will be noticed by the child. She may not know why you are angry, but she will know that you are. If your anger arises over attempts to discipline her, she may well feel that she is the cause of your anger. She will feel puzzled and confused; if the conflict persists, she may become anxious and insecure. A child of four can understand that people can disagree and still love each other. A child of two cannot.

The only reasonable course of action is to come to a family decision. However difficult, you must do it. Suppose, for instance, you disagree on when to smack a child for getting out of bed. One of you says smack the first time, the other says let her downstairs for five minutes, then, having got her back to bed, only one more chance.

How do you compromise? The realistic answer is probably that you cannot. In this kind of deadlock, it is generally best to try to solve the conflict by entirely different means. For instance, why not agree both to spend say ten out of 14 evenings during the next fortnight at home, establishing a new routine: letting the child stay up a little later than usual perhaps, and rewarding her for co-operation?

Quarrels cannot be forgotten when a baby arrives, but it is better not to quarrel in front of a child. This is especially true as she approaches the terrible twos. While she is saying no to you, she needs you to be saying yes to each other.

815 Not like an adult

In reflecting on 814, bear in mind that she will not think as you do for many years. Her world is seen only from her point of view. She will talk to you as if you share her thoughts, as if you are always with her, as if you look out of her eyes.

At three, a child is likely to come home from playgroup and say "You know that

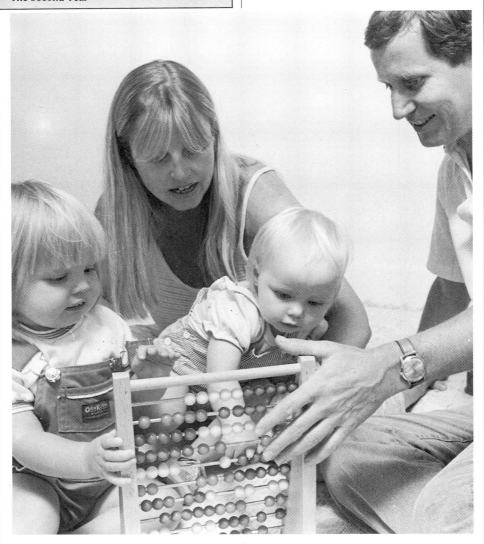

boy?" assuming that you do. Or ask out of the blue "Is it a red car?".

She will sit looking at a book and assume you see what she sees, even when you are in the next room. She is egocentric: she sees herself as the centre of all things.

Another characteristic of her thinking is that she behaves as if objects are alive. Her toys 'would like to go in the bath', a chair 'is naughty' when she bangs her knee, the moon can peep at her through the gap in the curtains.

She thinks that crimes can be measured by the extent of the damage, not the intent. So a girl who drops a bottle of milk while helping her mother is much naughtier than a girl who deliberately spills a little milk from her cup.

816 Confusions

She will think:

● There is more playdough when it is rolled into a ball because it looks like more. If you bang the ball down flat, she will think there is less.
● She will think there is more water in a tall glass than a short, fat one. Even if you pour the water from the short glass to the tall, she will not see that it is the same amount. She may not even see this at six years.
● She will think six buttons in a long line are more buttons that six in a short line.
● She knows that objects are constant, but she does not yet realize that some things can change, yet remain essentially the

same. That if you pour water from one glass to another of a different size, for instance, the amount of water stays the same.

Her reasoning is primitive and intuitive. If she sees two things happen, she assumes that one causes the other. She may think that the sunshine makes her leg hurt, or that because she has not had breakfast, it cannot be morning.

817 Emotions

She can feel loss and sadness, love and security, pleasure, assertiveness, anger, and curiosity. Watch her express them in her play:

● Dependency and security as she cares for her dolls and teddy bears.
● Pleasure as she laughs and smiles.
● Curiosity as she opens every door.
● Assertiveness as she says "No" for the tenth time this morning.
● Anger as she throws a block across the room because her tower has toppled over yet again.

One consequence of her not thinking as you do is that she does not always understand your explanations.

If you say "Please be quiet, I have a headache", can she understand? To do so, she has to put herself in your shoes, something she cannot do before she is about four or five.

It would be better to say "Shouting makes my head hurt" or "Jenny, shouting makes my head hurt" since children seem to understand better when their name is used.

Because children under four cannot do things in a systematic way, there is no point in asking them to search systematically for a lost glove or shoe. And there is no point in expecting them to understand that throwing a cup on the floor is just as naughty whether the cup breaks or not.

818 Second birthday

She is probably naming objects, and may even begin to lure you into conversations with "What's that?" Her language is no longer a novelty.

She plays with a new sophistication. She can have objects stand for other things, as words do. She begins to pretend. She sits

on the bus (really a kitchen chair), guided by her brother and drives them to town.

She will climb the steps to go down the slide, or perhaps climb out of her cot. She is no longer a baby; she is a talking, thinking child.

819 Parenthood at two

Many women feel that motherhood divides them from the person they were before, but at the same time brings them completeness. For many, it means far more time spent in the society of other women; a society based on closeness and support. Sisterhood is a word understood by many women with small children: the social and emotional tie produced by shared experience.

There is no equivalent brotherhood of men. Few ever mention the emotional aspects of their relationship with their children or, indeed, discuss fatherhood with other men.

The world at large goes on, as ever, by taking parenthood for granted. "What do you do?" "I'm a mother." And the conversation moves on to another topic. Those without children cannot know that raising them is a job – and moreover one with as great a potential for fascination as any other.

820 The talisman

Family life changes slowly, as you would expect of such an ancient institution. But evolving it is, and fatherhood in particular is today a more wholehearted affair than it was a generation ago. How far it may still develop is hard to tell, for society is not organized for complete sharing of parental roles. It does seem, however, that modern ideas on fatherhood are slowly but surely eating away at the taboo on tenderness as a masculine emotion.

One thing about families no one, I believe, would ever want to change: their way of being, and bringing, all things: joy, sorrow, pleasure and pain. Raising a family is the most creative thing that most of us do, although it is, at times, the most banal. It is certainly extravagant in time and money, yet to regret it is absurd.

The ability of family life to reconcile these contradictions is surely its most formidable strength – one you can hardly fail to pass on to your children. A gift to the future which your parents passed to you, and which they received from countless generations before them.

Medical Section

Advice is given in most entries on when to call to doctor. If still in doubt, see page 285.

Cross references simply as numerals refer to numbered paragraphs in the book's four main sections. Where cross references are given as page numbers they refer to text boxes, illustration panels or features in the four main sections.

Adenoids
Lymphoid tissue which 'stands guard' at the nose to keep infection at bay. Enlarged adenoids can make breathing difficult and lead to repeated ear trouble.

Symptoms
- Breathing through the mouth.
- Repeated middle ear infections.
- Permanently blocked nose.

What to do
- Ask to be referred to an ear, nose and throat specialist.
- Removal of the adenoids may be recommended. This may be carried out with or without the removal of the tonsils.

Allergy
Our bodies protect us from the millions of potentially harmful micro-organisms in the atmosphere by manufacturing antibodies to keep the invaders at bay.

An individual who is allergic makes antibodies which fight harmless as well as harmful substances.

Any substance which the body treats as harmful is called an allergen and it causes an allergic response. Fluid builds up in tissue causing swelling and sometimes muscle spasm. Grass pollen and the house dust mite are common allergens.

Asthma and **hay fever** are perhaps the commonest allergic responses in children. A few children have more than one allergy and there is a strong tendency for allergic responses to run in families, although the type of allergy may differ. You may have hay fever, your child **eczema**, your sister asthma. Allergic response can also change within your lifetime. You may have eczema as a baby, asthma as a child and hay fever as an adult. The allergens which start these responses can change too. An allergy can develop without warning after exposure to an allergen.

Infections play a part too; many young children have attacks of asthma every time they have a cold but remain relatively free of attacks between illnesses. Emotional stress also plays a role in some allergic responses.

Appendicitis
An inflammation of the appendix, a small, dead-end tube on the right-hand side of the lower abdomen, at the point where the large and small intestine meet.

Appendicitis is the most common reason for an emergency operation in children; the operation is called an appendicectomy.

Symptoms
- Abdominal pain, which starts around the navel and moves to the lower right-hand side of the abdomen.
- Fever.

- Vomiting.
- Loss of appetite.
- Sometimes diarrhoea or constipation.

What to do
- If you suspect appendicitis, call the doctor immediately. It is not dangerous in itself, but if it is left untreated an appendix can burst, causing peritonitis, which is more serious.

Asthma
An allergic condition which affects the lungs. It occurs because of the reaction of the child's antibodies to an allergen or allergens in the bronchi, which become blocked with mucus and go into spasm, causing breathing problems.

The allergen (see **allergy**) is usually breathed in but can be produced by allergic responses to foods or by other factors including exercise and emotional upset. In young children, asthma frequently occurs when the child is suffering from a cold or some other illness.

Common allergens are: house dust mite; pollen; animal hair; feathers; food; infections; air-borne spores.

Asthma was rarely diagnosed in the past and was often called 'wheezy bronchitis'. It is diagnosed more commonly today.

Symptoms
- Breathing difficulty.
- Wheezing.
- Using both chest and stomach in the attempt to push air out.
- Labouring over each breath.
- Pale face and blue lips. Breathing difficulties can be aggravated by the child panicking.

What to do
Attacks often take place at night and can vary from a slight wheeze to a dramatic gasping for breath. You should seek medical advice:
- On the first occasion your child has an attack.
- If the attack is more severe than normal.

The doctor will prescribe a bronchodilator, which works by relaxing the walls of the air passages. This is usually given first as a syrup, then, if this is ineffective, via an inhaler. In cases of severe asthma in a child too young to use an inhaler, you may be advised to obtain a portable nebulizer, which delivers a substantial dose in the form of a fine mist through a face mask. The doctor may also prescribe drugs taken orally to help prevent further attacks.

If the attack is severe the child will go into hospital for a few days. A physiotherapist can help with breathing and relaxation exercises.

Asthma is a chronic illness, but there is a fair chance that a child will grow out of it. Or asthma may be replaced by hay fever as the child reaches puberty.

See also **bronchitis**.

Anaemia
Anaemia is caused by a reduction in the number of red blood cells in the body, by a change in their shape, or by a reduction in haemoglobin. It may be caused by lack of iron, poor diet, or excessive blood loss. Ir it may be due to the bone marrow producing inadequate red blood cells, as in a disease such as **leukaemia** or by the inherited anaemias (sickle cell anaemia and beta-thalassaemia).

Both sickle cell anaemia and thalassaemia are genetic disorders in which the red blood cells are an abnormal shape and are thus inefficient carriers of oxygen. Sickle cell anaemia is found most often in people of Afro-Carribean origin, thalassaemia in those of Cypriot, Italian and Greek origin.

Symptoms
• Pale skin, most noticeable on fingertips, lips, around the eyes and on the tongue.
• Extreme tiredness, often weakness.
• Breathlessness after exertion.
• Dizziness.
• Raised pulse rate.

What to do
• Anaemia always needs attention. You should see a doctor, who will take a blood sample to confirm the diagnosis and may then refer your child to a specialist.
• You may be advised to increase the child's intake of iron, both in the diet and by supplements.
• In severe cases your child may have to go into hospital for investigation and perhaps a blood transfusion.

Appetite loss
Loss of appetite is not in itself an illness, but it is generally a sign of impending ill health. If your child has been 'off her food' for 24 hours, she is almost certainly sickening for something.

What to do
• Feel her forehead or take her temperature.
• Examine her throat – eating may hurt her if she has tonsilitis.
• Has she got a runny nose or other cold symptoms?
• Check her abdomen for pain.
• After 24 hours without eating, see a doctor even if there are no other symptoms (unless there is an obvious cause, such as diarrhoea, vomiting or flu, which you feel capable of treating yourself).

Arthritis
An inflammation of the joints caused by injury, infection, some viruses (such as German measles or glandular fever) or, more rarely, by rheumatic diseases such as Still's disease or rheumatic fever. Arthritis only occasionally affects children.

Symptoms
• Any painful inflammation of a joint.
• Aches and pains all over the body (similar to those with influenza).

What to do
• If your child has a high or fluctuating temperature, or painful or swollen joints, see a doctor. If the symptoms persist, he or she will refer the child to a specialist.
• The pain of arthritis is soothed by keeping the joint warm, say with a hot water bottle.
• A cold compress will reduce swelling. ·
• Help your child with any special exercises suggested by the consultant.
• Swimming is often recommended.

Athlete's foot
Athlete's foot is a fungal infection that affects the soft areas of the foot between the toes. It is contagious and is usually picked up by walking with bare feet in a public place. The fungus grows best in warm, damp conditions; sweaty feet are the ideal environment.

Symptoms
• Particularly white skin at the base of, or underneath, the toes which peels off in lumps.
• These areas are itchy and, if rubbed, will leave raw red patches.
• Thick yellow toenails, especially in advanced cases.

What to do
• Treat the area with an antifungal cream and foot powder.
• Change your child's socks every day and don't let other children use her towel.

Bedwetting
A common childhood problem: as many as one in four children aged between four and 16 wet the bed at some time or another, though less frequently after the age of ten. The problem is more common in boys than girls.

It is thought that in some children the problem is caused simply by bladder control being slow to mature. There is often a family history in such cases. In other children, who do not usually wet the bed, there is either an organic cause, such as a urinary tract infection, or an abnormality of the urinary system, or, more commonly, a psychological cause, such as stress at home or school. If bedwetting is accompanied by increased thirst and frequent urination, this could indicate diabetes.

What to do
• Reduce stress, give cuddles and comfort before bedtime. Read stories, and do everything to make bedtime relaxed.
• Put a rubber sheet on the bed and cover it with a light top sheet that can be washed easily.
• Try to make light of the problem: making your child anxious will only make the problem worse. See 796.
• Make sure she empties her bladder before going to bed. Reducing fluid intake after 6 pm can sometimes help.
• Check whether the urine has a fishy smell, as this is a sign of a urinary tract infection. If it does, see a doctor. See page 207.
• You can have a pad fitted to the bed that sets off an alarm when she begins to urinate. This can be successful in teaching a child to recognize a full bladder.
• Sometimes the problem arises because the child cannot retain urine. Encourage her to hold on for as long as possible after she feels she needs to go. Measure how much urine she passes. Once she can hold 12-14 fluid oz (300-350 ml) bedwetting should be reduced.
• The child may lack control of her pelvic floor muscles. Teach her to stop urinating in mid-flow and then start again. As her muscles strengthen, so her night-time control may increase.

Bites
In general, bites are not serious although they can be extremely painful and often distress the child. Animal bites tend to leave puncture marks, while insect bites leave a weal with a white centre and red base, similar to that found with hives.

What to do

● Wash the site of an animal bite under cold running water, dry it and apply a dry adhesive dressing. In areas where rabies exists, take the child to hospital if she is bitten by a wild or stray animal.
● Inspect the site next day to ensure no infection has developed. If it has, see a doctor.
● For insect bites, calamine lotion can reduce the swelling and irritation. Watch for severe allergic reaction.
● If you suspect that your child has been bitten by fleas, use an anti-flea powder to dust around the house, especially on carpets, and dust your pet too.
● Use an insect repellant if your child gets bitten by mosquitoes.
● If an animal bite has punctured the skin, see a doctor; if deep, the child may need a tetanus injection.
● She will also need medical attention if a wound is bleeding heavily, or if it becomes swollen and infected.

Bleeding

If the blood vessels are damaged in any way, bleeding will result. How heavy the bleeding is depends upon the vessel that is damaged – cutting a major vein or artery is extremely serious, whereas cutting a tiny capillary vessel is trivial. Bleeding can also be internal, in which case there may be no immediate symptoms apart from thirst and weakness.

Severe bleeding is, of course, an emergency: ring for an ambulance at once. It can rapidly lead to physiological **shock**.

What to do

● Apply pressure directly to the wound with a clean pad, to help stem the bleeding.
● Raise the wound as high as you can above the heart, which will slow down the bleeding.
● Lie the child down, so that blood will still flow easily to major organs and to the brain.
● Tie a dressing securely over the wound. If bleeding is severe, use anything you have on hand: a tie, a cloth belt or a scarf.
● Get to hospital as quickly as possible.
For minor injuries, see **cuts and grazes**.

Blepharitis

See eye infection.

Blisters

Blisters are an accumulation of fluid under the skin, often caused by burning or rubbing. They are nature's form of protection while the body repairs itself. The outer layer of skin separates from the inner, and fluid from the inner layer seeps out, to be reabsorbed later. The dead outer layer then falls away, leaving a new layer of skin beneath.

What to do

● A blister should be left intact.
● Simply cover it with gauze and a plaster.
● If it bursts, keep it clean and cover with a gauze dressing.
● If blisters becomes infected or are the result of a scald or sunburn, see a doctor.

Boils

Skin hair grows from a root to the skin surface along a hair follicle. When this becomes blocked, an infection can develop. Near the surface this causes a spot or pimple, but when it occurs at the root it produces a boil. A boil comes to a head within three days, and bursts to allow the pus to escape.

A single boil is not serious, but if the infection spreads a whole area can be affected. And if the bacteria get into the bloodstream, blood poisoning can result.

Symptoms

● A large, painful red lump, which may or may not have a head.
● A growing tenderness, especially if the boil develops over a bony area such as the jaw.

What to do

● Don't let your child touch the affected area.
● Wash the area gently with either surgical spirit or lightly salted warm water.
● Don't squeeze the boil, however tempting it may be, as this could lead to bacteria entering the bloodstream, or could spread the infection to the surrounding area.
● Once the boil has burst, keep the area as clean as possible.
● If the boil does not come to a head, or if your child seems in much pain, see a doctor, who may lance it.
● If red streaks radiate out from the boil, this could mean the infection is spreading. See a doctor, who may: prescribe an antibiotic if the infection has spread; prescribe an antiseptic to add to a bath if there are several boils; if the boils are recurrent, do tests to discover if there is an underlying cause.

Broken bones

The most common type of break in young children is a greenstick fracture, where the bone bends but does not actually break. A simple fracture is when the bone breaks in one place only; in a compound fracture, there is damage to surrounding tissue and the bone may even protrude through the skin.
It is not always obvious that a bone is broken.

Symptoms

● Check for swelling or bruising around any injury.
● Check that a child is able to move the affected area without pain: excessive pain may indicate problems. If there is reason to suspect damage, take her for an X-ray.
● Any deformation should be X-rayed.

What to do.

● If the bone is sticking through the skin, don't attempt to move her. Call an ambulance.
● If there is a wound, just put a sterile cloth over it.
● Where the bone is not sticking through the skin, try and immobilize the joint by using a sling for an arm or tying the knees and ankles together.
● Keep your child as warm and calm as possible. But don't give her anything to eat or drink as she may require a general anaesthetic. If there is a compound fracture a general anaesthetic *will* be necessary, as the bone will need to be manipulated into place.
● If the leg is badly broken the child may need to stay in hospital for traction.
● If plaster is applied, try and keep it as dry and clean as possible.

Bronchiolitis

This is caused by a virus inflaming the smallest airways of the lungs, the bronchioles. It usually occurs in babies under a year old and can often start as a cough or common cold. The lining of the bronchioles swells up and begins to produce mucus, which causes breathing difficulties. It can be a serious condition, in which breathing becomes badly strained.

Symptoms
- Rapid, laboured breathing.
- Difficulty taking feeds from breast or bottle.
- Drawing in the skin between the ribs and the stomach muscles with each breath.
- Sometimes, noisy breathing or wheezing.
- Cough.
- Fever.
- Blue around mouth.
- Drowsiness.

What to do
- Soothe your baby, as crying worsens the breathing problems.
- Make sure she has plenty of fluid.
- Check temperature and control fever by sponging and giving paracetamol syrup.
- If there is any blueness about the lips, or breathing becomes laboured, call the doctor urgently.
- If you think your baby may have bronchiolitis she should in any case be checked by a doctor. Hospital admission may be necessary.

Bronchitis

Bronchitis is an inflammation of the membranes of the larger airways, the bronchi. The lining of the bronchi swell and produce mucus, and it is the presence of the mucus which makes breathing difficult. The infection can be caused by a virus or bacteria and often follows other infections.

Symptoms
- Fever.
- Cough that produces phlegm.
- Rapid breathing and wheezing.
- Loss of appetite.
- Vomiting if much phlegm is swallowed.

What to do
- Call a doctor.
- Control fever by sponging and giving paracetamol syrup.
- Encourage her to cough up the phlegm. This may be easier if you put her, face down, across your knee and pat her back when she coughs.
- Don't suppress coughing with cough mixtures.
- Keep the air moist by boiling an electric kettle with the lid off every hour.
- Give plenty of liquids.
- Keep her propped up in bed. This makes breathing easier.
- Keep calm, and keep her relaxed.
- Bacterial bronchitis can be treated with antibiotics.
- Occasionally a child with bronchitis will need hospitalization.
  See also **asthma**.

Bruise

A bruise appears when the blood vessels under the skin are broken by a blow. The area at first looks red, then turns a bluish-black. After ten to 14 days the bruise disappears: escaped blood is broken down and reabsorbed.

Symptoms
- A purplish or red mark that eventually fades to yellow/green.
- Tenderness.
- Swelling, especially if over a bone.

What to do
- Minor bruising needs no treatment.
- Apply a cold compress to extensive bruising in order to reduce the swelling.
- If pain increases over the injured area after 24 hours, this could indicate a broken bone: see a doctor.
- If bruising occurs frequently, and without apparent cause, it could be due to leukaemia or haemophilia: see a doctor.

Burns

Superficial burns damage the top layers of skin; intermediate and deep burns involve the blood vessels and nerves below, causing serum to escape. In a minor burn a blister will appear, filled with this serum. In cases where the skin is completely burnt off, the serum weeps freely from the wound. This can cause rapid dehydration and physiological shock if the area is extensive. It is most important that burns are treated quickly, but the actual treatment depends on the severity of the burn.

Symptoms
- Blistering of the skin.
- A raw, sticky red area.
- In an electrical burn, a small blackened area will appear where the current touched the skin.

What to do
Superficial burns:
- Cool the burnt area by placing it under cold running water for a few minutes.
- Don't burst the blister.
- Don't apply cream or ointment to the affected area.
- Cover the area with a sterile dressing. Hold a cold compress over the area to reduce pain.
- Give paracetamol syrup to ease the pain.
- If a superficial burn has not healed within a week, see a doctor.

Deep burns
- Flood the burnt area by holding it under a cold running water for several minutes, or as long as the child can stand it.
- Remove clothes contaminated by chemicals as soon as possible. Remove clothing soaked in boiling fluids after it has started to cool under the running tap. BUT IF ANYTHING STICKS TO THE BURN, DO NOT REMOVE IT.
- If a child gets an electric shock, turn the mains off or knock her away with a non-conducting material such as a wooden broom handle.
- Call an ambulance if it is impractical to get the child to hospital yourself.
- Cover the area to prevent infection. Don't apply any creams.
- Lie your child down with her legs raised and her head to one side. This keeps the blood flowing to the vital organs and reduces shock.
- If a superficial burn has not healed in a week, see a doctor.

Catarrh

During a cold, measles or influenza, there is a build-up of mucus in the nose and throat properly called catarrh. This runs down into the throat, perhaps causing the child to cough, and if much is swallowed, the child may vomit.

Symptoms
- Nasal congestion, causing the child to breath through her mouth.
- A discharge from the nose.
- Vomiting when the mucus is swallowed.

What to do
- Encourage the child to blow her nose regularly.
- Prop your child up on pillows if catarrh running into her throat causes her to cough at night: this will reduce the amount she swallows.
- Don't try to clear her nose with a cotton wool swab.
- Don't use decongestants unless your doctor prescribes them.

Chapping

Skin that dries out with exposure to cold or hot air often starts to crack, and this is known as chapping. It most commonly affects areas exposed to the elements such as lips, fingers, hands and ears.

Symptoms
- Small cracks, redness and roughness on exposed areas of skin.

What to do
- Be especially careful to dress the child properly for cold, windy weather. Use lip salve and petroleum jelly or moisture cream on the face.

Chickenpox

A common, highly contagious disease, caused by a virus and marked by an itchy rash on the skin. The chickenpox virus is the same as that of shingles and can be reactivated during adulthood.

Chickenpox can start as fever but in very young children the rash is often the first sign. It appears in waves over three to four days and the child will be infectious until all the spots have dried up and formed scabs (about a week).

The rash usually covers the trunk, then moves to the face, scalp, arms and legs. It may also be found in extreme cases in the mouth, vagina and anus.

Although chickenpox is not serious, it can very occasionally lead to **Reye's syndrome** or **encephalitis**.

Symptoms
- A high temperature.
- Small blisters appearing on the trunk, then spreading to other parts of the body.
- Itchiness.

What to do
- It is most important to stop your child from scratching the spots as this can lead to permanent scars. Calamine lotion will reduce the itchiness.
- Your child is infectious as long as she has spots that have not dried up and formed scabs.
- Change a baby's nappies frequently, and leave them off when possible.
- A sedative may be necessary in some cases to help a badly infected child to sleep.
- Consult your doctor if scabs become infected.
- If after the scabs have all disappeared she complains of neck ache or has a fever, call the doctor immediately.

Chilblains

Small, pale, numb areas of skin experienced during cold weather. They become red, swollen and itchy when the area is warmed up. Chilblains are due to sensitive skin being exposed to cold and damp.

Symptoms
- Skin which is numb or red and itchy, especially on toes and fingers in winter.

What to do
- It is difficult to stop some children getting chilblains. Take special care to keep hands and feet warm and dry in cold, damp weather. Thermal mittens and lined boots will help.
- In extreme cases, your doctor may prescribe a drug to improve circulation.

Choking

The body's method of clearing an obstruction such as food, drink or a swallowed object from the airway to the lungs. If the object completely or severely blocks the airway, a child will turn blue and lose consciousness.

Symptoms
- Coughing and spluttering.
- Gasping.
- Blueness around the mouth.
- Loss of consciousness.

What to do
- If a child is spluttering and coughing but is not blue, she is getting enough oxygen and there is no real need to worry.
- Lie her across your knee and give her several sharp slaps on the back. This should help her to cough up the obstruction.
- If you can see something in the throat, try to hook it out with a finger but only if you are sure you will not push it further in.
- If the object cannot be dislodged by slapping the back, and if the child is blue or unconscious, find an open space and swing the child around, upside down, holding her firmly by the knees. The centrifugal force should dislodge the blockage.
- Once the blockage is cleared, lay an unconscious child in the **recovery position**. If she stops breathing give **mouth-to-mouth resuscitation**.
- Call an ambulance if your child is unconscious or blue.
- A child who is unconscious, even for a moment, should be checked by a doctor.

Coeliac disease

This is caused by a sensitivity to gluten, a protein found in cereals. The gluten causes an allergic reaction in the small intestine, with the result that it stops absorbing important nutrients from food. These are passed straight out of the body as faeces, which in coeliac disease are extremely foul-smelling.

The symptoms of this disease generally appear a few weeks after the introduction of cereals into a baby's diet.

Coeliac disease is potentially serious. If not

treated properly, it can permanently stunt your child's growth.

Symptoms
● Frequent, pale and foul-smelling faeces that do not flush away easily.
● Loss of appetite.
● Poor weight gain. The child will look malnourished.
● Lethargy.
● Pale skin, due to **anaemia**.

What to do
● See a doctor if your child is not thriving, or produces foul-smelling motions for more than a day or so, particularly if you have recently weaned her on to cereals.
● If a gluten allergy is suspected your child will be admitted to hospital for tests to confirm the diagnosis.
● The hospital will advise you which foods to avoid.
● Always check prepared foods carefully: many use flour as thickening.

Cold sores

Cold sores occur around the nostrils and lips. They are caused by the Herpes simplex virus. Once established, the virus tends to stay within the system causing recurrent sores. It is activated by cooling and heating of the skin: children are most susceptible when they are run down but exposure to the sun also produces sores.

What to do
● Apply surgical spirit, alcohol or perfume to the sores to dry them out. Petroleum jelly will soothe the irritation.
● The sores are infectious, so try to prevent your child touching them.
● Antibiotic cream can be prescribed if the cold sores become infected.

Colic

See 543.

Colour blindness

See **vision, problems with**.

Common cold

A viral infection affecting the linings of the nose and throat, causing a runny nose, a sore throat and possibly swollen tonsils or glands. Secondary, bacterial infections can occur and may need antibiotic treatment.

Symptoms
● Running nose.
● Nasal congestion with catarrh.
● Fever.
● Sore throat.
● Coughing and sneezing.
● Aches and pains.

What to do
You can only treat the symptoms, not the cold itself.
● Lower the child's temperature by tepid sponging and giving paracetamol syrup.
● Give children's cough medicine to relieve a cough.
● Prop her up if she is having difficulty breathing at night.

● Give plenty of fluids.
● Keep the atmosphere humid by boiling an electric kettle in the child's room. It reduces throat irritation.
● If you think your child has a secondary infection, see a doctor.

Conjunctivitis

An inflammation of the lining of the eyeball, making the eye red and weepy. The condition can be caused by a virus, bacteria, a foreign body, a chemical or an allergic reaction. One or both eyes can be affected and it is sometimes contagious.

Symptoms
● Sore, itchy eye.
● A red eye that discharges pus, causing the eyelids to be coated and to stick together after sleep.

What to do
● Inspect the eye for a foreign body that you can remove.
● Try to stop the child touching the eye.
● If you suspect conjunctivitis, see a doctor. He or she will probably prescribe antibiotic drops or ointment for an infection or an anti-inflammatory treatment for an allergic reaction.
   See also **foreign bodies**.

Constipation

Children do not need to open their bowels every day: bowels move when the need arises. Constipation or hard, pebble-like faeces often occur when a baby first goes on to a solid diet. Sometimes during a fever extra water is absorbed from the gut and the faeces become unusually hard.

Symptoms
● Hard, small faeces like pebbles.
● Pain in the lower abdomen on passing faeces.
● Blood in nappy or pants.

What to do
● Don't use laxatives.
● Keep up your child's fluid level.
● Keep her diet as varied and include as many unprocessed foods, fresh fruit and vegetables as possible.
● If your child is passing blood or seems in pain, see a doctor.
   See also **appendicitis**.

Convulsions

If a child runs a high temperature, or has a severe reaction to an immunization (see 623-625), don't panic. It will all be over in about five minutes.

Symptoms
● Sudden rise in temperature.
● Child is listless and looks vacant; may be jittery.
● Possibly blue in face.
● The child's body may stiffen.
● Limbs twitch.
● Loss of consciousness.

What to do
● Don't leave her. You can call for help when the convulsion is over. It will only last a minute or two. Accept that no one could get to you in time to help.
● Turn her on her stomach or side in case she is sick. If she starts being sick, try to lift her

head or turn it so the vomit runs out of her mouth and not down her throat. The real danger of a convulsion is not the fit itself but inhaling vomit. This can kill: the fit will not.
- Get her on to the floor, move furniture out of her way and loosen her clothes; move anything she could bump into.
- Don't restrain her.
- Leave her mouth alone; there is no need to prop it open, she is very unlikely to bite her tongue.
- Call the doctor as soon as she is resting peacefully.
- Sponge her with a tepid, damp sponge and remove extra clothing to reduce her temperature.

Cot death
Sudden, unexplained death of a baby while unattended – having been apparently well when put down to sleep. Also known as 'SIDS' or Sudden Infant Death Syndrome, it occurs most often in babies between two months and two years.

This is the nightmare every parent fears; publicity has driven its reality home. The only reassurance is that cot deaths really are uncommon: you hear about them because they are so tragic, and so inexplicable.

Research has not yet uncovered the cause of cot death, or indeed what happens. It has been established that there are more cot deaths among bottle-fed babies than breast-fed; and that there are more cot deaths in winter than summer. There is the suggestion that the baby's breathing mechanism fails, possibly in response to some trigger. The higher incidence of cot death in winter could mean that infection (or possibly allergy) are implicated as triggers. There appears to be a tendency for cot deaths to run in families.

But this is all speculation.

What to do
- To put your mind at rest about accidental suffocation, if nothing else, never give a baby a pillow until she is at least a year old. Likewise, provide a proper baby mattress with ventilation holes when the baby moves to a cot.

Cough
Coughing is the body's reaction to an irritant in the throat or the airways to the lungs. It clears the passages of mucus or phlegm. There are several kinds of cough, but the two main types are the unproductive cough and its opposite, the 'loose' cough. Coughing at night may be an early sign of **asthma**.

What to do
- Don't give your child a cough suppressant if she is producing phlegm: she is coughing because she needs to clear her lungs. If phlegm builds up, the chance of infection is increased.
- To help your child bring up phlegm or an obstruction, lie her across your knee and pat her back.
- Lie a baby on her stomach to sleep.
- Prop an elder child up at night on pillows to ease the coughing.
- Coughing makes a child's throat sore. To soothe it, give hot lemon and honey or blackcurrant drinks and pastilles.
- Keep the child calm: exertion can bring on a coughing fit.

- Humid air reduces throat irritation: boil a kettle in the room.
- If she starts to 'whoop', or if she is not sleeping, see a doctor.
   See also **asthma, bronchitis, croup, whooping cough**.

Cradle cap
Yellowish-white scales on the scalp. They are not serious and require simply a special shampoo. Oiling the baby's head will loosen the cradle cap before washing her hair or scalp.
   See also **dandruff, eczema**.

Croup
This is an acute inflammation of the area around the vocal chords occuring most commonly in children between two and four, but it can also occur in older children. An infection from a cold moves down the throat to affect the larynx and trachea. In older children, the condition may just cause **laryngitis**.

Symptoms
- Stridor – a distinctive hoarse wheeze on breathing in.
- In severe cases, a grey or blue face: get immediate medical attention.
- A barking cough.
- Laboured breathing.

What to do
- Keep the air moist as this will soothe the constricted air passages. Boil a kettle or run a hot bath and sit the child in the steamy atmosphere.
- Don't let the child lie on her back: this tends to exaggerate the obstruction.
- See a doctor.
   See also **bronchitis, common cold**.

Cuts and grazes
A cut breaks the skin and exposes the underlying tissue. Cuts bleed, which helps to clean the wound of germs. A graze is an injury that does not break the full thickness of the skin.

Deep cuts and extensive grazing may be prone to further infection such as tetanus.

What to do
- Simply hold the damaged area under a running cold water tap for a minute or two to cleand the wound.
- Place a sterile dressing on the cut or graze.

Serious cuts:
- Elevate the affected area to restrict blood flow.
- Tie a sterile bandage tightly over the wound to further reduce blood loss.
- Check for infection when the dressing is changed.
- If bleeding is heavy, or if the wound gapes, call a doctor at once or take your child to the nearest hospital casualty department: stitches may be needed.

Dandruff
A build-up of dead skin cells which get trapped by the hair and appear as white flakes. Treat with a dandruff shampoo.

Dehydration
This occurs in a number of illnesses: see

diarrhoea, dysentery, fever, food poisoning, gastroenteritis and **vomiting**.

Diabetes
Diabetes occurs in two forms, one of which begins in childhood or young adulthood and the other during middle age. It is due to a lack of insulin, a hormone produced by the pancreas. Insulin breaks down carbohydrates in the diet so that the body can use them for energy. A lack of insulin means that carbohydrates collect in the blood, causing fat and protein to be metabolized instead. This causes weight loss and a build-up of toxic waste products.

Diabetes is readily treatable. Your child can lead a normal life if she has daily insulin injections.

Symptoms
- Weight loss.
- Increased thirst.
- Hourly urination, possibly with bedwetting.
- Breath smelling of pear drops. This signifies the presence of ketones, one of the toxic products.
- Irritability and lethargy.
- Decreased resistance to infection.

What to do
- You and your child will have to learn how to administer the correct dose of insulin by injection.
- You will need to give your child a special diet (the doctor will advise) which keeps glucose levels constant. She will also have to eat at regular intervals.
- It is sensible for your child to wear a bracelet stating that she is a diabetic.
- You should always see a doctor when a diabetic child is ill: she is especially susceptible to infection.

Diarrhoea
In true diarrhoea, the intestines force food through at an increased rate, so that normal uptake of nutrients and absorption of water is restricted. This causes runny faeces, and eventually **dehydration**. Dehydration occurs rapidly in babies and is potentially grave.

Diarrhoea has a number of causes including: an infection by bacteria or virus; a non-intestinal infection such as **otitis media; influenza**; and **some fevers**.

What to do
- Don't give your child anything to eat. Give as much clear fluid as possible, little and often. Half-strength cola may be more acceptable to a small child than water, and has about the right amounts of sugar and salt. You can also give diluted fruit juice or water with one teaspoonful of glucose and a pinch of salt added. Don't give milk. After 24 hours, reintroduce food slowly.
- Ensure that the infection does not pass to the rest of the family by taking special care over hygiene.
- After the diarrhoea has finished, start the child on bland foods such as rice and soups.
- See a doctor if: a child is under a year and has had diarrhoea for several hours; there is blood in the faeces; there is **fever** and **vomiting** with the diarrhoea; the child has a high fever, or abdominal pain. The doctor may

prescribe a glucose and salt powder to add to cold drinks. See also **coeliac disease, influenza**.

Dizziness
This is quite common when a child has a raised temperature. It may also occur with breathlessness after exertion; and it could mean anaemia or concussion (see head injury), or it could be a prelude to a convulsion.

What to do
- Keep the child calm, sit her down and put her head between her knees to increase blood flow to her head.
- If the child experiences a number of dizzy spells or regularly complains of feeling dizzy after exercise, see a doctor.

Drowning
Having rescued a child from the water:
- If she is not breathing, start **mouth-to-mouth resuscitation**. If you can, start while the child is still in the water.
- Small children can go for long periods without breathing. Don't give up until help arrives.
- If she is unconscious but breathing, put her in the **recovery position**. Cover her to keep her as warm as possible. Check pulse and breathing at regular intervals.
- If she is conscious, get her out of the water, wrap her and treat her for **shock**.
- Get help. Call an ambulance or ask someone to drive you and the child to the nearest hospital.

Drowsiness
A symptom of several conditions: see **chickenpox, encephalitis, fever, measles, meningitis, mumps, Reyes' syndrome**.

Dysentery
Dysentery produces the same symptoms as a fever with diarrhoea and is due to the inflammation of the large intestine. It is caused by bacteria and is easily passed on by contact.

Symptoms
- Diarrhoea.
- Fever.
- Nausea.
- Painful abdominal contractions.
- Weakness.
- Blood, mucus or pus in the stools.

What to do
- If you live or travel in an area with poor sanitation, check your child's faeces if any symptoms of dysentery appear.
- See a doctor if faeces remain loose for 12 hours.
- Call a doctor at once if there is pus or blood in the faeces.

Earache
The most common reason for earache is an ear infection known as **otitis media**. This occurs especially in young children where the Eustachian tube is short and infections can easily travel from the throat to the middle ear. Earache can also occur if a child has a cold, **tonsilitis, toothache** or **mumps**. A foreign body in the ear can also cause infection.

Symptoms
- Deafness.
- Pain in and around the ear.
- Discharge from the ear.
- Swollen glands.
- Fever.

What to do
- Remove foreign object if possible, otherwise take the child to a hospital casualty department.
- Don't push anything into the ear and don't use ear drops unless advised.
- Clear any discharge with soap and warm water.
- Give paracetamol syrup to ease the pain.
- If the child complains of an earache and has a fever, or if there is a discharge from the ear, see a doctor.
- If the child is in severe pain, with fever and vomiting, call the doctor immediately.
- If your child has a middle ear infection, she will probably be given a course of antibiotics to clear it.

Eczema
Eczema is a dry, extremely itchy, red rash found on the face, neck, hands and the creases of the limbs. It comes and goes depending on the child's emotional and physical well-being.

Eczema is an allergic response and infant eczema is often associated with **asthma**. Most children grow out of eczema by the age of three but the tendency to develop allergies will remain.

Seborrhoeic eczema is caused by too many sebaceous glands; it can take the form of **cradle cap, blepharitis** and **otitis externa**.

What to do
- Consult your doctor, who may prescribe oral anti-histamines, anti-inflammatory creams, creams to moisturize the skin and soap substitutes.
- Check for a rash if you see your child scratching. Keep her fingernails short to reduce the risk of breaking the skin. You can put cotton mittens on a baby at night.
- Try to use soap as little as possible on your child's skin.
- Your anxiety will only make the condition worse.
- Dress her in cotton clothes, at least next to her skin, and use paper nappies on a baby.
- Avoid biological detergents and rinse clothes well. Avoid washing in soap powder any clothing worn next to her skin.

See **allergy**.

Electric shock
An electric shock can burn a child, make her **unconscious** or cause her heart to stop beating.

What to do
- Never touch a child until you have switched off the electricity, otherwise you may electrocute yourself. Switch it off at the mains.
- If you cannot switch off the electricity quickly, push the child away from the source, using a non-conductive material such as a wooden chair or plastic broom handle. Make sure your hands are dry and stand on a non-conductive material (such as a couple of cushions).
- When the contact is broken, examine your child. If she is unconscious, check that she is

breathing and whether she still has a pulse. If she is not breathing, begin to resuscitate her by **heart massage** and **mouth-to-mouth resuscitation**.
- If she is breathing, lie her in the **recovery position**.
- Burns should be treated by reducing heat, otherwise the tissue can go on burning even though the contact is broken. Place the burn under a running cold water tap if possible. Otherwise use a cold compress such as a large pack of frozen vegetables.
- Get the child to a hospital casualty department.
- If the burning is extensive she may go into **shock**.

See also burns.

Encephalitis
An inflammation of the brain which can be caused by a common childhood infection such as **chickenpox, mumps** or, occasionally, **whooping cough vaccine**.

Symptoms
- Severe headache.
- Pain when bending the neck.
- Intolerance to bright light.
- **Fever**.
- **Convulsions** and coma.
- Drowsiness.

What to do
- If your child develops fever and a headache when recovering from an infectious disease, get her to bend her neck. If this causes pain, call the doctor immediately.
- She will be admitted to hospital and will stay there until she has recovered, probably two to three weeks.

Epilepsy
The term means a tendency to have fits, seizures or convulsions – all three amount to the same thing. There are three types of epilepsy: 'grand mal', 'petit mal' and partial fits. The first is the most serious: there is loss of consciousness; the child falls to the ground and becomes rigid; the limbs jerk; she may froth at the mouth, and urinate. Petit mal fits, found mainly in children, are periods of interrupted or clouded consciousness, similar to day-dreaming, although the child cannot be roused. Partial fits vary greatly and may involve one or several of: transient involuntary movements; loss of speech; confusion; loss of concentration.

Fits are caused by abnormal electrical activity in the brain. Although disturbing, they are not life-threatening and with proper management a child should be able to lead a normal life. Petit mal fits usually cease in late adolescence.

What to do
- If your child becomes unconscious she should always see a doctor. Call the doctor after a first seizure. Once epilepsy is diagnosed, you can deal with fits unaided.

During an attack:
- Remove any objects on which she may hurt herself.
- Loosen her collar.
- Don't try to force anything between her teeth.
- Once the attack is over, put her in the **recovery position**.
- In a petit mal seizure simply ensure your

child comes to no harm while in the trance-like state.

• Treat your child as normally as possible and explain the condition to her teacher and her friends.

• Get her to wear a bracelet explaining her condition when you are not there.

• Teach your child to be aware of an approaching attack and to take precautions to avoid hurting herself.

• The condition can be treated with anti-convulsant drugs.

Eyes

The eyes have well-designed defences against accidental damage – which nonetheless may still be breached.

If a speck of dust enters an eye, it makes the eye weep, and the tears usually rid the eye of the dust. But if the foreign body gets embedded in the eye, or obscures the iris or pupil, there can be problems.

A blow to the eye can break the small blood vessels beneath the skin, making the surrounding area swell up and turn black. A toxic chemical splashed in the eye should be treated immediately.

Although soap in the eye can irritate and may frighten a child, it will not cause permanent damage.

What to do

• If there is an object in the eye, try to make your child blink repeatedly dislodge it.

• Try to flush the object out by pouring a glass of water across the eye.

• If the object does not come out, keep the eye closed and take the child to the nearest hospital casualty department.

• If the eye is injured by a blow, put a cold compress on the area to reduce the swelling. If the eye is very bloodshot, lie the child on her back and call a doctor.

• If a chemical gets into an eye, wash it out thoroughly with water. Ring your doctor for advice or take your child to the nearest casualty department as soon as possible. Household cleaners can cause burning and will need hospital treatment.

• If the eye is bleeding, put pressure on it with a sterile pad and go to the nearest hospital casualty department.

• If the eye is damaged, or you suspect damage, always seek medical advice.

See also **conjunctivitis**.

Fever

A fever is an abnormal rise in body temperature which is often a symptom of a viral or bacterial infection. Normal body temperature is 98.6°F or 37°C. A rise to 100°F is said to be a slight fever; 104°F is a high fever. It is normal for children to get hot after exercise, but raised temperature should drop within half an hour.

A child sometimes has a **convulsion** or fit during a fever. Although this is frightening at the time, it can be managed safely at home: see **convulsions**. Convulsions are almost unheard of in children over five.

Symptoms

• The child's forehead and body are unusually hot.

• Aching joints.

• Increased pulse rate.

• Loss of appetite.

• Constipation.

• Alternate sweating and feeling chilled.

What to do

• Call the doctor immediately: if the child has febrile convulsions; if the high fever is accompanied by a stiff neck; if the fever persists for 24 hours; if it is accompanied by a **rash, vomiting** or **diarrhoea**.

• If a child has a raised temperature, lie her down and cover her lightly; keep the room cool – 67°F (19°C) is ideal.

• To reduce her temperature, sponge her with a wet, tepid sponge or flannel. The water evaporating from her skin will reduce her temperature. (Don't use a cold sponge: it will close the blood vessels in the skin, so conserving heat in the blood.)

• Give paracetamol syrup to bring down her temperature. Don't give aspirin, as this is thought to play a part in **Reye's syndrome**.

• Change the bedclothes frequently and allow your child to sleep as much as possible.

• Give plenty of drinks as she will lose fluid through sweating.

Food poisoning

If a child eats infected food she will show signs of food poisoning within three to 24 hours. The bacteria release toxins into the intestines which cause inflammation. This in turn produces sickness and diarrhoea. The most common bacteria involved are *salmonella, shigella, E. coli* and *staphylococci.*

Food poisoning is a potentially grave condition in babies because it rapidly leads to dangerous levels of dehydration.

'Food poisoning' can be caused by chemicals, such as those in insecticides, or even by certain plants.

Symptoms

• Diarrhoea.

• Vomiting.

• Fever.

• Abdominal cramp.

• Loss of appetite.

What to do

• If you suspect your child has swallowed a chemical, take the bottle and the child to the nearest hospital casualty department.

• See a doctor if a baby is vomiting and has diarrhoea for more than three hours.

• Stop all food, but give the child plenty of fluids, a few mouthfuls at a time. Half-strength cola has the right balance of salts and sugar; or give diluted fruit juice or water with sugar and a pinch of salt. (If you have a soda machine, putting a few bubbles into the water may make it more attractive to the child.) Don't give milk: its fat content is relatively difficult for the stomach to absorb and increases the irritation.

• If this régime does not stop the diarrhorea after 24 hours, see a doctor.

• If she has a **fever**, cool her with a wet, tepid sponge.

• Food poisoning is contagious. Be sure to wash your hands and keep any cups she uses separate from those used by the rest of the family.

• Leave a bucket next to her bed so she does not have to get up to be sick.

- The doctor will probably prescribe a powder to help replace lost fluid and essential salts.
- In severe cases the child may be admitted to hospital for intravenous fluid treatment.

Foreign bodies

Children poke things into every possible orifice and sometimes they get stuck. Occasionally this is not noticed until infection occurs.

Symptoms
- Foreign body in ear, see **earache**.
- Foreign body in eye, see **eyes**.
- A foreign body in the nose may cause nose bleeds, a foul-smelling blood-stained discharge and a red, tender area over the nose.
- A foreign body in the vagina will cause soreness and a blood-stained discharge.

What to do
- An object pushed into the nose is not particularly harmful unless the child inhales it into her lungs. This can cause croup or choking.
- Cover the unblocked nostril and ask your child to blow. This sometimes dislodges the object.
- Look into her nose to see if you might reach the object with tweezers.
- If you cannot, take her to the nearest hospital casualty department.
- If your child has an object lodged in her vagina, take her to the doctor who will examine her, and may refer her to the hospital casualty department.

Gastroenteritis

An inflammation of the stomach and intestine caused by a virus, contaminated food or by bottles which are not properly sterilized.

Symptoms
- Vomiting.
- Nausea.
- Diarrhoea.
- Fever.
- Abdominal cramps.
- Loss of appetite.

What to do
See **food poisoning**.

German measles

This is a common viral infection, often referred to by its scientific name, *Rubella*. It is highly contagious and has an incubation period of 14-21 days. A rash first appears behind the ears before spreading to the rest of the body. However, German measles is usually mild and lasts only a few days.

The most worrying aspect of *Rubella* is its ability to cause defects such as blindness and deafness in an unborn baby if contracted by the mother in the first 12 weeks of pregnancy.

Symptoms
- Slight rise in temperature.
- A rash starting behind the ears and spreading to the rest of the body.
- Swollen glands at the back of the neck.

What to do
- Keep your child at home and inform any pregnant women that your child has German measles.
- If your child's temperature suddenly rises and her neck becomes stiff, call a doctor at once.

This could indicate encephalitis, a rare but potentially grave complication.

Glandular fever

This is also known as infectious mononucleosis and is a viral infection starting in much the same way as **influenza** or **German measles**. It is most commonly contracted by young adults and can be a debilitating illness. In a child it generally takes a milder form. There is no cure and it must therefore run its course, which will take at least a month. But it can be six months before your child is completely herself again.

Symptoms
- Swollen glands.
- Sore throat.
- Rash starting behind the ears.
- Depression.
- Aches and pains.

What to do
- See a doctor if your child has any of the above symptoms and seems to have a persistent cold, and to be run-down and low. A blood test can confirm glandular fever.
- Treat the symptoms as you would for a fever.

Glue ear

Glue ear is the presence of fluid, often of a thick, glue-like consistency, in the middle ear behind the eardrum. It is thought to be due to the middle ear failing to drain properly after **otitis media**. It is not painful, but if untreated it can lead to deafness in one or both ears. It does not usually cause permanent damage to hearing, however.

Symptoms
- 'Fullness' in ear.
- Earache.
- Partial hearing loss.

What to do
- If your child seems inattentive, especially following an infection, see a doctor to have her ears tested. The fluid will often drain of its own accord with time.
- In mild cases the doctor may prescribe an antibiotic. In more serious cases the fluid in the middle ear must be drained off surgically by making a tiny slit in the ear drum. Grommets will be placed in the child's ear(s) to facilitate the draining of any other fluid build-up.

Gum boil

A gum boil develops in the root of a decayed tooth and is filled with pus. It can be extremely painful.

Symptoms
- Swelling on the side of the face.
- A red lump at the base of the tooth.
- Pain.
- Swollen glands.

What to do
- Rinse the child's mouth to wash away pus.
- A hot water bottle on the affected side of the face may ease the pain.
- See a doctor. A course of antibiotics will be prescribed to clear the infection.
- Take the child to a dentist. The tooth may need to be removed if badly decayed.

Hay fever

Known also as allergic rhinitis (see **allergy**).

This allergic reaction occurs in the mucus membranes of the nose and eyelids. It is usually caused by pollen and occurs mainly in the spring and summer, but animal hair can produce a similar reaction. It is rare in children under five but quite often replaces **asthma** in a child as she grows up.

The pollen count is reported each day in many areas. You can check your child's reaction in relation to this. Some individuals have a response to a particular pollen. But if your child has hay fever symptoms at times when the pollen count is low, or during the night, check other possible allergens such as dust, animal fur and feather pillows.

Symptoms
• Sneezing.
• Runny nose.
• Watery, itchy red-rimmed eyes.

What to do
• Check possible allergens.
• Replace feather pillows with foam and feather duvets with polyester-filled ones. Air duvets in the sun as this reduces house dust mite.
• Keep carpets, rugs and soft toys to a minimum if the child is affected all year round.
• Vacuum mattresses regularly and keep covered.
• Do not have pets, or keep them to restricted areas of the house.

Head injuries and headaches
When a child complains of a headache it may be a simple headache or it may be due to a blow on the head or equally it may be a symptom of **sinusitis, tonsilitis, toothache** or **fever**.

Symptoms of concussion
• Headache.
• Vomiting.
• Stunned, dazed state.
• Drowsiness, pallor.
• Unconsciousness.

What to do
If the child has had a head injury:
• Watch carefully for signs of concussion. If she is running about and unaware of the blow ten minutes later, there is nothing to worry about. If she loses consciousness or becomes pale and drowsy, take her to hospital at once. Even if she is only unconscious for a few moments, she needs to be seen by a doctor.
• If her eyes become unco-ordinated, her speech muddled or she becomes clumsy or loses the use of a limb, go to hospital at once.
• If there is a discharge of blood or fluid from the ears, or bleeding from the nose, following head injury, take the child to hospital at once.
• Vomiting following head injury should be treated seriously. Take her to hospital at once.

Headaches not caused by injury:
• If the headache is accompanied by a stiff neck and fever, this could indicate **encephalitis** or **meningitis**. Call the doctor at once.
• Some children suffer from recurrent headaches and their cause is hardly ever found. Most children eventually grow out of them.
• Particularly painful recurrent headaches are

known as **migraines**.
• Headaches can be due to tension, so find out if your child is worried about anything.
• If your child has persistent headaches have her eyes tested.

Head lice, see **lice**.

Heart massage, see **mouth-to-mouth** resuscitation.

Heat problems
These include heat exhaustion, heat stroke and heat rash. When a baby or small child is too hot, the body's regulatory system tries to cool it down by producing sweat. In cases where the sweat glands cease to function because the body has already lost too much fluid, heat exhaustion sets in. If this is not treated quickly, heat stroke can occur, which is more serious and can be fatal.

Heat rash occurs in babies and young children when too much sweat is produced. The slight red rash is generally found on the face, neck and where there are creases in the skin. It is not serious and is easy to treat.

Symptoms
The following are symptoms of heat exhaustion; for heat stroke the symptoms are more severe and the child will eventually become unconscious.
• Slight temperature.
• Headache.
• Nausea.
• Dizziness.
• Clammy skin.
• Increased pulse.

What to do
• Immediately remove your child from the sun or hot place.
• Sponge her all over with tepid water, or place her in a tepid bath. On the beach, take her into the sea unless the water is very cold. Her temperature should be brought down slowly, so splash water over her or gradually immerse her rather than plunging her straight into the water. Loose, damp clothes will reduce her temperature.
• Give plenty of drinks.
• A heat rash can also be treated by placing the child in a tepid bath. Don't rub dry: instead, let the water evaporate to cool her down further.

Heat stroke is serious and needs immediate medical attention.

Symptoms
• High temperature.
• Hot dry skin.
• No sweating.
• Drowsiness, leading to confusion and unconsciousness.
• Rapid pulse.

What to do
• Get your child into the shade. Undress and fan her while someone calls an ambulance, or take her to the nearest hospital.
• If she is sweating, sponge her with tepid water. Place ice against her forehead and wrists.

Hepatitis
Inflammation of the liver. Hepatitis A, the common type in children, is a highly contagious

disease passed on from a carrier through poor hygiene, via food or drink.

It causes **jaundice** in most cases, but is rarely serious.

Symptoms
- **Influenza**-type symptoms.
- Yellowing of the skin, dark brown urine and pale stools.
- Loss of appetite.

What to do
- See a doctor immediately. He or she will take a blood sample to test for hepatitis. If positive the child will have to be isolated until the 'flu symptoms disappear.
- Be aware that hepatitis is contagious and be scrupulously hygienic.
- Lethargy, moodiness, and difficulty in concentrating may persist for up to six months after hepatitis.

Hernia
The most common type is the umbilical hernia, where the muscles in the abdominal wall allow a piece of intestine to protrude. An umbilical hernia in a baby usually disappears of its own accord by the age of four.

An inguinal hernia appears lower down the abdomen and is most commonly found in boys. Again, the intestine protrudes through the muscle wall and it is usually there from birth due to a congenital weakness. But it will not disappear on its own. With this type of hernia there is a danger that the protruding intestine will become trapped and it therefore always needs surgery.

What to do
- Try to push the hernia back inside the muscular wall. If it will do this and does not harden, there is no immediate danger.
- If the hernia becomes hard or will not go back inside the muscle wall, see a doctor. It may need surgery straight away. The operation is a simple one.

Hiccups
Contractions of the diaphragm which are beyond voluntary control. They draw air sharply through the larynx, so that the opening at the top of the larynx suddenly closes – making the 'hic' noise.

Babies get hiccups often, and come to no harm from them. An older child may find them irritating, just as an adult does.

Tricks for stopping hiccups involve making the lungs work overtime in an attempt to displace the involuntary activity. You can thump her, without warning, on her back, to make her gasp; or make her breathe in and out of a paper bag for about 30 seconds. The reduced oxygen content of air in the bag makes the lungs work harder. Many claim that this is the most effective remedy.

Hives
This rash can be caused by skin contact with a number of allergens, most commonly nettles, certain types of food such as strawberries or shellfish, and drugs such as penicillin or aspirin.

In serious cases the child may have an allergic reaction known as angioneurotic oedema which can spread to the tongue and throat, causing severe breathing difficulties.

Symptoms
- Classic nettle rash weals take the form of white lumps on a red base. These last up to an hour, and are replaced by another crop, often in a different area of the body.
- Itchiness.

What to do
- Soothe itchiness with calamine lotion.
- A warm bath containing washing starch may relieve the itching in severe cases.
See **allergy, rash.**

Hyperactivity
Hyperactivity is a diagnosis used very differently in Europe and the United States. Children classified as hyperactive in the United States include those with attentional, emotional and behavioural disorders. In Britain the term is used more strictly for a clinical condition in which the child is extremely restless, has poor concentration and needs little sleep. Some research has detected a link between food additives and hyperactive behaviour, but its reliability is questionable.

Symptoms
- Inappropriate and undirected activity. Being 'all over the place' but achieving little.
- Restlessness.
- Inability to focus attention or concentrate on anything for long.
- Behavioural problems.
- Sleeplessness.
- Disruptive behaviour (especially at school if the child is old enough).
- Aggression.

What to do
If you feel that your child might be hyperactive, ask your doctor to refer her for assessment. Many doctors in Britain do not 'believe' in hyperactivity, but even if he or she chooses a different name for the problem, they should refer you either to a psychotherapist or to a clinic which deals with behavioural disorders.

Hypothermia
A young baby cannot control her temperature. A room quite warm enough for an adult may be far too cold for a new-born baby; see 536.

The ratio of body surface to body volume makes it easy for a baby to lose heat rapidly. If body temperature falls below 95°F (35°C) she has hypothermia which is potentially fatal.

Symptoms
- Cold to the touch.
- Pale, sometimes blue skin.
- Shivering in a child (babies do not shiver).
- Drowsiness.
- Floppiness in babies.
- Extreme lethargy.
- Slurred speech.
- Confusion.
- Temperature below 95°F (35°C).

What to do
- Call the doctor immediately if your baby is under six months.
- Remember that it is dangerous to warm her too quickly: do it gradually.
- If out of doors cover her (especially if wet) and get her inside as soon as possible.
- Give her your body heat. Cuddle up closely to her, wrap blankets around you both.

- Once inside, take off any wet clothes and wrap her in a blanket.
- Call a doctor.
- Once she begins to warm up, you may put her into a warm bath: 98°F (36°C).
- Give warm, not hot, sweet drinks.
- If her temperature does not begin to rise, take her to hospital immediately.

Impetigo
A highly contagious bacterial skin infection caused by the staphylococci bacteria, with small, red, watery blisters around the mouth that eventually break to form scabs.

Symptoms
- Tiny red spots with watery heads around the nose, mouth or ears which burst, ooze and form crusts.

What to do
- See a doctor who will prescribe an antibiotic cream and a course of antibiotics.
- Stop your child touching the scabs.
- Wash the affected area with warm water to remove the crusts. Wear rubber gloves to prevent the bacteria spreading.

Influenza
Known commonly as 'flu, this viral infection is very like the common cold. There is no cure and the infection has to run its course.

It lasts about a week and is rarely serious. (Occasionally a more serious strain of 'flu occurs: there was one in 1916 and another in the 1950s, both of which killed large numbers of people.) However, the infection can leave the child low and susceptible to secondary infections such as **pneumonia** or **bronchitis**.

If your child suffers from **asthma** or **diabetes**, 'flu can cause complications: see a doctor.

Symptoms
- High temperature.
- Aches and pains in the limbs.
- Sore throat, runny nose and a cough.
- Diarrhoea and vomiting.
- Shivering, with weakness and lethargy.

What to do
- Control **fever** with paracetamol syrup and tepid sponging.
- Give plenty of drinks.
- Encourage rest.
- If, after your child has apparently recovered, she starts to vomit and run a high temperature, seek medical help immediately: this could be a sign of **Reye's syndrome**.
- If there is a secondary infection a doctor will be able to prescribe a course of antibiotics to clear it.

Ingrowing toenail
A painful condition caused by a toenail growing at an angle and penetrating the skin. It most commonly occurs in the big toe. An infection enters the wound causing swelling and build-up of pus.

What to do
- Cut a small V in the toenail to relieve the pressure at the edges.
- Apply an antiseptic cream to the affected area to reduce the infection.

- Cut toenails straight across and not too short.
- Have the child's shoes carefully fitted.
- If this is a recurrent problem, see a doctor.

Infected wounds
These need careful monitoring. If they do not get better within 24 hours, see a doctor.

Symptoms
- Red, weeping wound.
- Yellowish scab.
- Pain.

What to do
See a doctor if:
- Reddish streaks are seen centring on the wound.
- The skin around the wound is tight, hot and glossy.
- The wound throbs with pain.
- Pus oozes continuously.
- The area around the wound is swollen.

Itching
This is more a symptom than an illness; commonly found with skin complaints.

What to do
- Investigate the underlying problem. If there is no apparent reason for the itching, see a doctor who will diagnose the complaint and treat it accordingly.
- Use calamine lotion or bicarbonate of soda to reduce the itching.

See also **athlete's foot, chickenpox, chilblains, eczema, hives, ringworm, scabies, thrush, worms**.

Jaundice
The red blood cells, which carry oxygen around the body, have a life of about three months. Then they are broken down by the liver into bile, which is excreted via the intestine. It is bile which gives stools their characteristic yellow-brown colour. If the liver is not working efficiently, or if the blood cells are being broken down abnormally quickly, bile pigment accumulates in the blood and gives a yellow tinge to the skin and the whites of the eyes. The child's stools become pale.

Blood is filtered by the kidneys, turning waste products into urine. If a child has jaundice, these waste products include bile pigments, so the urine changes colour too. One in three babies have jaundice in the first days after birth. Usually there is no underlying disease; it happens because the liver takes time to start working properly. The hospital will check the baby regularly, because occasionally it can become more serious.

Later, jaundice is always a symptom of underlying disease. Possible causes are **hepatitis** and certain forms of **anaemia**, and in young babies a variety of infections can eventually cause jaundice.

Symptoms
- Yellowish colour to the skin.
- Dark brown urine.
- Yellowish colour to whites of eyes.
- Pale coloured stools.
- Nausea and loss of appetite.

What to do
- Jaundice is potentially serious: always see a doctor. The cause needs to be identified.

- Your child may be low, tired, and depressed for some weeks.
- Your child may need a special diet.
  See also **hepatitis**.

Kidney disease, see nephritis.

Kiss of life, see mouth-to-mouth resuscitation.

Laryngitis
A number of viruses can infect the larynx, causing laryngitis.

Symptoms
- Loss of voice, hoarseness.
- Dry cough.
- Raised temperature.
- Sore throat.

What to do
- Laryngitis is rarely serious.
If the child is feverish, shows signs of more general infection, or develops signs of **croup**, see a doctor.
- If the doctor thinks there is a bacterial infection he or she may prescribe antibiotics.
- Give plenty of warm soothing drinks such as lemon juice sweetened with honey.
- Reduce fever with a tepid wet sponge.
- Keep the air moist. If you have an electric kettle, boil it in the room with the lid off. Stay with the child while you do this.
  See also **bronchitis, tonsilitis**.

Leukaemia
A malignant condition involving the white blood cells. In the past the prognosis for childhood with leukaemia was poor, but today there is a very good chance of a complete recovery.

Leukaemia is caused by the cancerous growth of primitive white blood cells which prevent the growth of normal cells. There is a reduction in the child's immunity to disease, and a disruption of blood clotting.

Symptoms
- Failure to recover from an illness.
- Anaemia.
- Bruising.
- Purpura (a purplish-red rash).
- Nose bleeds.
- Pain in limbs or limping.

Treatment
- If leukaemia is suspected the child will be referred to a specialist for diagnosis.
- Cytotoxic drug therapy is the mainstay of treatment, combined with radiotherapy.
- Blood transfusions may be given.
- You will be advised on keeping your child away from sources of infection.

Lice
Few children get through their school days without an infestation of head lice. The adult louse lays its eggs in the hair, close to the scalp. The 'nits' hatch 14 days later and the young lice break the skin of the scalp to feed on the blood. This is what causes the itching.

Symptoms
- Itchy scalp.
- Tiny white eggs where the hair grows out of the scalp, especially behind the ears. You may also see adult lice.

What to do
- If you find nits, keep the child away from school, and inform a teacher of the infestation. Don't be embarrassed, most schools encounter the problem frequently.
- Buy a shampoo containing malathion from the chemist. Use it to treat the infected child and the rest of the family. Follow the instructions carefully.
- Use a fine comb to remove dead eggs.
- Repeat the treatment after seven days in case any eggs remain.
- Clean brushes or combs using either the shampoo or a lotion.

Liver disease, see hepatitis.

Long-sightedness, see vision, problems with

Masturbation
Children start to explore their genitals as they explore everything else in the world about them. When they find that it feels nice, they tend to use masturbation, as adults do, to relieve tension and to soothe. It does no more harm to a child than it does to an adult. Children are capable of masturbating to orgasm, and when they discover this are likely to repeat the experiment. If you find your child panting and red-faced in bed, this is almost certainly what she is doing.

It is important to keep a sense of proportion. If your child masturbates compulsively, she may need help: it could reflect an underlying emotional disturbance.

Measles
A highly contagious childhood viral infection. It is a killer in the Third World, and in the developed world it is still an unpleasant illness with the potential for serious complications, though they are uncommon. It can easily be prevented by making sure your child is immunized at around 15 months.

Measles begins something like a **common cold**. The incubation period is 14 days.

Symptoms
- Runny nose and dry cough.
- Fever, which can be as high as 104°F (40°C).
- Child feels ill.
- Koplik's spots. These look like grains of salt, and appear on the inside of the cheeks on day three or four.
- A dark red-brown rash follows about a day later. This usually starts behind the ears and spreads over the face and body.
- Eyes red and sore; your child may say that light hurts them.
- She may be very ill, even delirious.

Possible complications
- **Encephalitis**.
- Acute conjuctivitis.
- Sore throat.
- Secondary infections such as **bronchitis, pneumonia**, or an ear infection (see **earache**) can develop.

What to do
- Your child will want to lie down if she feels really ill so there is no need to force the issue.
- Prepare to nurse constantly: she may feel very sorry for herself.

- Reduce fever by sponging with tepid water.
- Bathe eyes if sore with cool salty water or eye lotion.
- Give plenty of drinks.
- Report any signs of complications to the doctor. If the child seems to get better and then relapses, this should be reported. Secondary infections may be treated with antibiotics.
  See also **meningitis**.

Meningitis
The brain is covered by thin but tough membranes called meninges. Meningitis is an inflammation of these membranes.

Viral infection of the meninges can occur after mumps (particularly in adults), but is not serious. Bacterial infection is more serious; there is a risk of it leading to brain damage in severe cases.

Symptoms
- Headache.
- High fever.
- Lethargy.
- Intolerance of bright light.
- Bulging fontanelles.
- A reddish-purple rash covering most of the body.
- Drowsiness and confusion.
- Stiff neck.
- Vomiting.

What to do
- Call the doctor as soon as you suspect meningitis.
- Check reactions to light, and the neck for stiffness; look at a baby's fontanelles.
- Your child will be referred to hospital.
- The diagnosis will be checked, and the type of meningitis determined, by taking a sample of fluid from the spine.
- If she has bacterial meningitis she will be treated with antibiotics, usually given intravenously in high doses.
- Viral meningitis clears up without treatment.
  See also, **mumps, encephalitis**.

Middle ear infection, see earache.

Migraine
Migraine is a recurring, often severely debilitating headache. The tendency to suffer from it runs in families. Often the headache is preceded by a series of strange sensations such as flashing lights, certain smells, strange feelings or numbness.

Symptoms
- Severe headache, sometimes only on one side.
- Pallor.
- Strange sensations prior to headache.
- Occasional vomiting.
- Abdominal pain (quite frequent in children).

What to do
- If your child suffers from frequent headaches, you should see a doctor to rule out more serious possibilities. A headache with abdominal pain should also be reported unless it recurs frequently: it could indicate **appendicitis**.
- Put the child to bed in a cool dark room.
- If migraine attacks happen often, keep a diary of your child's diet: attacks can be induced by certain foods. Chocolate is a common culprit.
- Drugs to treat attacks are available.

Milia
A rash of tiny white or yellowish spots which appear over the nose and cheeks of newborn babies. It is not serious, needs no treatment, and will go away when the sweat glands mature.

Mouth-to-mouth resuscitation
If you find your child unconscious without sign of breathing you should start mouth-to-mouth resuscitation at once. Every second counts.

- Tilt back the child's head.
- Check the airways are clear.
- Wipe away anything which could be poisonous from inside and around her mouth. (It may be safer to breath through her nose if you suspect she has been poisoned.)
- Support her jaw with one hand, but do not push on her neck.
- Pinch her nostrils tight.
- Close your mouth around hers and breath gently from the bottom of your lungs into her mouth. Her chest should lift.
- The chest should then fall.
- Repeat.
- With a baby, close your mouth over the nose and mouth. Don't pinch her nostrils.
- If the chest does not rise and fall, check again for a blockage, then make sure that the nose is pinched tight and that you have a proper seal around her mouth.
- Wait for the chest to fall between breaths.
- Give three or four breaths; then check her pulse. It is easiest to feel this in the neck: find the child's windpipe, then move round towards the ears and you will find a groove. The carotid artery runs along this groove. Feel the pulse at the top of the neck just below the jaw: you should feel a beat within five seconds.
- If the heart is beating, continue mouth-to-mouth resuscitation until she starts to breathe normally. Give 15-20 breaths per minute. Count two as you breathe out, one as you take a breath.

Heart massage
If the heart is not beating you will need to stimulate it:
- Lie her down on the floor and kneel beside her.
- Compress her chest by pushing down hard on her breastbone. See below for different procedures with different age groups.
If the child is two years or more: Place your hand so that the heel of your palm just covers the breast bone, and the rest of your hand is across the chest but your fingers don't push on the ribs. The top of your hand should rest half way down the breastbone about level with the nipples. Push down directly on to the heel of your hand with your weight directly above. Be careful – it is quite a fine balance between giving enough pressure and crushing her. You need to press the bone in about 1-1½ in (2.5-3.5 cm). Push with a rhythm of 'Push-and-one-and-push-and-one-and. . .' Do this for about a minute, then stop and give mouth-to-mouth resuscitation. Then give five compressions and one breath until her heart begins to beat.

Under two: Finger pressure should be sufficient. Lie the baby on the floor. Place one arm under her shoulder and grip the far arm. This should push her chest up. Now, using two fingers, press down on the breastbone between the nipples. Depress between ½-1 in (1.25-2.5 cm).

• Check every two or three minutes to see if the heart is beating, and stop the compression as soon as you feel the pulse.
• Continue with the resuscitation until she begins to breathe.

Mouth ulcers

There are several kinds of mouth ulcers; they are always painful.
• White blister-like spots on the roof of the mouth, the gums and the cheek probably indicate a primary attack of *Herpes simplex* (the cold sore virus), especially if accompanied by fever. Children affected with this can be quite ill, and the mouth so sore that eating is difficult. Later attacks of herpes will produce **cold sores**.
• White salt-like spots inside the cheeks could be Koplik's spots. She may have **measles**.
• Aphthous ulcers are small, painful, creamy-white bumps which appear throughout the mouth. They are often associated with stress.
• Traumatic ulcers are large, single red ulcers with yellow heads which the child may have inside the cheeks. They are often caused by injury. Check that her teeth are not rubbing; in bottle-fed babies check that the teat is not causing the damage. They heal slowly.
• White patches on the inside of the cheeks could mean that the child has **thrush**. The patches look like milk, but if you wipe them you will find that the cheek is raw underneath.

What to do
• If the child is in pain, see a doctor.
• If traumatic ulcers recur, check for possible causes. Smear the ulcer with petroleum jelly to protect it.
• Smear antiseptic jelly over the ulcers using the tip of your finger. Your doctor may prescribe an anti-inflammatory cream.
• Liquidize food and feed the baby or child through a straw if necessary.
• Ice-cold drinks can soothe a sore mouth.
• Avoid salty and acid foods and drinks.
• Try to discourage your child from biting the ulcers.
• Anaesthetic gels can cause allergic reactions. Always check by giving a tiny amount to the child first. If there is a history of **allergy** in your family, it is probably wise to avoid these.

Mumps

A common viral infection with an incubation period of 14-28 days. Your child will feel unwell for a few days before the symptoms appear. Immunization against mumps is now being introduced in combination with the innoculation against **measles**. Mumps is usually mild, although **encephalitis** is a serious complication. Mumps can cause sterility in adult men, but this is rare. Deafness is another possible complication.

Symptoms
• Feeling 'off colour'.
• Swelling of the saliva glands on either side of the face below the ears and beneath the jaw.
• Fever.
• Dry mouth.
• Acute pain on swallowing anything acid.
• Swelling of the face.
• Headache.
• Painful swelling of the testes may occur in boys, though it is uncommon. Lower abdominal pain (caused by swollen ovaries) can occur in girls.

What to do
• See a doctor to confirm the diagnosis.
• If the child complains of a stiff neck and headache ten days after the diagnosis, consult your doctor immediately: she could have **meningitis**.
• Tepid sponging to reduce fever.
• Liquidize food.
• Give plenty of drinks.
• A hot water bottle may soothe.
• Don't laugh at her face, or let others laugh unless she thinks it is funny.

Nail biting

Many children bite their nails. Most of them show no signs of insecurity and eventually grow out of the habit. Keep nails smooth and cut them frequently.

If nail biting is combined with **bed wetting**, frequent nightmares (see **sleep problems**) or other signs of stress you should look for the underlying cause. Ask for help if your child seems to need it.

Nails, infection of surrounding skin

Children who bite or pick their nails sometimes suffer from paronychia, which is an infection of the skin around the finger- or toenails. Nail biting often breaks the skin around the nail, allowing bacteria to enter. The swelling is caused by gathering pus.

Symptoms
• Redness and swelling of the skin around the nail.
• Soreness, then throbbing pain.
• Pus under or next to the nail.

What to do
• Don't squeeze out the pus: this can damage the nail bed.
• Apply a protective pad of cotton wool.
• Cold compresses may reduce the pain.
• The pus should drain naturally. If it does not you may need to ask the doctor to lance the swelling.
• Antibiotics may be prescribed if the infection is severe.

Nappy rash, see eczema.

Nephritis

A kidney disease which, if left untreated, can be serious. It usually develops after an infection such as **tonsilitis**, and can appear very suddenly.

Symptoms
• Reddish, dark-coloured urine.
• Not passing much urine.
• Slight oedema (swelling of ankles, face and abdomen).
• Headache.
• High blood pressure.

What to do
- See a doctor immediately.
- Remember that red-coloured food such as beetroot and blackcurrants can darken a child's urine.
- If your child's face looks puffy, check her ankles and abdomen.
- The doctor will take the child's blood pressure and check her urine. If nephritis is confirmed, she will be admitted to hospital.
- Complete recovery usually takes about two weeks.

Nettle rash, see **urticaria**.

Nightmares, see **sleep problems**.

Nits, see **lice**.

Nose, foreign body in, see **foreign bodies**.

Nose bleeds
Nose bleeds caused by a blow to the head or nose should be investigated by a doctor. Minor nose bleeds can be caused by a child picking her nose, or by accidental rupture of a tiny blood vessel.

What to do
- If the nose bleed follows a head injury, go to hospital immediately.
- Reassure your child and keep her calm; nose bleeds can be frightening.
- Put her head over basin. Swallowing blood will make her sick.
- If bleeding continues for more than two minutes, pinch the nostrils together and hold firmly. The blood should then clot.
- Don't block nostrils with tissue or cotton wool.
- Don't let the child fiddle with her nose. It may restart the bleeding.
- If the nose bleed does not stop after 30 minutes, take your child to a doctor.
- If your child suffers from frequent nose bleeds, ask your doctor to refer her to an ear, nose and throat specialist.

Nose picking
The old rhyme "Everybody's doing it, picking their nose and chewing it," is certainly right as far as most children are concerned. Besides being an unsightly habit, it can make the nose sore.

Keep your child's nails short and clean.

Otitis externa, see **eczema**.

Otitis media, see **earache**.

Paronychia, see **nails, infection of surrounding skin**.

Penis, tight foreskin
A baby's foreskin should be left alone. Don't try to push it back: if you force it repeatedly, you may cause small lesions which can eventually fix the foreskin to the penis. This will make it painful and difficult to retract the foreskin later.

Sometimes a boy's foreskin is abnormally tight. If it is, you will notice that the foreskin will swell into a balloon when the child is urinating, or that the urine just dribbles rather than flows out. By the age of five you should be able to draw back the foreskin: if this is not possible, circumcision may be advised. Consult your doctor.

Penis, caught in zipper
How serious this is will depend on whether the child is circumcised or not: catching the end of the penis is obviously more serious than catching the foreskin.

If he is circumcised and therefore the head of the penis is caught:

- Keep him absolutely still and either call an ambulance or carry him carefully to the car and rush him to hospital. Do not try to free the penis: wait until this can be done under local anaesthetic.
- A cold compress (a packet of frozen peas) will reduce the pain and inflammation on the journey to hospital.

If the foreskin or the loose skin of the shaft is caught:

- Lie the child down.
- Cut trousers from waistband on each side of the zip. Unpick the base of the zip and see if you can free the skin. Have one try, if that does not free the penis, take the child to hospital.

In hospital, the child will be given a local anaesthetic. The penis will remain sore and swollen for some days. To assist healing:

- Leave the penis open to the air as much as possible.
- Coat it with antiseptic cream.
- To reduce the pain, apply cold compresses and give him paracetamol syrup.
- If he has difficulty urinating, put a cold compress on to the penis before urinating and run a tap.
- Immerse the penis in a toy bucket or pot of warm (or cold) water while urinating.
- There will be no lasting damage.

Phimosis, see **penis, tight foreskin**.

Phenylketonuria
A biochemical disorder affecting only one in 10,000 children. If untreated it can cause severe mental retardation. However, if a baby is given a special diet, all its effects are prevented. All babies are tested for this six days after birth.

Pneumonia
Pneumonia can be caused by a viral or a bacterial infection. In young children, the cause is usually an infection of the upper respiratory tract. Pneumonia is always serious: you should see a doctor immediately.

Symptoms
- Breathing difficulties and noisy grunts when breathing.
- Pain in chest.
- Possibly vomiting or nausea.
- Possibly fever.

What to do
- Reduce fever by sponging with tepid water.
- Give plenty of fluids.

- Prop the child up with pillows to make breathing easier.
- Keep the room ventilated.
- The doctor may advise transferring her to hospital where she will be treated with antibiotics.

Poisoning

If a child eats or drinks anything poisonous, it is important to act quickly. The longer the poison stays in the stomach, the more will be absorbed into her bloodstream, with increasingly serious consequences.

The treatment for poisoning is frightening and unpleasant: be sure that she *has* eaten or drunk the poison before you rush her to hospital.

Pills and medicines

It is safest to assume that anything she has taken from the medicine cupboard is poisonous. A few sleeping pills or tranquillizers can kill a child. So can moderate doses of many painkillers, antihistamines or travel sickness pills, and large doses of vitamin pills.

Cigarettes and alcohol

Eating a cigarette can kill a one-year-old. So could drinking a glass of neat spirits.

Poisonous plants

- Garden berries such as yew, laburnum and deadly nightshade can kill. Privet berries and laurel berries are poisonous. So are rhododendron, crocus, lily of the valley, hydrangea and many other plants. If you are uncertain, ring the hospital casualty department.

What to do

- Ask the child what she has eaten. Get her to point if she does not know the name. It is important to act quickly, as she may become unconscious.
- Ring for an ambulance if your child is unconscious, or if you are certain that she has eaten something poisonous.
- If you know she has eaten something, but she looks well, ring the doctor or the nearest casualty department and ask their advice. If she is drowsy or acts strangely, don't waste time checking. Get her to hospital.
- Take the packet or a sample of berries with you to hospital.
- If she has swallowed any of the above, and you are certain that she has not taken anything corrosive (see below), clear any bits from her mouth, put her face down across your knee and try to make her sick. The easiest way to do this is to put two fingers down her throat and move them about until she vomits.
If nothing happens, give her some milk or salty water and try again. But do not waste time. It is important to get to hospital.
- Don't try to make an unconscious child sick.

Household cleaners

It is safe to assume that all household cleaners are dangerous, both alkalis such as bleach or acids such as disinfectants. Both burn the throat. Liquid polish and dry cleaning fluids give off poisonous fumes.

Garden products

These are particularly dangerous: tiny quantities of some weedkillers can kill.

Paints

Most paints, paint strippers, oils, petrol, and car polishes are extremely dangerous.

What to do

- Ring for an ambulance or get her to hospital at once.
- Do not make her sick: with corrosives this will worsen the damage.
- Give milk to dilute the poison.
- Try to rinse out her mouth, and wash her face with a sponge.
- Take the poison with you to hospital.

If she is unconscious:

- Call an ambulance.
- Place in the **recovery position**. Check that she is breathing; give **mouth-to-mouth resuscitation** if necessary, taking great care not to get any of the poison on your mouth. Wash her face if possible, and breath into her nose. You will need to keep her lips sealed as you do this.
- Take anything you find near the body, such as a container, to the hospital: it may help them decide how best to treat her.

Poliomyelitis

An infection of the spinal cord and nerves, now rare because it is preventable by immunization.

Pyloric stenosis, see projectile vomiting.

Rash

A rash is a temporary skin disorder, usually taking the form of an area of redness, sometimes with spots. Children often have rashes, sometimes quite dramatic ones, and there are many causes.

Some rashes accompany infectious diseases such as **chickenpox, German measles, measles, *Roseola infantum* and scarlet fever**.

Some rashes are allergic reactions, for example **eczema**, nettle rash (see **urticaria**) and nappy rash (see page 209). Sprays containing local anaesthetics can also cause allergic reactions.

Other rashes are reactions to heat, such as prickly heat rash (see **heat rash**), or to skin infestation, such as **ringworm** and **scabies**.

Purpura looks like a rash but is not. These tiny areas of bleeding beneath the skin can indicate a serious disorder, but may simply reflect a sensitivity to a drug. It should always be reported to a doctor, but test first by pushing a glass against the skin: if the rash remains visible, it is *purpura*.

Many rashes go away as suddenly as they arrive. Those which are more persistent hardly ever have a sinister underlying cause, but they should not be ignored.

What to do

- If a rash persists, see a doctor.
- A purpuric rash with **fever** could indicate **meningitis**.
- Itchy rashes can be soothed with calamine lotion, or a cold compress. Or put the child in a bath containing a handful of bicarbonate of soda or laundry starch.
- Discourage scratching.
- Keep the child cool: overheating will worsen the irritation.

Identifying rashes

- Thick, creamy-yellow scales over part of baby's scalp: probably **cradle cap**.

- Itchy pimples with tiny black spots, often between fingers or in groin: possibly **scabies** (you should be able to see the line the mite has taken to burrow into the skin).
- A circle of tiny bumps around a red or grey scaly ring on any part of the body, including the scalp: probably **ringworm**.
- Itchy white lumps surrounded by reddened areas; the lumps (called weals) can be tiny or become large, swollen white patches. Spots can disappear within hours, but are often replaced by another crop: probably **urticaria** or **hives**.
- Isolated weals or white lumps on a red background that are itchy and painful but fade within hours: probably insect **bites**.
- White (or yellowish) spots on nose and cheeks of a newborn baby: possibly **milia**.
- White spots resembling grains of salt inside the cheeks: possibly **measles**.
- White milky flecks, inside cheeks and on tongue, which look red and raw if you scrape them: possibly **thrush**.
- White itchy blisters between, and possibly under, the toes: probably **athlete's foot**.
- Single (or multiple) small white or brown growths on sole of foot: probably **verruca(s)**.
- Red pimply spots around anus: possibly **thrush**.
- Tiny red spots on exposed skin (face, hands, legs) that become watery, ooze, and finally develop scabs:possibly **impetigo**.
- Tiny blisters under the skin, which become dry, red and scaly and itch badly: probably **eczema**.
- Red scaly skin inside ear: possibly **otitis externa**.
- Faint red rash over neck and face, especially in creases of neck, groin and armpits, and flushed appearance: possibly **heat rash**.
- Small, dark red-brown spots starting behind the ears, spreading and becoming blotchy: possibly **measles**.
- Flat pink spots starting behind the ears and spreading to forehead and then the rest of the body; spots quickly merge so that child looks blotchy and flushed: possibly **German measles**.
- Pimply red rash on baby's nappy area: possibly **nappy rash**.
- Tiny red dots on a red flushed background, starting on the chest and neck and spreading to the whole body except around the mouth: probably **scarlet fever**.
- Flat red or pink rash, starting on trunk and then spreading, accompanied by high fever: probably *Roseola infantum*.
- Tiny, localized itchy blisters, appearing on one area of the lips or perhaps the nostrils: possibly **cold sore**.
- Purple-red rash of irregular spidery spots, which do not itch; spots remain when you press a glass against them: a purpura rash (see above). This may be caused by a reaction to a new drug, or by an infection. In conjunction with high fever it could indicate **meningitis**. It is also a symptom of **hepatitis** and **leukaemia**.
- Itchy small blisters, starting on trunk and spreading to rest of the body: possibly **chickenpox**.

Recovery position

If your child is unconscious, dizzy or in shock, or if you feel she may be sick, it is best to put her in the recovery position. In this position the tongue falls forwards and the child cannot inhale vomit. A sick baby is always safest lying in this way.

What to do
- Lie the child on her stomach.
- Bring her arms from under her body.
- Turn her head to one side.
- Bend the arm on that side and place the hand beside the head.
- Bend the knee on the same side and pull her leg up.
- The other arm and leg should be straight.

Reye's syndrome

Reye's syndrome is a rare but serious form of liver failure. If a child recovering from **influenza** or **chicken pox** suddenly develops a high fever and vomits uncontrollably, call a doctor immediately. Never give aspirin to children under 12 as Reye's syndrome can be a rare side effect.

Symptoms
- Sudden onset of uncontrollable vomiting.
- Fever.
- Unconsciousness or drowsiness, with delirium. Sometimes followed by coma.

What to do
- If your child has a fever and suddenly becomes drowsy or unconscious, call for an ambulance or rush her to the nearest hospital.
- While waiting for help, sponge with tepid water to control fever.
- The child will be admitted to hospital, where a liver biopsy will be performed. She will be looked after in the intensive care unit.
- Be prepared for a long convalescence.

Rheumatic fever

A rare allergic response to a streptococcal infection. It usually occurs after a bout of **tonsilitis**, or an **ear infection**.

Symptoms
- Fever.
- Swollen, painful joints.
- Feeling depressed and listless.
- Occasional blotchy rash.
- Possible chest pains.

What to do
- If any of these symptoms occur in a child recovering from 'flu or tonsilitis, call a doctor immediately.
- She will almost certainly have to go into hospital.

Ringworm

A contagious fungal infection which gets its name from the ring of scaly skin it produces (see **rash**). When it occurs on the scalp you will find a small bald patch. **Athlete's foot** is a form of ringworm.

Symptoms
- Red or grey scaly circles of skin with small itchy bumps around the edges.
- Small bald patches, round or oval in shape.

What to do
- See a doctor who will prescribe an antifungal cream.
- Throw away any brushes, combs and

headgear your child has used as infestation will be spread through these. Disinfectant does not kill fungi.
• Try to stop your child scratching: it spreads the infestation.
• Keep the child away from school.
• Give the child a separate towel and a new hairbrush.
• Examine your pets and get them treated too.
• Wash your hands carefully after treating your child's ringworm.
• Encourage your child to wash after she touches the affected areas.

Roseola infantum
This is often confused with **German** measles. It starts with a sudden inexplicable high fever, the rash following once the fever has subsided. The condition is not serious.

Symptoms
• High fever lasting about three days.
• A rash of small, separate spots appears all over the body. The spots start on the trunk and spread to the legs but they vanish so quickly that they can be missed, unless you happen to look at the right time.

What to do
• See a doctor if you want the diagnosis confirmed.
• There is nothing you can do except control the fever by sponging and giving paracetamol syrup.
• If the child is susceptible to febrile convulsions, the doctor may prescribe something to control these.

Roundworm, see worms

Runny nose
After **fever**, this is probably the most common symptom in children. In winter it is usually a sign of the **common cold**. In summer it may be an indicator of an allergic reaction such as **hay fever**.
Some small babies with immature immune systems have colds almost continuously in their first year. A cold should not last more than about ten days.
Other possible causes of a runny nose are a **viral infection, influenza**, or a **foreign body in the nose**.

What to do
There is no cure, but see **common cold** and **hay fever** for ways to ease a runny or blocked nose. Petroleum jelly reduces soreness of the nose, and moist air helps to keep the mucus flowing.

Rubella, see German measles.

Scabies
This is a minor skin complaint, but it is irritating and contagious. The *Sarcoptes* mite burrows under the skin and lays eggs, which cause irritating pimples. The mite favours the area between the fingers, but also likes warm areas such as the groin. When the eggs hatch, the mites can be passed on by contact.

Symptoms
• Itchiness.
• You may be able to see the line of the mite's burrow and the black spot of the eggs.
• Small pimples and scabs form on the itchy areas.

What to do
See a doctor who will prescribe a lotion to kill the mites and eggs. All the family should be treated.
• You should all have a bath, then paint the whole body below the neck with the lotion. Don't wash again for 24 hours. Repeat about two days later.
• Wash all the infested child's bedding and towels, and any clothing worn while infested. The mite can live for about five or six days off the human body.

Scarlet fever
This used to be a serious disease, but now that it is possible to control the bacteria responsible with antibiotics or sulphonamides it rarely causes problems. The incubation period is about five days.

Symptoms
• Sore throat with inflamed tonsils similar to **tonsilitis**.
• High fever.
• Loss of appetite.
• Vomiting.
• Abdominal pain.
• Furry tongue with red patches.
• On day two or three, a rash of tiny red dot-like spots appears and the child's skin is flushed red. The rash starts on the chest and neck and spreads to the whole body, except the area around the mouth, which looks pale by comparison. Complications include middle ear infection (see **earache**), **kidney infection** and **rheumatic fever**.

What to do
• Call a doctor.
• Control the child's fever by tepid sponging and giving paracetamol syrup.
• Liquidise her food to make swallowing easier.
• Give soothing drinks for the throat.
The doctor will prescribe antibiotics or sulphonamides to prevent complications and to control the illness.

Shock
Shock can be mild or severe. *Mild shock* can be caused by a fright, a minor injury or even bad news. It brings about an automatic set of responses which make the child go pale and shake. See below for severe shock.

Symptoms
• Constricted blood supply to the skin makes the child go pale.
• Increased heart rate.
• Sweating and/or shivering.
• The child will look pale and clammy and will fee uneasy and 'odd'.
• She may vomit.

What to do
• Lie the child down and loosen her clothes.
• Get her head lower than her feet.
• Turn her head to one side in case of vomiting.
• Cover her with a blanket and comfort her.
• Don't give hot sweet drinks until she has recovered.
• Watch her carefully: she should recover quickly and may go into a peaceful sleep. If

after half an hour she has not recovered, call a doctor.

Severe shock is a potentially fatal condition caused by severe injury. There is heavy loss of body fluids, and progressive failure of circulation and breathing. This could be the result of **vomiting** and **diarrhoea**, heavy internal or external **bleeding, or severe burns**. Brain damage can also disrupt control of the heart and circulation.

Symptoms
- Pale, greyish-blue skin, especially around lips and fingernails.
- Cold, clammy skin.
- Sweating.
- Weak and rapid pulse.
- The child may collapse and become unconscious.
- Dizziness, faintness and blurred vision.
- The child may ramble, not recognize you, and could become delirious.
- She may be restless and anxious, rather as if she has had a nightmare.

What to do
- Get medical help quickly.
- Reassure the child.
- Treat any bleeding.
- Lie her down with her feet higher than her heart. Loosen tight clothing, and turn her head to one side.
- Keep her warm but beware of overheating.
- If she is unconscious, lie her in the **recovery position** and check her breathing until help arrives.

Short-sightedness, see vision, problems with.

Skull fracture, see head injuries.

Smothering
Babies will not be smothered by bedclothes, but they can be smothered by pillows or plastic bags. Never give a baby under one year a pillow to sleep on. If a baby puts a plastic bag over her head, the bag will cling to her face as she breathes in; after a few breaths she will no longer be able to get any air.

What to do
- Act quickly.
- Rip off the plastic.
- If she then takes a large breath, all is well.
- If she does not breathe, start **mouth-to-mouth resuscitation** at once. Give her six or eight breaths, then carry her to the telephone, still breathing into her mouth, and call for an ambulance between breaths.
- Continue breathing until help arrives.
- If you don't know how to do mouth-to-mouth resuscitation, call for an ambulance immediately.

Child covered by sand, mud or earth:
- Dig her out, clearing her chest as well as her face. The weight of sand on the ribcage will stop her breathing.
- Clear her mouth, throat and nose. If she splutters, all is well. But rush her to hospital, as there may be sand in her lungs.
- If her colour is normal, take her straight to hospital.

- If she is blue, give mouth-to-mouth resuscitation if you know how to do it. Clear her mouth first to reduce the risk of blowing sand into her lungs.
- If you don't know how to do mouth-to-mouth resuscitation, go straight to hospital.

Soiling
By the age of four, children should have bowel control by day, if not by night, and apart from the occasional accident. If a child starts to soil her pants during the day (having once had control) there is probably some underlying cause such as a new baby, or parental disharmony. Soiling is probably a cry for help and will almost certainly stop when things are more settled.

Sometimes persistent soiling is the result of retaining faeces: prolonged retention produces a distended bowel, the bowel movements become infrequent, and the child has dry stools which are large and painful to pass. Parents may not realize the child is constipated, noting only the leakage of faeces-stained mucus into the pants, which occurs because the bowel is so impacted with faecal matter.

Although the initial cause of soiling may be emotional upset, if the child's bowel becomes chronically distended the physical condition can persist even after the emotional cause has been treated.

There is some evidence that the tendency runs in families.

What to do
- Constipation is best treated by increasing the roughage in the child's diet, and by allowing fewer sweets and cakes. Give her plenty of citrus fruits, and add small quantities of bran to her meals. Brown rice, pasta and wholemeal bread should replace white varieties.
- In learning (or relearning) control after three, it is sometimes helpful to give a child a star chart. For example, give her one gold star each time she has a motion, and a red star for every five hours without soiling her pants. She can use her stars to buy privileges or small presents.
- Be matter-of-fact about soiling. Don't scold or try to shame the child and never ridicule her.
- Try to establish a routine time for the child 'to go'.
- Try not to worry too much: soiling is exceedingly rare in adolescents and young adults unless they are severely retarded or psychotic.

Snakebite
Children are often afraid of snakes: even if they have never seen one the thought of snakes can be frightening. A snake bite, even if not venomous, could be a major drama. It is important to establish what sort of snake inflicted the bite. An accurate description will help the hospital to give the appropriate antivenom.

Symptoms
- Snake bites usually leave one or two puncture marks.
- Swelling and pain.
- Gradual spreading of pain and numbness through the rest of the limb.

What to do
- Get as accurate a description of the snake as

you can from the child.
- Clean and dress the site of the wound.
- Rush the child to the nearest hospital casualty department.
- Don't try to suck out the poison and don't apply a tourniquet.

Sore throat
A sore throat is a symptom of several illnesses, including **common cold, influenza, mumps, tonsilitis**, or of a number of respiratory tract infections.

What to do
- See a doctor if the sore throat lasts over 24 hours and is getting worse or if the child seems generally unwell. Streptococcal infections need immediate treatment to prevent complications.
- Check for a red throat (saying 'Ah' really does give a helpful view of the throat).
- Give warm, soothing drinks, such as honey and lemon. Ice cream and iced juice soothe pain too.
- Check there is no fever, and feel her neck to see if the glands are swollen.
- Liquidize food to make eating easier.
- Paracetamol syrup will ease pain.
- An older child can gargle with diluted antiseptic.

Splinters
- If the splinter is standing proud of the skin, you can remove it by catching the end with a pair of eyebrow tweezers.
- To remove more deeply embedded splinters, place a lump of ice over the splinter before operating: this will reduce the pain.
- If there is no end sticking out, try squeezing. This may cause the splinter to protrude enough to catch the end with tweezers.
- If the splinter has penetrated just below the skin, sterilize a fine needle by passing it through a flame and try to tease the splinter out. You should be able to free enough to catch it with tweezers.
- Place a little antiseptic cream over the wound.
- If the splinter has penetrated more deeply, it is best to leave it alone, unless it is causing much pain. Splinters often work themselves out, or can remain harmlessly under the skin. It may be prudent to check that the child's tetanus immunization is up to date. Soaking in the bath will often loosen a splinter so it can be removed easily.
- Splinters of metal or glass should be removed by a doctor.
- If you think the splinter is contaminated in any way, take the child for an anti-tetanus injection.

Spots, see rashes.

Sprains and strains
All joints are supported by tough strappings called ligaments. If you fall awkwardly, you sometimes make a joint exceed its normal range of movement, resulting in a torn ligament. Such a tear, known as a sprain, causes bleeding into the joint, which in turn gives rise to swelling and pain.

The joints of the ankle, knee and wrist are those most likely to be sprained. Sprains are rare in pre-school children because their joints are still very supple.

What to do
- Check the joint. If it is misshapen take your child to the hospital casualty department: it is probably not a sprain, but a fracture or dislocation.
- Apply a cold compress (such as a packet of frozen peas); this will reduce pain and swelling.
- Make your child rest.
- If the swelling and bruising do not subside, and if she cannot put her weight on the foot (or hand) after 24 hours, see a doctor. You need to check that it is a sprain and not a dislocation or a fracture.
- She may need an X-ray.
- Once she can take some weight on the joint, support it with a cr
pe bandage. Check that swelling does not make the bandage too tight.
- Continue to make her rest as much as possible.

Squint, see vision, problems with.

Stammering
Most small children stammer occasionally as they rush to get out their words. Nearly all children will grow out of this occasional stammering. Over concern is likely to aggravate the situation.

It is difficult not to be concerned about persistent stammering. This tends to run in families and if you, or a close relative, suffer, you will naturally be sensitive to the problem. Never ridicule the child, or fill in her sentences for her. But don't pretend the stammer is not there: help her gain confidence instead.

If stammering persists, ask to have your child referred to a speech therapist. If therapy is started early, there is a reasonable chance of eliminating the child's stammer.

Sticky eyes
Many babies have a yellowish discharge from their eyes in the first days after birth. You may see it as a slight crusting on the lashes and lids, possibly causing the eyelids to stick together. This is mild inflammation, usually caused by something (such as amniotic fluid or blood) getting into the eye during the birth.

What to do
- Let a doctor see the eye. It is almost certainly not serious, but occasionally antibiotics are needed to clear the infection up.
- Clean the eye with cotton wool dipped in sterile water. To reduce cross-infection, use a separate swab for each eye.
- Lie the baby down with the infected eye uppermost, and change bed linen frequently until it has cleared.

Stings
Stings are rarely serious, though they are initially painful and most children make a dreadful fuss about them. Occasionally, children have a violent allergic reaction to stings, or receive multiple stings. The latter may be dangerous. Treat more than two or three stings as an emergency.

Symptoms
- A wasp sting leaves a small puncture mark with swelling and irritation.

• A bee sting usually remains in the puncture. The sting is a small sac on the end of a barb.
• A jellyfish sting leaves a red swelling; parts of the jellyfish can stick to the skin.
• In a serious case, the child may develop breathing difficulties or show signs of **shock**.

What to do
• Bee stings should be removed with tweezers: don't try to squeeze them out. Avoid sqeezing the poison sac at the top of the sting. Treat the area of the sting with a thick paste of bicarbonate of soda and water. Apply a cold compress.
• Wasp stings are best treated with an acid cold compress: use a pad of vinegar- soaked cotton wool, held in place with a lump of ice.
• Jellyfish stings should be washed and treated with calamine lotion or a cold compress.
• If your child shows signs of shock or develops breathing difficulties after a sting, take her to hospital immediately.

Stomach ache
Stomach ache is a symptom of which the underlying cause could be anything from wind to a serious abdominal problem.

Symptoms
• Babies will scream and draw up their legs.
• Young children often cannot localize pain: a tummy ache could mean almost anything. But if stomach pain is severe, she will cry, lie curled up and walk bent double. Call a doctor if this happens.
• If a baby screams with stomach pain, becomes pale and grey, and repeats this about 20 minutes later, she may have acute intussusception or a severe obstruction: if so, her stools will look like redcurrant jelly. Call a doctor immediately.

Stye
A stye is an inflammation of one of the eyelash follicles.

Symptoms
• A swollen red area, usually on lower lid, which grows and fills with pus. It usually bursts on the fourth or fifth day.

What to do
• Discourage the child from touching the stye.
• Soothe the area with a cool compress.
• When the pus comes to a head, bathe with warm water. If you can pull out the eyelash from the centre of the stye, this will help the pus drain.
• See a doctor if the whole eyelid begins to swell, or if the stye does not clear within five or six days.

Sudden infant death syndrome (SIDS), see cot death.

Sunburn
It is easier to prevent than to cure.
Remember:

• Babies' skins are delicate. Fair- skinned children take time to build up a protective tan. You should always protect them with high sun protection factor cream.
• Sun is reflected off water and off sand. Take special care at the seaside.
• Wind can disguise the power of the sun: the drying effect is likely to accelerate the sunburn.
• Skin rarely exposed to the air is most likely to burn. Your toddler will love to run on the beach without a nappy: but her bottom will need high sun protection factor cream.

Symptoms
• Red, hot, sore skin.
• Blisters.
• Slight temperature.

What to do
• Apply a soothing cream such as a proprietary after-sun cream or calamine lotion. A cold compress will soothe if the burn is localized.
• Leave skin uncovered indoors, but loosely covered outside. Cotton is best for covering.
• Give paracetamol syrup to ease the pain.
• Check for fever. Slight fever is fairly normal, but if her temperature rises appreciably, see a doctor.
• If she is confused or drowsy she may have heatstroke – see **heat problems**. Get medical help immediately.

Swallowing foreign bodies
Providing the object is not sharp or poisonous, and has gone down rather than lodging in the throat, there is no danger. Watch for it in the child's faeces.

Symptoms
• Sharp objects will usually stick in the throat. Check her mouth, hands and the floor to make sure it has been swallowed. If you cannot find it, take her to hospital where she will be X-rayed.
• If you are uncertain whether the swallowed object is poisonous, play safe: ring the nearest hospital casualty department or take her along.

Swollen glands
The lymph glands which lie in the neck, armpits and groin become tender and swollen as they fight off infection. You can feel the swellings as lumps. If all the glands swell, she probably has a viral infection.
• Swollen glands in the side of the neck may indicate **tonsilitis**.
• Swollen glands in the back of the neck may indicate **German measles**.
• Swollen glands just in front of the ear and below the jaw may indicate **mumps**.

Tapeworm, see worms.

Temperature
Normal body temperature is 96.8°F (36°C). But a child's temperature is rarely exactly this: it varies according to the time of day and on how active she is. Slight variations are nothing to worry about. A temperature of over 100°F (37.7°C) is properly described as a **fever**, and a temperature below 95°F (35°C) is called hypothermia. Neither should be ignored. A fever needs to be controlled whether it is 100°F (38°C) or 102°F (39°C).

A child's temperature fluctuates more than an adult's. A child can rapidly develop a fever, and almost as rapidly lose it. Her temperature can also reach alarmingly high levels. The quickest way to check your child's temperature is to feel her forehead (compare it with your own if you are unsure). If she feels unusually hot or cold, check with a thermometer.

• The easiest way to take a child's temperature is with a liquid-crystal forehead thermometer or 'fever strip'. These only have to be placed against the child's forehead for a few seconds before they react. Liquid-crystal thermometers are, however, less accurate than conventional mercury thermometers. But while doctors often need precision, parents rarely do.
• If you feel happier knowing her exact temperature, a mercury thermometer will give an accurate reading. If your child is under six, take her temperature by the under-arm method. Shake the thermometer first. It makes sense to have the child sitting on your lap. Place the thermometer under her arm against the skin, and hold her arm down. Leave for two minutes, then read the thermometer.

To take a child's temperature orally, shake the thermometer and ask the child to open her mouth. Place the thermometer under her tongue and tell her to hold it in place with her tongue. Leave it for two minutes, then read the thermometer.
• Don't take the thermometer out too soon, or leave a child alone with a thermometer.
• Don't take a child's temperature orally after she has had a warm or a cold drink; don't attempt it by any method after she has been active.
• If the thermometer breaks in her mouth, take out the glass with a tissue and check she has not swallowed any mercury. Call a doctor if you suspect she has.

For treatment of a high temperature, see **fever**.

Testes, undescended
A boy's testes develop within the body cavity and only descend into the scrotum in the months before birth. After descent, they remain hanging in the scrotal sac.

In some boys, the passage through which the testes descend fails to close, and the testes can thus move up and down, in and out of the scrotum. Occasionally, the testes don't descend at all.

Symptoms
• A retractable testicle nearly always moves permanently into the scrotum in the child's first few years; it will disappear into the body cavity when touched, especially if the touch is cold.
• If the testes have not descended, the scrotum is always empty. If sperm are to be produced when your son is adult, the testes must be in the scrotum. He will need a small operation. This should take place before he is about seven.

Tetanus
Tetanus is a potentially fatal bacterial infection which no child should be allowed to catch. It is entirely preventable through innoculation. Children will need booster injections every five years if full protection is to be maintained.

Symptoms
• The bacteria usually enter through a cut, typically when the cut comes into contact with rusty metal or garden rubbish.
• The muscles become stiff.
• Sore throat.

• Difficulty in breathing.
• Difficulty in swallowing.

What to do
If a child shows any of these symptoms following an accident where tetanus infection is possible, take her to hospital immediately or call an ambulance.

Threadworms, see worms.

Thrush
An infection of the skin, mouth and some other parts of the body caused by the fungus *Candida albicans*. The fungus normally lives in the mouth, intestines and vagina and most of the time is kept in check by some of the many bacteria to which we are host. Occasionally, when this balance is disrupted, thrush is manifests itself as a rash.

Babies can catch thrush as they pass through the vagina at birth.

Symptoms
• Creamy-white, milk-like curds in the mouth or vagina.
• Red raw patches under the curds if they are scraped off.
• A red rash around the anus.

What to do
• Change nappies frequently to prevent infection around the anus.
• See a doctor, who will prescribe antifungal medicine and/or cream.

Tonsilitis
An acute infection of the tonsils.

Symptoms
• Sore throat
• Difficulty in swallowing.
• Red, enlarged tonsils, often with white or yellow spots.
• Feeling low.
• Fever
• Smelly breath.
• Swollen glands.
• Breathing through the mouth.

What to do
• See a doctor. Tonsilitis is not serious, but if untreated can lead to serious complications such as **rheumatic fever** or deafness. The doctor will prescribe an antibiotic if it is caused by a bacterial infection.
• Treat the symptoms of fever and soreness by tepid sponging, soothing warm or ice-cold drinks, paracetamol syrup and liquidised food. Ice cream both soothes and nourishes.
• Repeated attacks of tonsilitis and ear infections may suggest that the child's tonsils and adenoids need removing. You should be referred to an ear, nose and throat specialist.

Toothache
The problem occurs when a child's teeth decay.

Symptoms
• Pain in teeth.
• Occasionally, referred pain to ears or jaw. The pain can be located by tapping the teeth in turn with the back of a teaspoon.

What to do
• Take her to the dentist.
• Give paracetamol syrup to ease the pain.

341

Toxocara and toxocariasis, see worms.

Travel sickness
Motion sometimes upsets the balance organs of the inner ear and this produces travel sickness. Children seem to be more prone than adults, but they often grow out of it by adolescence.

Symptoms
• Suddenly going quiet.
• Pallor.
• Nausea.
• Dizziness.
• Vomiting, often with little warning.
• Cold, clammy forehead.
• Faintness.

What to do
• Give a susceptible child travel sickness medication before starting any journey.
• Travel with towels, and give the child a strong paper bag in which to be sick. If it is a car journey, stop frequently.
• Take along something to drink so that the child will not become dehydrated if she vomits.
• Give her a light meal before the journey, but avoid fatty foods.
• If you are in a car and notice that she has suddenly gone quiet and looks pale, stop the car so she can get some air and walk about.
• If you cannot stop, get her to lie down and close her eyes.
• If on a boat, encourage the child to lie down if she feels seasick. If she wants to be up and about, tell her to keep her eyes on the horizon.

Tuberculosis
An infection of the lungs that can do severe damage if left untreated. It can affect not only the lungs, but also the spine, kidneys and meninges, which cover the brain.

'TB' used to be a common killer in most countries, but has now almost been eradicated in the West. If your child comes into contact with anyone who has the disease, see a doctor. Children are now innoculated against TB at the age of 13: an essential precaution.

Umbilical cord, infection of
Usually the umbilical cord withers after birth and drops off, but occasionally it becomes infected.

Symptoms
• Redness and swelling of the umbilical stump.
• Discharge (sometimes pus) from stump.

What to do
• Consult your midwife who will advise on how to clean the cord and what to apply. She will advise you to see a doctor if necessary.
• Clean the cord at each nappy change.
• Occasionally, infection from the cord can spread. Your baby may need a course of antibiotics if this happens.

Urinary tract infection
Urinary tract infections affect the urethra, bladder, ureter and sometimes the kidneys; they can be serious. Girls are more prone than boys.

A new-born baby who has a dry nappy after two hours needs watching. All babies should urinate frequently. If she remains dry or the urine is concentrated, give extra drinks. If she remains dry and the urine remains strong or takes on a fishy smell, see a doctor. Do so immediately if there is blood in the urine.

Older children sometimes get urinary infections.

Symptoms
• Frequent passing of water.
• Possibly bed wetting.
• Burning sensation on passing urine.
• Cloudy urine (sometimes with an unpleasant fishy smell).
• Feeling 'low'.
• Abdominal pain.
• Low back pain.
• Fever.

What to do
• See a doctor immediately.
• Give plenty of fluids to flush out the kidneys. Let her drink as much as she can.
• A hot water bottle will comfort her if she is in pain.
• Sometimes a minor abnormality in the urethra leads to frequent infection. You will probably be referred to a specialist if this is suspected.

Unconsciousness
If your child is unconscious, even momentarily, she must see a doctor.
Take her to the nearest hospital casualty department or call an ambulance.

What to do
• If a child looks unconscious, shake her gently or pinch her. Talk to her. If she does not respond:
• Check that she is breathing. If she is, put her on her side in the **recovery position**.
• If she makes odd sounds, check that the airways are free.
• Call an ambulance.
• If she has fallen, don't move her.
• If you are sure there are no bones broken, turn her over into the *recovery position*.
• Never leave an unconscious child alone.

Undescended testes, see testes, undescended.

Urticaria, see hives.

Vagina, foreign bodies in, see foreign bodies.

Verrucas, see warts and verrucas.

Vision, problems with
The eye is a complex organ, and many people do not have perfect vision.

Short- and *long-sightedness* are essentially defects in the shape of the eyeball, usually congenital. Short-sightedness rarely develops before the child is about nine or ten, and long-sightedness often develops later in life. Both can, of course, be corrected with spectacles.

Colour blindness occurs because a certain pigment is missing from the eye's light-sensitive apparatus, usually the one concerned with perceiving either red or green. It is much more common in boys than in girls. Nothing can be done to correct the problem: the child will see colour, but the colours will be different from normal. Total colour blindness is rare.

Squint: Babies' eyes often wander in the first weeks of life, but the pupils should be 'fixed' by three months. Squints after this age should be reported to a doctor. Squints happen because the vision of the two eyes is very different (ambylopea) or because of weak muscles supporting one of the eyeballs.
Squints need treatment. A 'lazy eye' is just as the phrase implies: an eye which is not being used. Without use, it will become incapable of working. For a successful outcome, this problem needs to be treated before the child reaches four.

What to do
● Have your child's eyes tested at regular intervals.
● If she needs glasses, get ones with plastic lenses; they are safer and lighter than glass lenses.

Vomiting
Forcible expulsion of the stomach contents. It is usually preceded by nausea, the sensation of sickness. Some children are often sick, others rarely so.
Vomiting is a symptom of many different illnesses, some of them serious, others trivial.

See a doctor immediately if:
● Vomiting follows a head injury.
● A newborn baby does projectile vomiting (487) with each feed.
● A young baby passes frequent, watery stools as well as vomiting.
● A young baby vomits and is in severe, though possibly intermittent, pain, especially if her stools contain mucus and blood.
● She vomits and has abdominal pain (especially if it is around the navel and to the lower right side – it could be due to **appendicitis**).
● She is vomiting and cannot move her neck forward without pain.
● Don't give food to a child who is vomiting. Give clear fluids in small amounts (see **diarrhoea**).

See a doctor if:
● She vomits more than twice in a day except in cases of obvious travel sickness.
● Vomiting is accompanied by diarrhoea. In this case treat as for diarrhoea, but if she vomits repeatedly and cannot keep even clear fluids down, call a doctor.

Warts and verrucas
These are harmless small growths on the skin, caused by a virus. Warts often grow on the hands and face, verrucas appear on the feet. Both are contagious. A child will occasionally have a crop of warts; they can spread from one site to another.

Symptoms
● Hard lumps of raised, dry-looking, thickened skin.
● Hard lumps (often with a dark centre) on the sole of the foot.

What to do
● If you are uncertain whether the lumps are

warts, see a doctor.
● See a doctor if the warts are on the face or genitals. Otherwise they are best left alone unless the child finds them irritating.
● Most warts eventually go away.
● If the child finds the wart or verruca irritating, try using one of the patent wart cures that can be bought at a chemist. Don't use these on the face or genitals. They are acid, and work by burning.
● If the warts persist, and make the child unhappy (or they are in a place where he keeps catching them), you may be referred to a hospital wart clinic.

Wax in the ears
It is normal to have some wax in the external ear canal. Occasionally it builds up to a level at which it can cause a temporary hearing loss.

Symptoms
● Visible build-up of wax.
● Hearing loss.
● The child complains of ringing in her ears.

What to do
● Never poke anything into your child's ear to clear wax.
● Ask the doctor if her ears should be syringed.

Wheezing
Babies often make wheezing sounds as if there were phlegm on their chests when they simply have mucus in the back of their throats which has dripped down from the nose during a cold. If there is wheezing from the chest in response to an infection, this may well be because the baby (or child) has **asthma** or **bronchitis**. If in doubt, ask a doctor to listen to her chest.

Whooping cough
Unless you are advised by your doctor or health visitor that there are medical indications for not having your child innoculated against whooping cough, she should have this vaccination. Because children are innoculated less frequently, this disease is now on the increase. It can be serious, especially for babies.
If your child has been in contact with whooping cough and develops the symptoms of a cold, tell the doctor immediately, especially if she is under a year.

Symptoms
● Cold symptoms, which drag on for some days; she will cough quite 'normally' at first.
● The cough then becomes excessive, especially during the night. The child will cough several times on one breath, and because she becomes breathless will develop the characteristic 'whoop'. The sound is made by air being drawn past the swollen larynx.
● Young babies with whooping cough often don't whoop: they just cough in spasms and may turn blue/grey during an attack; this can be dangerous.
● Vomiting can occur after the child coughs.
● Sleep deprivation, due to coughing.
● Whooping cough can last up to ten weeks.
● Because the child may vomit frequently, there is a danger of dehydration.
● There is a high risk of secondary infection of the middle ear, **bronchitis** or **pneumonia**.

What to do
● See a doctor, and keep the child away from

other children, especially babies.
● Don't leave the child alone at any time. The coughing can be frightening for the child and fear makes each bout worse. There is also a danger that the child will inhale vomit.
● During a coughing bout sit with her, and make her lean forward a little. You should have a bowl ready in case she is sick.
● Give her a little to eat and drink immediately after a coughing bout; it is the best way to ensure nourishment.
● Don't give cough medicines except on the doctor's advice.
● The doctor may prescribe antibiotics, though these are not a cure. However, they may reduce the illness's severity and they do stop it being infectious. Otherwise your child may be infectious for a month.
● You may be advised to take a baby with a severe attack of whooping cough into hospital, where oxygen can be given quickly if needed.
● Keep your child as quiet as possible: exertion can bring on a coughing attack.

Worms
A number of different types can infest children.

Threadworms are the mildest and commonest.

Symptoms
● Itching around the anus.
● The worms are seen either in the faeces or around the anus. They come out of the anal passage in the dark and when the child is warm; you may be able to see them if look at your child's anus while she is sleeping. They look like tiny threads, and you can remove them by picking them up on adhesive tape.

What to do
● Stop your child scratching herself. Since the worms lay eggs around the anus, she can reinfect herself if she puts her fingers to her mouth.
● Treat your child with a worming powder: these are available from any pharmacy. As worms are very infectious, all the family should be treated at the same time. A second dose should be taken after two weeks.

Roundworms are rare, except in tropical countries.

Symptoms
● Worms, like long white earthworms, in the faeces.
● Worms in vomit.

What to do
● Inspect your child's faeces if you have travelled in an area where infestation is common.
● If you find worms in her faeces, take a sample with you to the doctor, who can prescribe an antiparasitic drug.

Tapeworm infestation is also rare.

Symptoms
● White flat moving segments in stools. See a doctor, who will prescribe an antiparasitic drug.

Toxocara is caught from the faeces of animals. The eggs of the parasite are in animal faeces. If the child swallows the eggs (by touching infected faeces and putting her hand in her mouth), they can hatch in her intestines and then burrow out into the body. They often lodge in the lungs where they are coughed up and can reinfest the child.

Symptoms
● Loss of appetite.
● Possibly fever.
● Abdominal pain.
● Loss of sight. In rare cases a worm can lodge in the eye and cause blindness.

What to do
● See a doctor who can prescribe an antiparasitic drug.
● Never leave the cat's litter tray where a toddler or baby can play with it.
● Encourage a child to wash her hands after playing with the cat or dog.
● Worm your pets at frequent intervals.
● Cover the sand pit to stop cats or dogs using it as a litter tray.

X-rays
Having an X-ray can be a frightening experience for a child: the machinery is large, moves and makes strange noises.
   If your child needs an X-ray, explain as fully as you can what will happen. You may be asked to hold a child while she is being X-rayed.

Index

The numerals in this index refer to the numbered paragraphs, except where page numbers are specifically mentioned. See also the medical section.

Q

R

S

Picture Credits